India Live 2017

Update in
Interventional Cardiology

India Live 2017

Update in
Interventional Cardiology

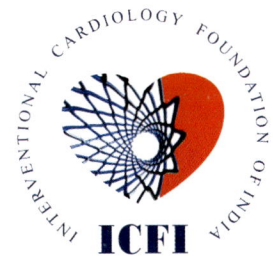

Editor-in-Chief

Ashwin B Mehta MD FACC
Director of Cardiology
Jaslok Hospital and Research Centre
Mumbai, Maharashtra, India

Co-Editors

Nihar Mehta DNB (Cardiology)
Consultant Cardiologist
Jaslok Hospital and Research Centre
Mumbai, Maharashtra, India

Rahul Chhabria DNB (Cardiology)
Associate in Cardiology
Jaslok Hospital and Research Centre
Mumbai, Maharashtra, India

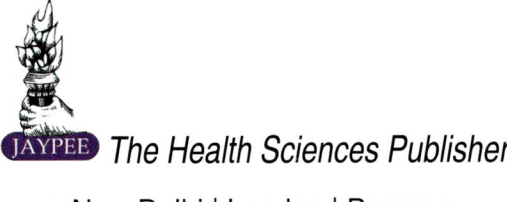

JAYPEE *The Health Sciences Publisher*

New Delhi | London | Panama

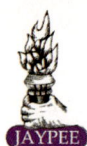

Jaypee Brothers Medical Publishers (P) Ltd

Headquarters
Jaypee Brothers Medical Publishers (P) Ltd.
4838/24, Ansari Road, Daryaganj
New Delhi 110 002, India
Phone: +91-11-43574357
Fax: +91-11-43574314
E-mail: jaypee@jaypeebrothers.com

Overseas Offices

J.P. Medical Ltd.
83, Victoria Street, London
SW1H 0HW (UK)
Phone: +44-20 3170 8910
Fax: +44(0)20 3008 6180
E-mail: info@jpmedpub.com

Jaypee-Highlights Medical Publishers Inc.
City of Knowledge, Bld. 235, 2nd Floor, Clayton
Panama City, Panama
Phone: +1 507-301-0496
Fax: +1 507-301-0499
E-mail: cservice@jphmedical.com

Jaypee Brothers Medical Publishers (P) Ltd.
17/1-B, Babar Road, Block-B, Shaymali
Mohammadpur, Dhaka-1207
Bangladesh
Mobile: +08801912003485
E-mail: jaypeedhaka@gmail.com

Jaypee Brothers Medical Publishers (P) Ltd.
Bhotahity, Kathmandu, Nepal
Phone: +977-9741283608
E-mail: kathmandu@jaypeebrothers.com

Website: www.jaypeebrothers.com
Website: www.jaypeedigital.com

© 2017, Jaypee Brothers Medical Publishers

The views and opinions expressed in this book are solely those of the original contributor(s)/author(s) and do not necessarily represent those of editor(s) of the book.

All rights reserved. No part of this publication may be reproduced, stored or transmitted in any form or by any means, electronic, mechanical, photocopying, recording or otherwise, without the prior permission in writing of the publishers.

All brand names and product names used in this book are trade names, service marks, trademarks or registered trademarks of their respective owners. The publisher is not associated with any product or vendor mentioned in this book.

Medical knowledge and practice change constantly. This book is designed to provide accurate, authoritative information about the subject matter in question. However, readers are advised to check the most current information available on procedures included and check information from the manufacturer of each product to be administered, to verify the recommended dose, formula, method and duration of administration, adverse effects and contraindications. It is the responsibility of the practitioner to take all appropriate safety precautions. Neither the publisher nor the author(s)/editor(s) assume any liability for any injury and/or damage to persons or property arising from or related to use of material in this book.

This book is sold on the understanding that the publisher is not engaged in providing professional medical services. If such advice or services are required, the services of a competent medical professional should be sought.

Every effort has been made where necessary to contact holders of copyright to obtain permission to reproduce copyright material. If any have been inadvertently overlooked, the publisher will be pleased to make the necessary arrangements at the first opportunity.

Inquiries for bulk sales may be solicited at: jaypee@jaypeebrothers.com

Update in Interventional Cardiology

First Edition: **2017**

ISBN: 978-93-86322-22-7

Printed at Sanat Printers

Course Directors of India Live

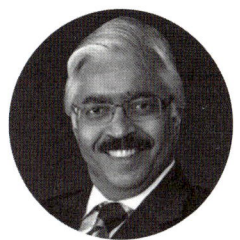

Ashok Seth
Chairman
Cardiovascular Sciences and
Chief of Cardiology
Fortis Escorts Heart Institute
New Delhi, India

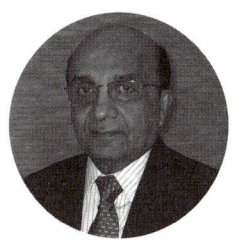

Ashwin B Mehta
Director of Cardiology
Jaslok Hospital and Research Centre
Mumbai, Maharashtra, India

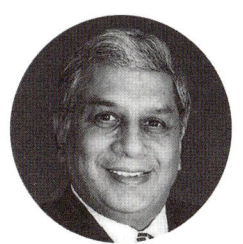

Mathew Samuel Kalarickal
Director
Interventional Cardiology and Cardiac
Catheterisation Laboratories
Apollo Hospital
Chennai, Tamil Nadu, India

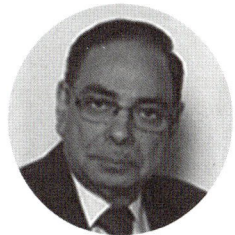

Upendra Kaul
Executive Director and Dean, Cardiac Sciences
Fortis Escorts Heart Institute
New Delhi, India

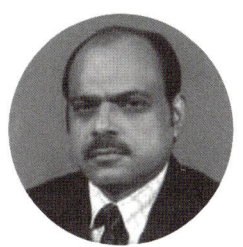

Vinay K Bahl
Professor and Head
Department of Cardiology
All India Institute of Medical Sciences
New Delhi, India

Contributors

Aamish Kazi MBBS DNB
Consultant Radiologist
Picture This by Jhankharia
Mumbai, Maharashtra, India

Ajit Desai MD DM (Cardiology)
Consultant Cardiologist
Jaslok Hospital and Research Centre
Mumbai, Maharashtra, India

Ajit S Mullasari MD DM (Cardiology)
Director
Department of Cardiology
Institute of Cardiovascular Diseases
Madras Medical Mission
Chennai, Tamil Nadu, India

Ameya Udyavar DM DNB (Cardiology)
Consultant Cardiac
Electrophysiologist
PD Hinduja National Hospital
Mumbai, Maharashtra, India

Amit Vora MD DM
Consultant Cardiologist and
Electrophysiologist
Arrhythmia Associates
Mumbai, Maharashtra, India

Andhalkar Bhagyashree MD
Cardiology Registrar
Smt. SR Mehta Cardiac Institute and
Sir KP Trust Hospital
Mumbai, Maharashtra, India

Annapoorna Kini MD
Professor of Medicine
Director
Cardiac Catheterization Laboratory
Cardiovascular Institute
Division of Cardiology
Mount Sinai Hospital and
School of Medicine
New York City, New York, USA

Anunay Gupta MD DM (Cardiology)
Department of Cardiology
All India Institute of Medical Sciences
New Delhi, India

Ashok Seth FRCP (Lond) FRCP (Edin)
FRCP (Ire) FACC FESC FSCAI FIMSI FCSI
Chairman
Cardiovascular Sciences and Chief of
Cardiology
Fortis Escorts Heart Institute
New Delhi, India

Ashwin B Mehta MD FACC
Director of Cardiology
Jaslok Hospital and Research Centre
Mumbai, Maharashtra, India

Bharat Dalvi MD DM (Cardiology) FACC
Glenmark Cardiac Center
Mumbai, Maharashtra, India

Bharat Shivdasani MBBS
DNB (Cardiology)
Consultant Cardiologist
Jaslok Hospital and Research Centre
Mumbai, Maharashtra, India

Bhavin Jankharia MBBS MD
Consultant Radiologist
Picture This by Jhankharia
Mumbai, Maharashtra, India

CG Bahuleyan MD DM FRCP FSCAI
Chairman
Cardiovascular Centre
Ananthapuri Hospitals and Research
Institute
Thiruvananthapuram, Kerala, India

Dhiraj Kumar MBBS
MD (Internal Medicine)
Senior Registrar Cardiology
Department of Cardiology
KEM Hospital
Mumbai, Maharashtra, India

G Raghul MD DM
Associate Consultant
Department of Cardiology
Apollo Hospitals
Chennai, Tamil Nadu, India

G Sengottuvelu MD DM DNB
FRCP (Glasg) FSCAI FMMC
Fellowship in Interventional
Cardiology (France)
Senior Consultant and Interventional
Cardiologist
Apollo Main Hospitals
Chennai, Tamil Nadu, India

Hetan C Shah MD DNB Cardiology
FACC FESC
Associate Professor
KEM Hospital
Consultant Interventional Cardiologist
Jaslok Hospital
Mumbai, Maharashtra, India

Kajal Aggarwal MBBS Dip. (Cardiology)
Associate Consultant
Medanta—The Medicity
Gurugram, Haryana, India

Kirti Punamiya MD DM
Consultant Staff Cardiologist
Breach Candy and Saifee Hospitals
Mumbai, Maharashtra, India

Kshitij Sheth DNB (Pediatrics)
FNB (Pediatric Cardiology)
Sir HN Reliance Foundation Hospital
Mumbai, Maharashtra, India

Manjunath CN MD
DM (Cardiology)
Professor and Head
Department of Cardiology
Director, Sri Jayadeva Institute of
Cardiovascular Sciences & Research
Bengaluru, Karnataka, India

Mathew Samuel Kalarickal MD DM
Director
Interventional Cardiology and Cardiac
Catheterisation Laboratories
Apollo Hospital
Chennai, Tamil Nadu, India

Mithun J Varghese MD
Cardiologist
Cardiac Catheterization Laboratory
Cardiovascular Institute
Division of Cardiology
Mount Sinai Hospital and School of
Medicine
New York City, New York, USA

Nagaraja Moorthy
Associate Professor
Department of Cardiology
Sri Jayadeva Institute of
Cardiovascular Sciences and Research
Bengaluru, Karnataka, India

Nihar Mehta DNB (Cardiology)
Consultant Cardiologist
Jaslok Hospital and Research Centre
Mumbai, Maharashtra, India

Parang Sanghavi DNB DMRD MBBS
Consultant Radiologist
Picture This by Jhankharia
Mumbai, Maharashtra, India

Prafulla Kerkar MD (Internal Medicine)
DM (Cardiology) DNB (Cardiology)
FACC (US) FESC (Europe) FSCAI (USA)
Professor and Head
Department of Cardiology
KEM Hospital and Seth GS Medical
College
Mumbai, Maharashtra, India
Consultant Interventional Cardiologist
Asian Heart Institute
Mumbai, Maharashtra, India

Prattay Guhasarkar DM
Fellow of Cardiology
Jawaharlal Institute of Postgraduate
Medical Education and Research
(JIPMER)
New Delhi, India

Praveen Chandra MD DM
Chairman
Division of Interventional Cardiology
Medanta—The Medicity
Gurugram, Haryana, India

Rahul Chhabria DNB (Cardiology)
Associate in Cardiology
Jaslok Hospital and Research Centre
Mumbai, Maharashtra, India

Rashmi Xavier MD DM
Associate Consultant
Division of Interventional Cardiology
Medanta—The Medicity
Gurugram, Haryana, India

Rohit Goel MD DM (Cardiology)
Associate Consultant
Medanta—The Medicity
Gurugram, Haryana, India

Samin K Sharma MD
Cardiac Catheterization Laboratory
Cardiovascular Institute
Division of Cardiology
Mount Sinai Hospital and
School of Medicine
New York City, New York, USA

Sanjay Kumar Chugh MD
DM (Cardiology, AIIMS) D Cardiology (Cal)
FACC FSCAI FESC FCSI (India) FIMSA
Principal Consultant
Department of Interventional
Cardiology
Escorts Heart Institute
New Delhi, India
and
Fortis Escorts Kalyani Heart Centre
Gurugram, Haryana, India
Head
Department of Cardiology and
Chief Interventional Cardiologist
Jaipur Golden Hospital
New Delhi, India

Satishkumar S Kolekar MD (Medicine)
DM (Cardiology)
Consultant Interventional Cardiologist
Ruby Hall Clinic
Pune, Maharashtra, India

Satyendra Tiwari MD DNB
Fortis Escorts Hospital
New Delhi, India

Shifas Babu M MD DM DNB
Consultant
Cardiovascular Centre
Ananthapuri Hospitals and Research
Institute
Thiruvananthapuram, Kerala, India

Shirish (MS) Hiremath MD (Medicine)
DM (Cardiology)
Consultant Interventional Cardiologist
Director
Cathlab
Ruby Hall Clinic
Pune, Maharashtra, India

Shreepal Jain MD (Pediatrics)
FNB (Pediatric Cardiology)
Sir HN Reliance Foundation Hospital
Mumbai, Maharashtra, India

Srinivasan Narayan MD
DNB (Cardiology)
Fellow in Interventional Cardiology
Institute of Cardiovascular Diseases
Madras Medical Mission
Chennai, Tamil Nadu, India

Sunita Chugh MBBS DFM D Echo
MASE
Consultant
Non-invasive Cardiology
Tata Memorial Hospital
Mumbai, Maharashtra, India

Upendra Kaul MD DM FCSI FSCAI
FAPSIC FACC FAMS
Executive Director and Dean
Cardiac Sciences
Fortis Escorts Heart Institute
New Delhi, India

Vijay Trehan DM (Cardiology)
Director and Professor
Department of Cardiology
Jawaharlal Institute of Postgraduate
Medical Education and Research
(JIPMER)
New Delhi, India

Vijayakumar Subban MD DM FNB
Senior Consultant
The Madras Medical Mission
Chennai, Tamil Nadu, India

Vikram R Lele MD (Med)
DNB (Nucl. Med.) DRM
Director
Department of Nuclear Medicine and PET-CT
Jaslok Hospital and Research Centre
Mumbai, Maharashtra, India

Vinay K Bahl MD DM
Professor and Head
Department of Cardiology
All India Institute of Medical Sciences (AIIMS)
New Delhi, India

Yashasvi Chugh MBBS
Internal Medicine Resident
Jacobi Medical Center
Albert Einstein College of Medicine
Bronx, New York, USA

Preface

Perhaps no other discipline in medicine has seen such galloping strides as the field of interventional cardiology has. So fast is the evolution of the technology that it is difficult to keep pace with it. By the time you follow the recommended guidelines, the guidelines become obsolete in the light of new knowledge. Interventions in chronically occluded vessels, development of bioabsorbable stents—a new era, and intravascular imaging have changed the pattern of our practice.

The purpose of this update in interventional cardiology is manifold. It attempts at providing clear understanding of techniques from basic to beyond—to lay down principles that could allow the highest standards of safety and efficacy; to provide complete comprehensive run-down on any particular subject is beyond the scope of this book. What we have attempted is to emphasize the key points encompassing tips and tricks to fine-tune the skills of an interventional cardiologist.

With chapters on complications and high-risk PCI, the authors hope to provide wherewithal to bail out of a dreadful situation. The authors have poured in their years of experience to familiarize the reader with several practical methods of performing and troubleshooting the usual and unusual situations in the cathlab. In nutshell, the book will help in decision-making and executing the decisions in the cathlab.

This book has been possible with collaborative support of my co-editors and contributors. I hope the book empowers an interventionist with knowledge that would eventually acquire success, safety and efficacy while attempting the entire gambit of interventional procedures.

Ashwin B Mehta

Acknowledgments

This book is a culmination of consolidated efforts of a number of people. The most important ones are the contributors. Each one has made an outstanding contribution in their field, and despite their busy schedule, they have accepted our invitation and spared no efforts to come out with most illustrious and outstanding articles. We wish to deeply acknowledge their contribution from the bottom of our hearts.

Our sincerest thanks to the Directors of India Live, Dr Ashok Seth, Dr Upendra Kaul, Dr Mathew Samuel Kalarickal, and Dr Vinay K Bahl. Without their continuous encouragement and support, this task would not have been possible.

Several other members of our team have put in incessant efforts in correspondence, communication and synchronization amongst the various authors. Special mention for Mrs Kirti Talawadekar. Without her sincere efforts, the book would not have seen the light of the day within the specified time limit.

We would also thank the Jaypee Brothers Publishers team, especially Mr Sabarish Menon and Ms Kritika Dua for their continuous support and helping us in every way for timely publication of this book.

Ashwin B Mehta
Nihar Mehta
Rahul Chhabria

Contents

1. **Vascular Access** — 1
   Ajit Desai, Rahul Chhabria

2. **Coronary Stents: Evolution and Advances** — 11
   Praveen Chandra, Rashmi Xavier, Rohit Goel, Kajal Aggarwal

3. **Slender Transradial Interventions** — 26
   Sanjay Kumar Chugh, Yashasvi Chugh, Sunita Chugh

4. **Left Main Coronary Intervention** — 37
   Vinay K Bahl, Anunay Gupta

5. **Current Approach to Chronic Total Occlusions** — 45
   Kirti Punamiya

6. **Ostial Lesions** — 60
   Ajit S Mullasari, Srinivasan Narayan

7. **Coronary Bifurcation Lesions** — 70
   Nihar Mehta, Ashok Seth

8. **Calcified Lesions** — 97
   Mathew Samuel Kalarickal, Vijayakumar Subban

9. **PCI in Patients Post Coronary Artery Bypass Grafts** — 116
   Shirish (MS) Hiremath, Satishkumar S Kolekar

10. **Percutaneous Coronary Intervention in ST Elevation Myocardial Infarction** — 136
    Hetan C Shah, Ashwin B Mehta

11. **High-Risk Percutaneous Coronary Interventions** — 149
    Upendra Kaul, Satyendra Tiwari

12. **Complications during Percutaneous Coronary Interventions** — 162
    Vijay Trehan, Prattay Guhasarkar

13. **Intracoronary Assessment: Role of IVUS and OCT** — 179
    G Sengottuvelu, G Raghul

14. **Role of FFR in Evaluation of Coronary Artery Disease** — 197
    CG Bahuleyan, Shifas Babu

15. **Cardiac MRI and Cardiac CT: Indispensable Tools for the Diagnosis of Coronary Artery Disease** — 211
    Bhavin Jankharia, Parang Sanghavi, Aamish Kazi

16. **Radionuclide Studies in Cardiology**   218
    Vikram R Lele

17. **Balloon Mitral Valvuloplasty**   229
    Manjunath CN, Nagaraja Moorthy

18. **Pulmonary and Aortic Balloon Valvuloplasty**   247
    Bharat Dalvi, Kshitij Sheth, Shreepal Jain

19. **Transcatheter Aortic Valve Replacement (TAVR)—Current Status**   263
    Ashwin B Mehta, Nihar Mehta

20. **Transcatheter Closure of Congenital Heart Defects**   289
    Prafulla Kerkar, Dhiraj Kumar

21. **Interventions in Hypertrophic Cardiomyopathy**   304
    Samin K Sharma, Mithun J Varghese, Annapoorna Kini

22. **Interventions in Pulmonary Embolism**   315
    Bharat Shivdasani, Rahul Chhabria

23. **Recent Advances in Cardiac Electrophysiology**   328
    Andhalkar Bhagyashree, Amit Vora

24. **Newer Devices in Electrophysiology: Leadless Pacemakers and Subcutaneous ICD**   336
    Ameya Udyavar

Index   *347*

1

Vascular Access

Ajit Desai, Rahul Chhabria

Complications related to vascular access are most common and most dreaded ones during percutaneous interventions. It increases both morbidity and mortality related to them. Obtaining an appropriate vascular access is the basis of a successful procedure. If proposed interventional anatomy is available then decision regarding access can be taken more appropriately. Once decided, a proper technique to gain vascular access helps to avoid complication.

FEMORAL ACCESS

Femoral access is still remains the preferred technique for cardiac catheterization at many centers. Although radial route has gained huge popularity because of patient convenience and less access site compilations, femoral route has an edge over it in complex procedures, it is technically easier, can use dedicated hardware which gives better support for the procedure. A simultaneous venous access can be used for temporary pacing, monitoring pulmonary artery pressures, or infusing fluids or medications. Femoral arterial access is still the most common access site for cardiac catheterization in USA.[1] The technique of taking puncture is often underestimated but is a single most frequent cause of access site complications.[2]

Important considerations in evaluation before the femoral access
1. Absent/weak femoral pulse
2. Prior femoral arterial access site complications (dissection, pseudoaneurysm, ischemic limb)
3. Prior femoral arterial access and closure device used
4. Active groin infection
5. Prior groin surgery (excessive scarring)/radiation therapy
6. Morbidly obese

ANATOMY OF FEMORAL ARTERY AND IDEAL LOCATION OF PUNCTURE

Femoral artery is entered through the femoral triangle, which in the groin is bounded superiorly by inguinal ligament, medially by adductor longus and laterally by sartorius muscle. Structures of femoral triangle from lateral to medial include femoral nerve, femoral sheath and its content which include femoral artery, femoral vein and deep inguinal lymph nodes and associated lymphatic vessels (Fig. 1).

An ideal "landing zone" of femoral artery puncture is defined by vascular entry above the femoral bifurcation and below the upper margin, which is several centimeters below the inferior excursion of the inferior epigastric artery[3] (Fig. 2). Lower puncture can result in increased incidence of bleeding complications like hematoma and pseudoaneurysm because of lack of underlying bony structures to give adequate substrate for compression. Also the relatively smaller caliber of artery below the bifurcation makes it more prone for catheter related arterial occlusions.[4] Whereas higher cannulation is also associated with increased risk of retroperitoneal hemorrhage because of lack of underlying bony structure for effective compression.[5]

PRACTICAL LANDMARKS FOR PUNCTURE

1. *Skin/Inguinal crease*: It ideally signifies underlying inguinal ligament. An ideal arterial puncture (not skin puncture) should be 2–3 cm below the

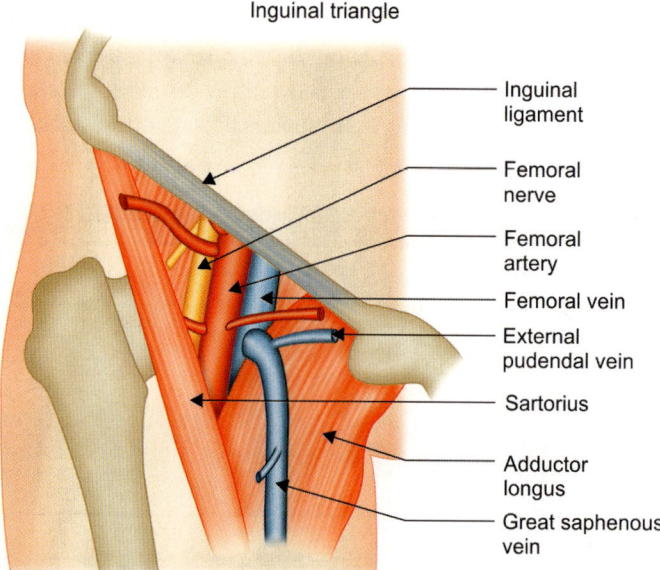

Fig. 1: Boundaries and contents of femoral triangle.

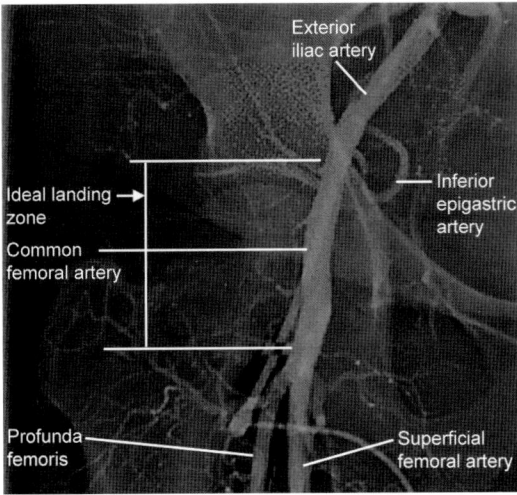

Fig. 2: Ideal site for cannulation of femoral artery.

mid-point of the crease. However, in obese patients the ligament is much lower.
2. *Bony landmarks*: Ideal point lies 2-3 cms below the mid-inguinal point which is the mid-point of a line drawn from anterior superior iliac spine and pubic tubercle.
3. *Maximal pulsation*: Site of maximal pulsation may help in easy cannulation but it may often lead to a higher or lower puncture especially in obese patients.
4. *Fluoroscopic landmark*: It is more appropriate method for cannulation of femoral artery and is used frequently in catheterization labs. In an AP view a metal clamp is used to mark the ideal point of arterial puncture. The ideal radiological location is 1 cm lateral to most medial aspect of femoral head, midway between its superior and inferior borders. The skin puncture is done 1-2 cm below that point at an angle of 30-45° from the skin. Target zone from the lower border of the head of femur to the mid portion of the head is ideal, whereas the safety spot (even in the 23% of cases with high femoral artery bifurcation) is at the mid-portion of the head of femur.[6]

Tips and Tricks
1. Position the thigh—abducted and external rotation
2. Never force the wire: if wire is not advancing then adjust the needle by a slight pull or rotate it a little; it may then be possible to insert the wire. If not, it is better to withdraw the needle and re-puncture the artery
3. Preferably use a J-tipped guidewire
4. Preferably anterior puncture

COMPLICATIONS

The overall incidence of complications of femoral access was around 6% in 1990s[7] but with advances in hardwares it is now around 2%.[8] Various factors that are associated with higher incidence of complications include inappropriate puncture technique, larger French sheaths, counter-puncture of artery, inadequate compression, repeat procedures, advanced age, peripheral artery disease, high doses of anticoagulation, use of GP IIb/IIIa inhibitors and obesity.[9] Analysis from the IMPACT II trial has identified modifiable risk factors, such as early sheath removal, avoiding placement of venous sheaths, and careful monitoring of heparin doses as potential ways of decreasing bleeding risk and complications.[10] The common complications include:

1. **Hematoma**: As per a series of 474 patients showed an incidence of 1.3% for a large hematoma (>10 cm) and 8.9% for a smaller hematoma (<5 cm).[11] It usually requires conservative management; even large hematomas rarely require surgical evacuation until there is an arterial connection or infected hematomas.
2. **Pseudoaneurysm**: Incidence of pseudoaneurysm varies from 0.5 to 7.7% in various series.[7] Factors associated with pseudoaneurysm are lower puncture, multiple punctures, and inadequate compression. Smaller pseudoaneurysms of 2-3 cm can be managed conservatively with close follow up or can be closed with ultrasound guided compression of the neck. Those larger than 3 cm rarely close spontaneously and requires either ultrasound guided compression or Doppler guided thrombin injection into the sac. Surgery is reserved if these measures fail.
3. **Arteriovenous fistula**: It is rare with an incidence of approximately 0.4%. It occurs when the artery is punctured through the vein or it overlies the vein. Most of them are small and close spontaneously but a large fistula causing symptoms of high-output failure need to be corrected surgically.
4. **Acute arterial thrombosis**: Occlusion of the femoral artery may occur due to thrombosis or local arterial injury.
5. **Retroperitoneal hematoma**: A higher puncture can cause a leak into the retroperitoneal space. It is a life threatening complication and the diagnosis requires high index of suspicion. The alarming features include unexplained hypotension which may be fluid responsive initially, unexplained drop in hematocrit, pain/discomfort in flanks. It can be sometimes missed even on ultrasound. An adequate evaluation of source of bleeding should be identified and corrected appropriately. Rarely, there can be a diffuse bleeding in retroperitoneal space which is result of coagulopathy and requires urgent correction of the same.

Closure Devices

Closure by manual compression is the gold standard, however, it has disadvantages of patient discomfort, prolonged bed rest, need of interrupting anticoagulation, and more time of healthcare providers. Vascular compression devices (VCD) improve patient comfort, shorten time for hemostasis, ambulation and discharge. However, studies have shown higher risk of infection and leg ischemia with closure devices. A large randomized trial comparing angio-seal with manual compression showed similar complication rates in both groups; with main advantage of angio-seal being patient comfort with shorter bed rest and immobilization.[12]

There are two types of closure devices active and passive. Passive ones like FemoStop provides a mechanical compression with a belt with a transparent inflatable bubble. Active VCDs results in immediate closure and includes suture devices, collagen plugs or clips.

Collagen Plug Device: Angio-Seal

It contains a small collagen plug at tip and an absorbable suture. First, the existing arterial sheath is exchanged for a specially designed 6F or 8F sheath with an arteriotomy locator. Once blood return confirms proper positioning within the arterial lumen, the sheath is held firmly in place while the guidewire and arteriotomy locator are removed. The Angio-Seal device is inserted into the sheath until it snaps in place. Next, the anchor is deployed and pulled back against the arterial wall. As the device is withdrawn further, the collagen plug is exposed just outside the arterial wall and the remainder of the device is removed from the tissue track. Finally, the suture which connects the anchor, the collagen plug, and the device is cut below skin level, leaving behind only the anchor, collagen plug and suture, all of which are absorbable.

Other devices include Collagen plug device—Mynx, Cardiva Catalyst (Boomerang), **Polyglycolic Acid (PGA) plug device: ExoSeal, Clip device: Starclose, Suture devices: Perclose**.

Transcatheter Aortic Valve Implantation (TAVI)

For TAVI, larger sheaths are required and hence the pre-procedure protocol for evaluation of the same involves the CT angiography of the peripheral vessels to evaluate the diameter, iliofemoral axis, tortuosity, calcification and extend of atherosclerosis. A diameter of femoral artery required should be more than or equal to 6 mm so as to accommodate 18F sheath. Closure devices are used post procedure to close the access.

Radial Access

Over the last decade, the radial access has gained lot of popularity as it is more comfortable to the patient, has very less complication rates as compared to femoral route. However, it has some limitations like frequent radial spasms, limitations of catheter size which restricts its use in complex cases. Studies have shown major advantage of radial access in patients with acute coronary syndrome where larger doses of anticoagulants, GP IIb/IIIa inhibitors and in some cases fibrinolytics are used. Use of radial route has shown reduction in access site complications, overall morbidity and mortality.[13] This is due to the superficial location of the radial artery, the extensive palmar collaterals, lack of adjacent veins or nerves, and hence easy and safe hemostasis, and no ischemic squeal or injury of surrounding structures.

Anatomy of Radial Artery

Radial artery is a branch of brachial artery and mostly the bifurcation occurs just below the elbow joint. It passes along the lateral margin of the forearm until it reaches the level of the wrist. The radial artery passes along the lateral margin of the forearm until it reaches the level of the wrist. In the upper forearm the vessel is deep to the body of the supinator longus muscle. In the mid forearm, down to the level of the wrist, it lies between the tendons of the supinator longus and the flexor carpi radialis. The radial artery is usually smaller than the ulnar artery at their origins, but is equal or larger at the wrist as the ulnar artery gives off numerous branches in the forearm.[14]

Absolute contraindications to radial artery cannulation include inadequate circulation to the extremity, Raynaud syndrome, thromboangiitis obliterans (Buerger's disease), and full-thickness burns or skin infection over insertion site.

Evaluation of palmar arch: When the radial artery is compressed complete, it is essential to have a good palmar arch so as to maintain adequate perfusion of hand.

Modified Allen's Test (Fig. 3)

- *Positive modified Allen's test*—If the hand flushes within 5-15 seconds, it indicates that the ulnar artery has good blood flow; this normal flushing of the hand is considered to be a positive test.
- *Negative modified Allen's test*—If the hand does not flush within 5-15 seconds, it indicates that ulnar circulation is inadequate or nonexistent; in this situation, the radial artery supplying arterial blood to that hand should not be punctured.

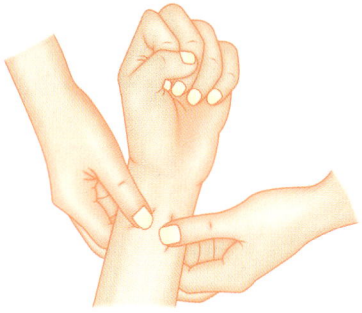
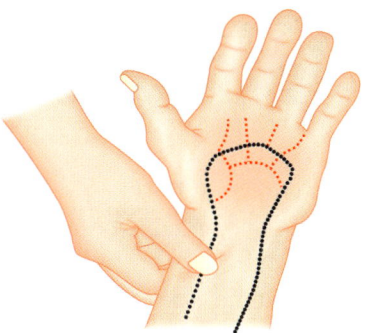

Thumbs occlude radial and ulnar arteries. Pallor is produced by clenched fist.

Thumb occludes radial artery while ulnar artery is released and patent. Unclenched hand returns to baseline color because of ulnar artery and connecting arches.

Fig. 3: Modified Allen's test.

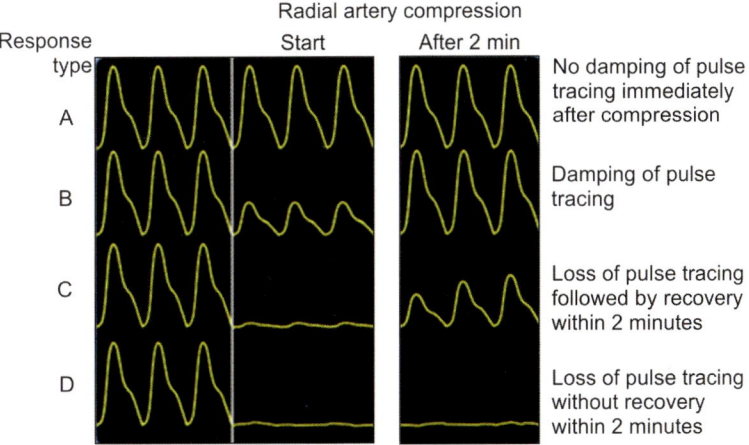

Fig. 4: The four patterns of ulnopalmar arch patency assessed by plethysmography and pulse oximetry as described by Barbeau et al. (2004). A, B, and C suggest adequacy of patency of palmar arch.

Plethysmography and Pulse Oxymetry for Evaluation of Palmar Arch

On the basis of the modified Allen's test ≤9 seconds criteria, 6.3% of patients were excluded from the transradial approach, whereas with plethysmography and pulse oxymetry types A, B, and C, only 1.5% of patients were excluded (Fig. 4).[15]

Puncture Technique

The patient's wrist is hyperextended and held in place with an arm board and gauze dressing so that the wrist is exposed (Fig. 5). Positioning of the

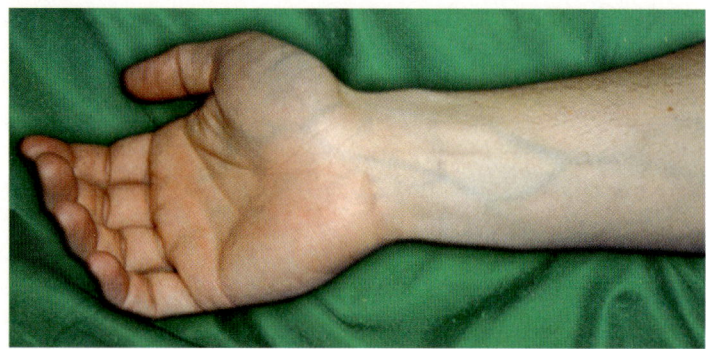

Fig. 5: Patient's wrist is hyperextended and stabilized with a roll of towel under the forearm.

patient's arm and wrist is one of the most important preparatory steps, as hyperextension of the wrist brings the radial artery more superficial and increases success rate.

The entry site is typically 1–1.5 cm above the junction of the arm and the hand (Typically at the level of second crease). Typically the best approach is to find the area of maximal arterial pulsation. An Angiocath or Jelco can be used to puncture the artery. Initial angle of the needle with the forearm should be between 30 and 45 degrees. Counter-puncture technique is preferred choice of puncture as it gives more chances of successful cannulation. Once pulsatile blood flow is noted the sheath is inserted by Seldinger technique.

Right or Left Radial Approach

The choice between right and left radial approach is more or less related to the operator's preference. The left radial approach (LRA) requires a different table set-up and logistics. The Judkins catheters can be used to cannulate the ostia while going by left radial approach. The LRA is certainly the approach of choice when the Allen's test is negative on the right radial or when a left internal mammary artery (LIMA) angiography is indicated.

Ulnar Approach

The ulnar artery as an access site was an acceptable alternative with lower success rates compared with transfemoral and transradial approaches. The mean success rates were between 38% in intention-to-treat patients and 100% in highly selected cases. The lower success rates can be explained by deeper location of the artery, close proximity to ulnar nerve which can lead to pain if punctured, and also it doesn't have a good bone support for compression.

COMPLICATIONS

Complications related to radial access are little different than those with femoral route. As the caliber of artery is smaller spams and occlusions are common. Most radial complications are preventable.

Spasm: It is the most frequent complication with radial route. It causes pain and discomfort to patient and also difficulty in manipulations of hardware through it. Risk factors for spasm are patient and operator bound, and include anxiety, age, female gender, improper sheath: lumen ratio, tortuosity, hematoma, and repeated puncture.

Tips for preventing radial artery spasm
1. First attempt is the best attempt
2. Adequate premedication and local anesthesia + intra-arterial vasodilators
3. Use of hydrophilic sheaths—less pain and spasm
4. Smaller catheters (5F vs 6F)
5. Less procedure time and fewer catheter manipulations
6. Use coronary wire to cross in case of radial loop

Radial occlusion: It occurs in 3–5% of cases and is asymptomatic as a rule; 50% of radial occlusions spontaneously recanalize over time. Predictive factors for radial occlusion include long duration of catheterization, high sheath: artery ratio, heparin dosage, longer sheath, and prolonged compression times.

Bleeding, iatrogenic radial artery perforation: One of the most common reasons for femoral crossover is iatrogenic perforation or dissection of the RA, which can usually be treated conservatively with a proximal pressure bandage. If undetected, perforation may lead to severe forearm hematoma.

Forearm hematoma: Hematoma most commonly results from perforation of a side branch or avulsion of small radial artery from a radial loop. A low threshold to perform a radial artery arteriogram when any resistance to guidewire or catheter insertion is encountered will help prevent this complication. Adequate compression is usually required.

Compartment syndrome is the most dreaded complication of radial artery hemorrhage. A large hematoma causes hand ischemia due to pressure-induced occlusion of both the radial and ulnar arteries. Fasciotomy with hematoma evacuation must be performed as an emergency procedure to prevent chronic ischemic injury. This complication is rare, occurring only once in our early experience; it should always be preventable.

Brachial and Axillary Artery Puncture

The indications of these accesses are similar to those of radial artery puncture. Few advantages of these accesses are these arteries are larger than radial but have disadvantage of higher local complication rates. In present scenario, these would be used as a rescue technique when radial and lower limb arteries are not available.

REFERENCES

1. Rao SV Ou FS, Wang TY, et al. Trends in the prevalence and outcomes of radial and femoral approaches to percutaneous coronary intervention: a report from the National Cardiovascular Data Registry. J Am Coll Cardiol Cardiovasc Interv. 2008;1:379-86.
2. Babu SC, Piccorelli GO, Shah PM, et al. Incidence and results of arterial complications among 16,350 patients undergoing cardiac catheterization. J Vasc Surg. 1989;10:113-6.
3. Cilingiroglu M, Feldman T, Salinger MH, et al. Fluoroscopically-guided micropuncture femoral artery access for large-caliber sheath insertion. J Invasive Cardiol. 2011;23:157-61.
4. Altin RS, Flicker S, Naidech HJ. Pseudoaneurysm and arteriovenous fistula after femoral artery catheterization: association with low femoral punctures. Am J Roentgenol. 1989;152:629-31.
5. Illescas FF, Baker ME, McCann R, et al. CT evaluation of retroperitoneal hemorrhage associated with femoral arteriography. Am J Roentgenol. 1986;46: 1289-92.
6. Turi ZG. An evidence-based approach to femoral arterial access and closure. Rev Cardiovasc Med. 2008;9:7-18.
7. Omoigui NA, Califf RM, Pieper K, et al. Peripheral vascular complications in the Coronary Angioplasty Versus Excisional Atherectomy Trial (CAVEAT-I). J Am Coll Cardiol. 1995;26:922-30.
8. Marso SP, Amin AP, House JA, et al. Association between use of bleeding avoidance strategies and risk of periprocedural bleeding among patients undergoing percutaneous coronary intervention. JAMA. 2010;303:2156-64.
9. Muller DW, Shamir KJ, Ellis SG, et al. Peripheral vascular complications after conventional and complex percutaneous coronary interventional procedures. Am J Cardiol. 1992;69:63.
10. Mandak JS, et al. Modifiable risk factors for vascular access site complcations in the IMPACT II Trial of angioplasty with versus without eptifibatide. Integrillin to Minimize Platelet Aggregration and Coronary Thrmobosis. J Am Coll Cardiol. 1998;31(7):1518-1524.
11. Anderson K Bregondalh M, Kaestel H, et al. Haematoma after coronary angiography and percutaneous coronary intervention via the femoral artery frequency and risk factors. Eur J Cardiovasc Nurs. 2005;4(2):123-7.
12. Hermanides RS, Ottervanger JP, Dambrink JH, et al. Closure device or manual compression in patients undergoing percutaneous coronary intervention. J Invasive Cardiol. 2010;22(12):562-6.
13. Agostoni P, Biondi-Zoccai GG, de Benedictis ML, et al. Radial versus femoral approach for percutaneous coronary diagnostic and interventional procedures: Systematic overview and meta-analysis of randomized trials. J Am Coll Cardiol. 2004;44:349-56.
14. Haerle M, Hafner HM, Dietz K, et al. Vascular dominance in the forearm. Plast Reconstr Surg. 2003.111:1891-8.
15. Barbeau GR, Arsenault F, Dugas L, et al. Evaluation of the ulnopalmar arterial arches with pulse oximetry and plethysmography: comparison with the Allen's test in 1010 patients. Am Heart J. 2004;147:489-93.

2

Coronary Stents: Evolution and Advances

Praveen Chandra, Rashmi Xavier, Rohit Goel, Kajal Aggarwal

Coronary angioplasty, conceptually described by Dotter and Judkins in 1964, was first performed by Andreas Gruntzig in 1977.[1] Coronary stents were developed in the mid-1980s and since then have seen major refinements in design and composition. There has been a huge shift in the management of coronary artery disease from the usage of pure old balloon angioplasty to the development of stents and now with the evolution of absorbable stents. The on-going studies are to refine the design, structure and material of stents to get better and improved outcomes. This article will review the development of coronary stents, their current status and the potential future directions.

PLAIN OLD BALLOON ANGIOPLASTY

Initially angioplasty only consisted of plain balloon dilatation however carried the complications of acute vessel closure due to dissection and elastic recoil. The usual incidence of elastic recoil was in 5–10% patients immediately (minutes-hours) after the procedure leading to a rebound occlusion of the artery, which often led to severe complications, including acute myocardial infarction (AMI) and the need for emergency coronary artery bypass grafting (CABG). Following plain old balloon angioplasty (POBA) there is endothelial cells denudation and medial tearing also exposing circulating blood cells to the sub-endothelial matrix leading to platelet aggregation and thrombosis, and hence leading to acute closure of the artery.[3] Balloon injury also initially induced medial smooth muscle cell necrosis,[4] followed by a phase of coordinated proliferation of medial smooth muscle cells and subsequent migration of these cells into the intima in response to the release of chemo-attractants such as the platelet-derived growth factor.[3] This neointimal proliferation leads to post-angioplasty Restenosis. This led to the development of coronary stents to overcome these issues of Coronary stents. Presently most of the percutaneous coronary intervention (PCI) procedures performed involve balloon angioplasty and stent deployment.

FIRST-GENERATION STENTS

The first coronary stent implanted in humans was the WALLSTENT by Sigwart in 1986. This was associated with difficulty with the delivery system hence was withdrawn from the market.[5] Palmaz-Schatz stent was developed in 1987 by Palmaz and co-workers which was the first FDA approved stent in USA.[2] This was the most widely used and studied stent in 1990s. This was followed by the development of multiple stents namely: Flexstentw (Cook), Wiktorw (Medtronic), Microw (Applied Vascular Engineering), Cordisw (Cordis) and Multi-linkw (Advanced Cardiovascular Systems). These stents were not free of problems due to high metal density which resulted in subacute stent thrombosis resulting in frequent failures due to embolization. Although as compared to POBA the risk if in stent restenosis (ISR) was lower they still carried a high risk of ISR. This limited their use and increased the search for newer stents with reduced complication rates. After the two landmark trialsl BENESTENT (the Belgium Netherlands Stent Arterial Revascularization Therapies Study) and the North American Stent Restenosis Study (STRESS), it was concluded that Bare metal stents were superior as compared to POBA in stenotic lesions and was the accepted standard of care in PCI eligible patients. However bare metal stents (BMS) had the risk of repeat revascularisation due to Restenosis.

This led to the revolutionary change in the development of drug eluting stents coated with antiproliferative material which prevented development of Restenosis and a dramatic reduction in the need for revascularization procedures. A few landmark trials like the RAVEL,[6] SIRUS[7] and TAXUS[8] had shown a reduction in the restenosis rates to less than 10% with need for repeat revascularisations. A permanent polymer coating was applied to release kinetics of the drug which is placed to reduce the chances of neointimal hyperplasia. Subsequently both first-generation drug eluting stents (DES), the SES (Cypher®, Cordis, Johnson & Johnson, Miami, FL USA), and the PES (Taxus®, Boston Scientific, Natick, MA USA) were rapidly approved by the regulatory bodies in Europe and the USA in 2002/2003.

Initially the DES was being used primarily for simple Type I lesions but this gradually expanded to being used for complex lesions[9] like chronic total occlusions,[10] bifurcation lesions, left main disease.[11] This initial enthusiasm was short lived till the announcements from the SCAAR trial (Swedish Coronary Angiography and Angioplasty Register), where it was seen that late stent thrombosis rates were high and fatal.[12,13] The autopsy studies showed a delay in arterial healing and impaired re-endothelialization that were associates strongly with fatal late stent thrombosis.[14] The development of neoatherosclerosis within the neointima led to development of late stent thrombosis as well.[15] The clinical cases of very LST were reported up to 4 years after the initial implantation of first-generation DES. These safety concerns led to a remarkable reduction of DES usage in 2007 and clinicians began to prescribe dual anti-platelet therapy for 1 year or longer to avoid LST. Around this time the US Food and Drug Administration (FDA) demanded that all DES manufacturers support the ongoing DAPT trial[16] in an effort to determine the optimal duration of dual anti-platelet therapy for DES. Interestingly, the 5-years follow-up of the SCAAR results did not suggest a long-term significant increase of LST in DES as compared with BMS.[17]

SECOND-GENERATION DES

Although, the first-generation DESs were another leap forward compared with BMS; there was still concern about LST and reduced deliverability with the 140 μm strut/polymer thickness. This led to the evolution of second-generation DESs which were designed to overcome these difficulties using thinner cobalt chromium alloys, new cell-cycle inhibitors (everolimus/zotarolimus), and more biocompatible polymers (fluoropolymers/phosphorylcholine). The first-generation DES continued to release drug for a prolonged duration, the release kinetics of the second-generation DES was generally shorter.

The Xience V® (Abbott Vascular, CA, USA) everolimus-eluting stent (EES) is also marketed by Boston Scientific as PROMUS® (Everolimus-Eluting Platinum Chromium Coronary Stent System) and is composed of a poly-vinylidene fluoride and hexafluoropropylene (PVDF-HFP) polymer that is loaded with everolimus at a concentration of 1 μg/m². EES release 80% of everolimus within 1 month and 100% release within 4 months after implantation. The clinical trial program included the SPIRIT I,[18] SPIRIT II,[19] SPIRIT III,[19] and SPIRIT IV trials[20] the open-label SPIRIT V registry,[21] and the all comer COMPARE trial.[22] The overall results of these studies consistently exhibited low major adverse cardiac event (MACE) rates, target vessel failure, and definite or probable stent thrombosis with the EES as compared with first-generation DES (PES) hence were found to be superior to first generation stents.

The contact angles (the angle between liquid/blood versus solid/stent) is what determines the biocompatibility of a stent and the hydrophilic nature of stent polymer. The following are the contact angles of various stents: PC (Endeavor,® Medtronic Vascular, Santa Rosa, CA, USA) 83°, BioLinx™ (Resolute, Medtronic, Santa Rosa, CA, USA) 94°, PBMA (Cypher) 115°, SIBS (Taxus) 118° and fluoropolymer (Xience) 129°. In vitro studies demonstrate that the more hydrophilic, the less macrocyte adhesion occur relative to other DES platforms. Endeavor stents have demonstrated the lowest inflammation and fibrin scores at 30 days in animal models. The Endeavor zotarolimus-eluting stent (ZES) was well studied in the ENDEAVOR,[23]

ENDEAVOR II[24] [ENDEAVOR III,[25] SORT OUT III,[26] and ZEST[27] trials, and in the E-FIVE registry,[28] which confirmed consistently low MACE rates and target vessel failure. The rates of late stent thrombosis was also rare with the second generation DES as compared to first generation DES]. The resolute ZES has a novel biocompatible hydrophilic polymer, termed BioLinx, that combines the biocompatible nature of the Endeavor stent with a hydrophobic core to allow for prolonged drug elution and improved long-term reductions in neointimal hyperplasia. The Resolute stent has 50 and 85% drug release at 7 and 60 days after stent implantation, respectively, versus the Endeavor, with 75% drug release at 2 days. This effect is correlated clinically with TLR rates of 12% of the Resolute versus 16% in the Endeavor group at 2 years.[29]

THIRD-GENERATION STENTS

The third generation stents namely the Promus element (Boston Scientific, Natick, MA, USA) was made of the same polymer, same drug elution property with the only difference of having a platinum alloy to improve fluoroscopic visibility of the stent. The backbone of the stent was also altered by reducing some of the interconnectors which led to improved deliverability although it led to longitudinal compression as compared to other stents. The clinical outcomes of the Promus Element versus the Xience VR stents were comparable up to 3 years in the PLATINUM studies.[30] Due to concerns about longitudinal compression, the stent has since been altered to allow for more support on the proximal and distal crowns.

Bioabsorbable Scaffolds

Due to the high thrombosis and restenosis rates which still are the main limitations of current permanent metallic stents which led to the development of bioabsorbable stents.[31,32] In contrast to BMSs, DESs have a reduced restenosis rate due to the presence of anti-proliferative agents in the coating layer of the stent surface and reduced rate of repeat revascularization. However, late and very late stent thrombosis remains the limitation of DES in spite of prolonged dual antiplatelet therapy.[33-36]

To overcome the problems associated with the available main treatment options, such as balloon angioplasty, BMS and DES, which were considered three revolutions in the field, the fully biodegradable scaffold technology was introduced as the fourth revolution in interventional cardiology.[37] Bioabsorbable scaffolds have been introduced to overcome limitations of permanent metallic stents, including
- Stent thrombosis requiring prolonged antiplatelet therapy
- Bleeding complications due to long-term dual antiplatelet therapy

- Rigid caging of a stented vessel
- Mismatch of the stent to vessel size resulting in a smaller lumen diameter after stent implantation
- Impairment of vessel geometry
- Impaired access and flow to side branches
- Endothelial dysfunction
- Prevention of lumen expansion associated with late favorable remodeling and vessel reactivity at the stented site
- Hindrance of any future surgical revascularization
- Impairment of noninvasive imaging with magnetic resonance imaging (MRI) and computed tomography (CT).[31,37-40]

Evolution of Bioabsorbable Stents

The Igaki-Tamai poly-L-lactic acid (PLLA) scaffold without any drug coating was the first bioresorbable device to be evaluated in humans in a first-in-man (FIM) study enrolling 15 subjects.[17] The FIM study of the scaffold showed no Major Adverse Cardiac Events (MACE) or scaffold thrombosis (ST) within 30 days and 1 repeat PCI at the 6 months follow-up. Late lumen loss (LLL) rate was 0.48 mm without inducing excess of neointimal hyperplasia.[17] Another study enrolling 50 subjects showed encouraging results with cardiac death, noncardiac death and MACE including all-cause death, non-fatal myocardial infarction (MI), and target lesion revascularization (TLR)/target vessel revascularization (TVR) as 2, 12 and 50%, respectively, at 10 years follow-up.[18] Only two definite scaffold thrombosis (one sub-acute and one very late) were observed. The latter case was due to the DES implanted proximal to the Igaki-Tamai® stent.

There are two drug-eluting bioabsorbable vascular scaffolds with a CE-mark on the market, ABSORB Bioresorbable Vascular Scaffold (BVS) (Abbott Vascular, Santa Clara, CA, USA) that received the CE-mark in January 2011 followed by DESolve (Elixir Medical, Sunnyvale, CA, USA) in May 2013, proofing the concept of drug-eluting bioabsorbable vascular scaffolds.

The first commercially available bioabsorbable scaffold, Absorb BVS, consists of a backbone of poly-L-lactide (PLLA) coated with poly-D-L-lactide controlling the release of an antiproliferative drug everolimus. The first-in-man ABSORB (Cohort A) trial was tailored to identify the safety and performance of the first generation scaffold with an enrolment of 30 subjects. This trial revealed a very good clinical safety as there was no cardiac death, ID-TLR or scaffold thrombosis during 2 years follow-up.[20] A 3.4% Ischemia-driven MACE (ID-MACE) rate with only one non-Q wave MI in the 2 years after index procedure was encouraging as well. Angiographic results such as an in-scaffold late lumen loss of 0.44 ± 0.35 mm and 0.48 ± 0.28 mm at the 6 month and 2 years follow-up, respectively, and a % diameter stenosis of

27% for both the 6 months and 2 years follow-up were equivalent to some of the permanent DESs[21,22] and less than BMS.[23]

As the ABSORB Cohort A trial revealed that the first generation of the scaffold had some problems such as a high rate of incomplete strut apposition and late acquired mal-apposition due to poor conformability, scaffold shrinkage, and chronic recoil problems,[19,20] all of these issues have been resolved with the second generation bioresorbable everolimus-eluting scaffold systems (ABSORB BVS). The ABSORB Cohort B trial enrolling 101 subjects (45 subjects in Cohort B1 and 56 subjects in Cohort B2) showed very good 6 months angiographic results with an in-scaffold late lumen loss of 0.19 ± 0.18 mm in Cohort B1 and 0.27 ± 0.32 mm in Cohort B2 at 6 months and 1 year follow-up, respectively. These results are similar to permanent DESs.[21,26,27] The MACE rate of 7.1% was observed for Cohort B2 at 1 year follow-up.[28] The first-in-man ABSORB Cohort A study and subsequently the Cohort B study preliminarily demonstrated the safety and efficacy of the scaffold under clinical study conditions.

As all available data of ABSORB are from small, non-randomized studies with short-term and mid-term follow-up, many clinical trials and registries were initiated to expand the experience with Absorb BVS system for a long-term follow-up with broader inclusion criteria for the treatment of complex lesions, subjects in real-world settings, and in different geographies.

Following the ABSORB Cohort A and B studies, a multicenter, randomized, single-blind, active-controlled ABSORB-II trial comparing ABSORB everolimus-eluting bioresorbable scaffold vs Xience everolimus-eluting stent was initiated. This trial is the first randomized controlled comparison of a bioresorbable scaffold with a metallic stent. The study, in which 501 subjects were enrolled, showed similar 1 year composite secondary clinical outcomes between Absorb and Xience arms.[29] The Target Lesion Failure (TLF) rate between the Absorb and Xience group was 5 and 3% ($p = 0.35$), respectively. The clinically indicated TLR (CI-TLR) rate was 1% for the Absorb arm and 2% for the Xience arm ($p = 0.69$). Definite and probable scaffold or stent thrombosis rate was 0.9 to 0% ($p = 0.55$) for the Absorb and Xience arms, respectively. This study showed similar results between new generation DES (Xience) and drug-eluting bioresorbable scaffold (ABSORB) arms.[41]

ABSORB III, a multicenter, randomized trial (2:1 Absorb vs Xience) with up to 2008 subjects at 220 US and non-US sites[30] revealed a 7.8 and 6.1% TLF rate in the Absorb and Xience groups, respectively, proving noninferiority for the primary endpoint of the study. Device thrombosis rate of the Absorb and Xience arm was 1.5 and 0.7 ($p = 0.13$), respectively.[42]

These studies[41,42] have proved the safety and efficacy of the BVS under clinical study conditions. The following registries have been initiated to also obtain a broad range of data for ABSORB BVS in the real world patient population:

- ABSORB EXTEND is a prospective single-arm study with an enrolment of up to 800 patients with more complex coronary disease at up to 100 sites.[31] Interim analysis of the first enrolled 512 subjects showed good safety and efficacy results with 0.4% of cardiac death, 2.9% of MI, 1.8% of ID-TLR, 0.8% of definite and probable scaffold thrombosis and 4.3% of ID-MACE at the 12 months follow-up.[43]
- GHOST-EU registry enrolled 1189 subjects showed acceptable rate of TLF at 6 months (4.4%) although early and midterm scaffold thrombosis rate were high.[44]
- GABI-R including over 5000 subjects from approximately 100 sites in Austria and Germany.[46]
- ABSORB FIRST with an enrolment of 1802 subjects at approximately 90 sites (ClinicalTrials.gov NCT01759290);
- ABSORB UK including 1000 subjects at 23 sites (ClinicalTrials.gov NCT01977534);
- IT-Disappears with 1000 subjects at 50 sites in Italy (ClinicalTrials.gov NCT02004730)

DESolve (Elixir Medical, CA, USA), a bioresorbable coronary scaffold (BCS) combining PLLA based scaffold with novolimus as an antiproliferative agent, is the second bioabsorbable scaffold which received the CE mark.[45] The FIM study of this new scaffold showed neither scaffold thrombosis nor major adverse cardiac events at the 12 months follow-up. At 6 months, in-scaffold LLL was 0.19 ± 0.19 mm, which is very similar to the LLL rate (0.19 ± 0.18 mm) of the ABSORB Cohort B1.[47]

Intravascular ultrasound (IVUS) analysis showed that no scaffold recoil or late malapposition occurred. This study demonstrated the initial feasibility and efficacy of the DESolve BCS. However, the number of subjects enrolled in the study, 16 subjects, is very low. Thus, this study provided only preliminary data for the design of larger studies to obtain substantiated safety and efficacy results for the device. Therefore, another trial, DESolve Nx enrolling 126 subjects was conducted.[46] The 6 months LLL was 0.21 ± 0.34 mm. MACE rate was 3.35% including one cardiac death, one non-Q wave MI and two TLR cases.[46] There was no definite scaffold thrombosis.

MAGMARIS STENT—PREVIOUS STUDIES

The Absorbable Metal Stent (AMS) consisting of absorbable magnesium (Mg) alloy was introduced to overcome the limitations of contemporary stents.[48] This scaffold has a high mechanical strength, low elastic recoil (<8%), high collapse pressure (0.8 bar), and minimum foreshortening (<5%), all of which are comparable to stainless steel stents.[48] Moreover, the degradation of Mg produces an electronegative charge resulting in a hypothrombogenic scaffold, which may be an important advantage to overcome the scaffold thrombosis issue. The initial preclinical study in a porcine model showed that the scaffold was rapidly reendothelialized and degraded into inorganic salts with little inflammatory response.[49,50] These results might be important preliminary signals to expect a good safety profile which needs to be proved in clinical studies.

After acceptable safety and patency rates of the first AMS trial for treatment of infra popliteal arteries in 20 subjects,[51] the Clinical Performance and Angiographic Results of Coronary Stenting with Absorbable Metal Stents[36] (PROGRESS-AMS) trial was performed to test the bare AMS in coronary arteries. This multicenter, single-arm FIM study assessed the efficacy and safety of the scaffold in 63 subjects with single *de novo* lesions. This study showed a good safety profile with no death, MI or scaffold thrombosis during the 12 months follow-up. Furthermore, IVUS analysis showed the absence of residual metal ensuring the unlike of late and very late stent thrombosis, which is a main disadvantage of the current DESs. However, in-scaffold late lumen loss and ischemia-driven TLR rates were high: 1.08 ± 0.49 mm and 23.8%, respectively, at 4 months. Intravascular ultrasound (IVUS) analysis showed that acute recoil was the primary cause of the high late lumen loss rate and restenosis which might be due to early loss of radial force of the scaffold. Despite the very good clinical outcomes, angiographic parameters were less promising, suggesting a need for slower scaffold absorption and addition of antiproliferative drug elution concept to prevent neointimal hyperplasia.[47,52] As a consequence, this study showed not only the safety and feasibility of an AMS but also a necessity for the modification of some of the scaffold properties. The AMS device was improved by using a different Mg alloy to prolong the degradation time to carry on scaffolding property and scaffold integrity. To improve radial strength, the cross-section shape of the strut was altered from rectangular to square. In addition, to inhibit neointimal proliferative response, the scaffold strut surface was coated with a drug-polymer matrix of the absorbable polymer carrier polylactic-coglycolic-acid (PLGA) and antiproliferative drug paclitaxel.[53]

DRug **E**luting **A**bsorbable **M**etal **S**caffold First Generation (DREAMS IG), an improved version of the AMS, was tested in the BIOSOLVE-I study. In this prospective, multicenter, FIM trial, subjects at five European centers were enrolled. The study results showed a good clinical safety profile as there was no cardiac death or scaffold thrombosis up to the 12 months follow-up. Only one periprocedural target vessel MI occurred following the treatment of a stenosis located at the circumflex artery after the 12 months follow-up angiography. As by definition, the target vessel also includes side branches, this MI was classified as target vessel MI even though it was not related to the original target lesion located in obtuse marginal artery treated with the scaffold. Due to this event, the TLF rate increased to 7% at the 1 year follow-up while the 6 months result was 4%. In comparison to its AMS precursor, the DREAMS demonstrated a significant improvement in the rate of clinically driven TLR (4.7%[13] vs 26.7%[36]) at 12 months postprocedure. The TLF rate for BIOSOLVE-I remained stable with no further TLF cases (7%) up to 3 years post-procedure,[54] while one additional TLR case was observed for BVS Cohort B between 2 and 3 year follow-up resulting in a total of 10% TLF rate. Additionally no cardiac death nor a stent thrombosis event had been observed in the BIOSOLVE-I study up to 3 years post procedure.[54]

With an in-scaffold LLL of 0.65 ± 0.50 mm at 6 months and 0.52 ± 0.39 mm at 12 months, DREAMS did not reach the excellent late lumen loss of ABSORB or other contemporary DESs.[55] However, the in-scaffold LLL at 6 months (0.65 ± 0.50 mm) and at 12 months (0.52 ± 0.39 mm) showed a reduction of 40 and 52%, respectively, compared to the LLL of 1.08 + 0.49 mm at the 4 months follow-up reported in the PROGRESS study.[47]

This study results showed that although the refinement of the device resulted in significant improvements compared to the bare AMS and the TLF rates were comparable to contemporary DESs and the ABSORB BVS, DREAMS 1G was not competitive regarding the late lumen loss observed for ABSORB or other commercially available DES. Therefore, this device needed to be improved to obtain better angiographic endpoint results.

The next generation of the scaffold, DREAMS 2nd generation (2G), addressed all limitations of DREAMS 1G. The scaffold backbone was modified to obtain a more flexible and stronger device, especially to improve acute and chronic radial strength to withstand the extra scaffold plaque for a longer time. Radiopaque markers were added for X-ray visibility of the scaffold. Furthermore, the drug-polymer coating has been changed to bioabsorbable PLLA and Sirolimus instead of Paclitaxel to decrease neointimal formation more effectively. The same coating is also successfully used in the commercially available Orsiro sirolimus eluting coronary stent system[56-58] (BIOTRONIK AG, Buelach, CH). DREAMS 2G is currently under investigation in the BIOSOLVE-II study (BIOTRONIK – Safety and Clinical Performance of the Drug Eluting Absorbable Metal Scaffold. DREAMS 2G in the Treatment of Subjects with de novo lesions in native coronary arteries).[59] It is the first study to assess the safety and performance of a novel sirolimus-eluting absorbable magnesium scaffold in symptomatic patients with *de novo* coronary artery lesions.

The primary endpoint of this prospective and multicenter single-arm study was in-segment LLL at 6 months post-procedure. 123 subjects have been enrolled in the study. Study subjects undergo a clinical follow-up at 1, 6, and 12 months and annually thereafter until 3 years post-procedure. An angiographic follow-up is performed at 6 months post-procedure for 113 implanted subjects. For a subset of up to 30 evaluable subjects, an intravascular ultrasound (IVUS), and optical coherence tomography (OCT) was performed at 6 months follow-up. At one center, vasomotion was assessed with acetylcholine followed by nitroglycerin in a subgroup of 25 subjects.

Mean in-segment LLL at 6 months was 0.27 ± 0.37 mm. In segment LLL decreased by 41.8% (from 0.52 to 0.27 mm) from BIOSOLVE-I to BIOSOLVE-II with DREAMS 2G. This result is better than the LLL of the ABSORB Cohort A 19 (0.36 ± 0.29 mm) whereas it is inferior to the LLL of the ABSORB Cohort B1 24 (0.11 ± 0.28 mm) at 6 months follow-up. As late lumen enlargement and favorable tissue response were reported for the absorbable scaffolds,[51-60] LLL value might not affect the long-term outcomes of the study. For instance, with a 0.44 mm LLL at the 6 months follow-up, the 5 years outcome of the ABSORB Cohort A was excellent without any additional MACE. However, this result needs to be confirmed in larger studies. The neointimal hyperplasia area was 0.08 and 0.30 mm^2 in BIOSOLVE-I and BIOSOLVE-II, respectively. This value is identical to the value recorded in the ABSORB Cohort B (0.08 mm^2) 24 and lower than in the ABSORB Cohort A (0.30 mm^2) and DeSolve (0.4 mm^2).[45] Decreasing radial strength during the absorption process might be the reason of the inconsistency between LLL and neointimal hyperplasia results of the study. IVUS analysis in a subgroup showed that degradation of DREAMS 2G is slower than DREAMS 1G whose degradation time was too fast as mean scaffold and mean lumen area decreased faster in BIOSOLVE-I than in BIOSOLVE-II 70 (mean scaffold area –11.1 vs –0.5%; mean lumen area –15.3 vs –2.4%).

No malapposed struts were detectable during the OCT analysis as the investigational device was fully embedded in the vessel wall. Furthermore, 80% of the vasomotion subgroup subjects showed vasoconstriction or vasodilatation with a threshold of change of 3.0% or more.[59] In BIOSOLVE-II study, Target Lesion Failure (TLF) was 3% at 6 months which is very similar to the TLF rate of new generation metallic stent.[55] During 6 months follow-up of the study, one target vessel MI occurred (<1%) and 2 subjects underwent clinically driven TLR (2%). One death of unknown cause (<1%) was classified as cardiac death. No definite or probable scaffold thrombosis was observed neither in BIOSOLVE-I[59] nor in the previous studies performed with precursor devices.[47] Recently the 12 months clinical results and angiographic findings of the BIOSOLVE-II study have been published.[61] Quantitative coronary angiography (QCA) parameters remained stable from 6 to 12 months [paired data of 42 patients: in-segment late lumen loss 0.20 + 0.21 vs 0.25 + 0.22 mm, P = 0.117, D 0.05 + 0.21 mm (95% CI: 20.01;0.12); in-scaffold late lumen loss 0.37 + 0.25 vs 0.39 + 0.27 mm, P = 0.446, D 0.03 + 0.22 (95% CI: 20.04;0.10), respectively]. Intravascular ultrasound and optical coherence tomography findings corroborated the QCA results. No additional Target lesion failure event occurred beyond the 6 months follow-up and during the entire follow-up of 12 months; none of the patients experienced a definite or probable scaffold thrombosis. In summary, the 6 and

12 months follow-up results of the BIOSOLVE-II study reveals that DREAMS 2G improves late lumen loss compared to its precursor devices while maintaining a favourable clinical and safety profile.[59,62] The ongoing BIOSOLVE-III study is a prospective, multicenter trial to be conducted in up to 61 subjects enrolled at up to 7 investigational sites. Clinical follow-up visits will take place at 1, 6, and 12 months and annually until 3 years post-procedure. All subjects will undergo angiographic follow-up at 12 months. This study will provide data for the deliverability and acute performance regarding procedure success of DREAMS 2G with an improved crossing profile.

CONCLUSION

We have gone a long way from POBA to absorbable stents but still research is ongoing to improve the deliverability, conformability, improving radial strength without increase in strut thickness, reduce rates of stent thrombosis, reduce rate of stent Restenosis. Despite the current generation DESs have dramatically improved the rates of adverse events in clinical practice, the ongoing quest to reduce the risk of late stent thrombotic events while maintaining maximal lumen diameters and retuning normal vessel physiology is ongoing. The biodegradable polymers and completely biodegradable stents represent the "cutting edge" in the evolution of DES technology. As substantiated by early clinical trials, these stents achieve temporary vessel scaffolding to obtain optimal vessel calibers, prevent vessel recoil, and stabilize dissections until the vessel has healed. Since, they get absorbed overtime they leave behind a normal healed vessel with return of normal vasomotor tone. Dual antiplatelet duration is not reduced and may be required for a longer time given the thicker stent struts with bioabsorbable stents. Several important features such as optimal polymer composition, degradation, drug release kinetics, impact of neoatherosclerosis, and stent fracture are the focus of current investigations. Ongoing "real world" clinical experience is needed to gain better evidence after promising initial results in order to confirm their advantage.

REFERENCES

1. Gruntzig A. Transluminal dilatation of coronary-artery stenosis. Lancet 1978; 1:263.
2. Garg S, Serruys PW Coronary stents: current status. J Am Coll Cardiol 2010;56:S1-42.
3. Chandrasekar B, Tanguay JF. Platelets and restenosis. J Am Coll Cardiol 2000; 35:555–62.
4. Clowes AW, Reidy MA, Clowes MM. Mechanisms of stenosis after arterial injury. Lab Invest 1983;49:208–15.
5. Sigwart U, Puel J, Mirkovitch V, et al. Intravascular stents to prevent occlusion and Restenosis after transluminal angioplasty. N Engl J Med 1987;316:701–6.

6. Morice MC, et al. A randomized comparison of a sirolimus-eluting stent with a standard stent for coronary revascularization. N Engl J Med. 2002;346(23):1773-80.
7. Moses JW, et al. Sirolimus-eluting stents versus standard stents in patients with stenosis in a native coronary artery N Engl J Med. 2003;349(14):1315-23.
8. Stone GW, et al. A polymer-based, paclitaxel-eluting stent in patients with coronary artery disease. N Engl J Med. 2004;350(3):221-31.
9. Chieffo A, Aranzulla TC, Colombo A. Drug eluting stents: focus on Cypher sirolimus-eluting coronary stents in the treatment of patients with bifurcation lesions. Vasc Health Risk Manag. 2007;3:441–51
10. Saeed B, Kandzari DE, Agostoni P, et al. Use of drug-eluting stents for chronic total occlusions: a systematic review and meta-analysis. Catheter Cardiovasc Interv. 2011;77:315–32.
11. Colombo A, Chieffo A. Drug-eluting stent update 2007: part III: technique and unapproved/unsettled indications (left main, bifurcations, chronic total occlusions, small vessels and long lesions, saphenous vein grafts, acute myocardial infarctions, and multivessel disease). Circulation. 2007;116:1424–32
12. Camenzind E, Steg PG, Wijns W. Stent thrombosis late after implantation of first-generation drug-eluting stents: a cause for concern. Circulation. 2007;115: 1440–55
13. Nordmann AJ, Briel M, Bucher HC. Mortality in randomized controlled trials comparing drug-eluting vs. bare metal stents in coronary artery disease: a meta-analysis. Eur Heart J. 2006;27:2784–814.
14. Joner M, Finn AV, Farb A, et al. Pathology of drug-eluting stents in humans: delayed healing and late thrombotic risk. J Am Coll Cardiol. 2006;48:193–202.
15. Nakazawa G, Finn AV, Vorpahl M, et al. Coronary responses and differential mechanisms of late stent thrombosis attributed to first-generation sirolimus- and paclitaxel-eluting stents. J Am Coll Cardiol. 2011;57:390–98
16. Mauri L, Kereiakes DJ, Normand SL, et al. Rationale and design of the dual antiplatelet therapy study, a prospective, multicenter, randomized, double-blind trial to assess the effectiveness and safety of 12 versus 30 months of dual antiplatelet therapy in subjects undergoing percutaneous coronary intervention with either drug-eluting stent or bare metal stent placement for the treatment of coronary artery lesions. Am Heart J. 2010;160:1035–41.
17. Sarno G, Lagerqvist B, Fröbert O, et al. Lower risk of stent thrombosis and restenosis with unrestricted use of 'new-generation' drug-eluting stents: a report from the nationwide Swedish Coronary Angiography and Angioplasty Registry (SCAAR). Eur Heart J. 2012;33:606-13
18. Tsuchida K, Piek JJ, Neumann FJ, et al. One-year results of a durable polymer everolimus-eluting stent in de novo coronary narrowings (The SPIRIT FIRST Trial). EuroIntervention. 2005;1:266–72.
19. Stone GW, Midei M, Newman W, et al. Randomized comparison of everolimus-eluting and paclitaxel-eluting stents: two-year clinical follow-up from the clinical evaluation of the Xience V Everolimus Eluting Coronary Stent System in the treatment of patients with de novo Native Coronary Artery Lesions (SPIRIT) III trial. Circulation. 2009;119:680–6.
20. Serruys PW, Ruygrok P, Neuzner J, et al. A randomised comparison of an everolimus-eluting coronary stent with a paclitaxel-eluting coronary stent: the SPIRIT II trial. EuroIntervention. 2006;2:286–94.
21. Grube E, Chevalier B, Smits P, et al. The SPIRIT V study: a clinical evaluation of the XIENCE V everolimus-eluting coronary stent system in the treatment of patients with de novo coronary artery lesions. JACC Cardiovasc Interv. 2011;4:168–75.

22. Kedhi E, Joesoef KS, McFadden E, et al. Second-generation everolimus-eluting and paclitaxel-eluting stents in real-life practice (COMPARE): a randomised trial. Lancet. 2010;375:201–9.
23. Waseda K, Miyazawa A, Ako J, et al. Intravascular ultrasound results from the ENDEAVOR IV trial: randomized comparison between zotarolimus- and paclitaxel-eluting stents in patients with coronary artery disease. JACC Cardiovasc Interv. 2009;2:779–84.
24. Fajadet J, Wijns W, Laarman GJ, et al. Randomized, double-blind, multicenter study of the Endeavor zotarolimus-eluting phosphorylcholine-encapsulated stent for treatment of native coronary artery lesions: clinical and angiographic results of the ENDEAVOR II trial. Circulation. 2006;114:798–806.
25. Kandzari DE, Leon MB, Popma JJ, et al. Comparison of zotarolimus-eluting and sirolimus-eluting stents in patients with native coronary artery disease: a randomized controlled trial. J Am Coll Cardiol. 2006;48:2440–7.
26. Maeng M, Tilsted HH, Jensen LO, et al. 3-Year clinical outcomes in the randomized SORT OUT III superiority trial comparing zotarolimus- and sirolimus-eluting coronary stents. JACC Cardiovasc Interv. 2012;5:812–8.
27. Park DW, Kim YH, Yun SC, et al. Comparison of zotarolimus-eluting stents with sirolimus- and paclitaxel-eluting stents for coronary revascularization: the ZEST (comparison of the efficacy and safety of zotarolimus-eluting stent with sirolimus-eluting and paclitaxel-eluting stent for coronary lesions) randomized trial. J Am Coll Cardiol. 2010;56:1187–95.
28. Jain AK, Meredith IT, Lotan C, et al. Real-world safety and efficacy of the endeavor zotarolimus-eluting stent: early data from the E-Five Registry. Am J Cardiol. 2007;100:77M–83M.
29. Tada T, Byrne RA, Cassese S, et al. Comparative efficacy of 2 zotarolimus-eluting stent generations: resolute versus endeavor stents in patients with coronary artery disease. Am Heart J. 2013;165:80–6.
30. Stone GW, Teirstein P, Meredith I, et al. Three-year results of the platinum randomized trial comparing platinum chromium promus element and cobalt chromium promus/xience v everolimus–eluting stents. J Am Coll Cardiol. 2013;61:61732–5.
31. Waksman R. Promise and challenges of bioabsorbable stents. Catheter Car_diovasc Interv 2007;70(3):407-14.
32. Nef H, Wiebe J, Achenbach S, et al. Evaluation of the short- and long-term safety and therapy outcomes of the everolimus-eluting bioresorbable vascular scaffold system in patients with coronary artery stenosis: Rationale and design of the German-Austrian ABSORB RegIstRy (GABI-R). Cardiovasc Revasc Med 2016;17(1):34-7.
33. Daemen J, Wenaweser P, Tsuchida K, et al. Early and late coronary stent thrombosis of sirolimus-eluting and paclitaxel-eluting stents in routine clinical practice: data from a large two-institutional cohort study. Lancet 2007;24;369(9562):667-78.
34. Lasala JM, Cox DA, Dobies D, et al. Drug-eluting stent thrombosis in routine clinical practice: two-year outcomes and predictors from the TAXUS ARRIVE registries. Circ Cardiovasc Interv 2009;2(4):285-93.
35. Lagerqvist B, James SK, Stenestrand U, et al. Long-term outcomes with drug-eluting stents versus bare-metal stents in Sweden. N Engl J Med 2007;356(10):1009-19.
36. Daemen J, Simoons ML, Wijns W, et al. Meeting report ESC forum on drug eluting stents, European Heart House, Nice, 2007. EuroIntervention 2009;4(4):427-36.

37. Onuma Y, Serruys PW. Bioresorbable scaffold: the advent of a new era in percutaneous coronary and peripheral revascularization? Circulation 2011;123(7): 779-97.
38. Haude M, Erbel R, Erne P, et al. Safety and performance of the drug-eluting absorbable metal scaffold (DREAMS) in patients with de-novo coronary lesions: 12 month results of the prospective, multicentre, first-in-man BIOSOLVE-I trial. Lancet 2013;381(9869):836-44.
39. Lu C, Filion KB, Eisenberg MJ. The Safety and Efficacy of Absorb Bioresorbable Vascular Scaffold: A Systematic Review. Clin Cardiol 2016;39(1):48-55.
40. Lind AY, Eggebrecht H, Erbel R. Images in cardiology: the invisible stent: imaging of an absorbable metal stent with multislice spiral computed tomography. Heart 2005;91(12):1604.
41. Ormiston JA, Serruys PW, Regar E, et al. A bioabsorbable everolimus-eluting coronary stent system for patients with single de-novo coronary artery lesions (ABSORB): a prospective open-label trial. Lancet 2008;371(9616):899-907
42. Meredith IT, Ormiston J, Whitbourn R, et al. First-in-human study of the Endeavor ABT-578-eluting phosphorylcholine-encapsulated stent system in de novo native coronary artery lesions: Endeavor I Trial. EuroIntervention 2005;1(2):157-64.
43. Serruys PW, Chevalier B, Dudek D, et al. A bioresorbable everolimus-eluting scaffold versus a metallic everolimus-eluting stent for ischaemic heart disease caused by de-novo native coronary artery lesions (ABSORB II): an interim 1-year analysis of clinical and procedural secondary outcomes from a randomised controlled trial. Lancet 2015;385(9962):43-54.
44. Ellis SG, Kereiakes DJ, Metzger DC, et al. Everolimus-Eluting Bioresorbable Scaffolds for Coronary Artery Disease. N Engl J Med 2015;373 (20):1905-15.
45. Abizaid A, Ribamar CJ, Jr., Bartorelli AL, et al. The ABSORB EXTEND study: preliminary report of the twelve-month clinical outcomes in the first 512 patients enrolled. EuroIntervention 2015;10(12):1396-401.
46. Capodanno D, Gori T, Nef H, et al. Percutaneous coronary intervention with everolimus-eluting bioresorbable vascular scaffolds in routine clinical practice: early and midterm outcomes from the European multicentre GHOST-EU registry. EuroIntervention 2015;10(10):1144-53.
47. Verheye S, Ormiston JA, Stewart J, et al. A next-generation bioresorbable coronary scaffold system: from bench to first clinical evaluation: 6- and 12 month clinical and multimodality imaging results. JACC Cardiovasc Interv 2014;7(1):89-99.
48. Nef H, Wiebe J, Achenbach S, et al. Evaluation of the short- and long-term safety and therapy outcomes of the everolimus-eluting bioresorbable vascular scaffold system in patients with coronary artery stenosis: Rationale and design of the German-Austrian ABSORB RegIstRy (GABI-R). Cardiovasc Revasc Med 2016;17(1):34-7
49. Serruys PW, Silber S, Garg S, et al. Comparison of zotarolimus-eluting and everolimus-eluting coronary stents. N Engl J Med 2010;363(2):136-46.
50. Onuma Y, Ormiston J, Serruys PW. Bioresorbable scaffold technologies. Circ J 2011;75(3):509-20
51. Heublein B, Rohde R, Kaese V, et al. Biocorrosion of magnesium alloys: a new principle in cardiovascular implant technology? Heart 2003;89(6):651-6.
52. Waksman R, Pakala R, Kuchulakanti PK, et al. Safety and efficacy of bioabsorbable magnesium alloy stents in porcine coronary arteries. Catheter Cardiovasc Interv 2006;68(4):607-17.
53. Peeters P, Bosiers M, Verbist J, et al. Preliminary results after application of absorbable metal stents in patients with critical limb ischemia. J Endovasc Ther 2005;12(1):1-5.

54. Waksman R, Erbel R, Di MC, et al. Early- and long-term intravascular ultrasound and angiographic findings after bioabsorbable magnesium stent implantation in human coronary arteries. JACC Cardiovasc Interv 2009;2(4):312-20.
55. Wittchow E, Adden N, Riedmuller J, et al. Bioresorbable drug-eluting magnesium-alloy scaffold: design and feasibility in a porcine coronary model. EuroIntervention 2013;8(12):1441-50.
56. Haude M, Erbel R, Erne P, et al. Safety and performance of the DRug-Eluting Absorbable Metal Scaffold (FREAMS) in patients with de novo coronary lesions: 3-year results of the prospective, multicentre, first-in-man BIOSOLVE-I trial EuroIntervention 2016;12(2):e160-e166.
57. Serruys PW, Ruygrok P, Neuzner J, et al. A randomised comparison of an everolimus-eluting coronary stent with a paclitaxel-eluting coronary stent:the SPIRIT II trial. EuroIntervention 2006;2(3):286-94.
58. Windecker S, Haude M, Neumann FJ, et al. Comparison of a novel biodegradable polymer sirolimus-eluting stent with a durable polymer everolimus-eluting stent: results of the randomized BIOFLOW-II trial. Circ Cardiovasc Interv 2015 February;8(2):e001441.
59. Waltenberger J, Brachmann J, van der Heyden J, et al. Real-world experience with a novel biodegradable polymer sirolimus-eluting stent: twelve-month results of the BIOFLOW-III registry. EuroIntervention 2016 February 20;11(10):1106-10.
60. Pilgrim T, Heg D, Roffi M, et al. Ultrathin strut biodegradable polymer sirolimus-eluting stent versus durable polymer everolimus-eluting stent for percutaneous coronary revascularisation (BIOSCIENCE): a randomised, single-blind, non-inferiority trial. Lancet 2014 December 13;384(9960):2111-22.
61. Haude M, Ince H, Abizaid A, et al. Sustained safety and performance of the second-generation drug-eluting absorbable metal scaffold in patients with de novo coronary lesions: 12-month clinical results and angiographic findings of the BIOSOLVE-II first-in-man trial. Eur Heart J 2016.
62. Karanasos A, Simsek C, Gnanadesigan M, et al. OCT assessment of the long-term vascular healing response 5 years after everolimus-eluting bioresorbable vascular scaffold. J Am Coll Cardiol 2014 December 9;64(22):2343-56.

3

Slender Transradial Interventions

Sanjay Kumar Chugh, Yashasvi Chugh, Sunita Chugh

INTRODUCTION

The transradial approach has gained popularity globally, for coronary diagnostic and therapeutic procedures, and has successfully emerged as an alternative to the femoral route.[1,2] Transradial access (TRA) carries the merits of decreased access site complications and major bleeding; lower costs and earlier patient ambulation.[3-8] Despite its increasing popularity, TRA has a steeper learning curve,[9] in part contributed by failures in radial artery punctures[6] and arterial anatomical variability encountered during the procedure;[10,11] contributing to prolonged procedural time,[5] crossover rates[6] as well as patient discomfort.

Transradial (TR) primary angioplasty has been shown to reduce all -cause mortality compared to transfemoral procedures.[7,12-14] In the RIVAL study,[7] there was a reported 40% relative reduction in the risk of death, MI, stroke, or non-CABG-related major ACUITY bleeding and a significant 61% relative reduction in the 30-day mortality (1.3 VS 3.2%, p = 0.006, Hazard ratio = 0.39) among ST elevation myocardial infarction (STEMI) patients treated via the radial artery.

In the RIFLE STEACS,[12] the largest randomized study on primary percutaneous coronary intervention (PCI) study in which 1001 STEMI patients were randomized to either radial or femoral access (1:1), there was a significant reduction in mortality (30 day cardiac mortality 5.25 vs 9.2%, p = 0.02) and MACE. In the HORIZONS-AMI[13] trial 200 pts underwent transradial primary PCI. One year death and re-infarction for transfemoral versus transradial access was 7.8 vs 4.0%, p = 0.06; with reduction in major non-CABG bleeds. The ESC 2012 updated STEMI guidelines state that for Primary PCI for STEMI: Transradial access is recommended, if performed by experienced operators. Recently, the RIVAL investigators[14] have reported significant reduction in fatality and major bleeds in ACS when angioplasty was performed through radial artery in a multicenter randomized European study. Transradial primary angioplasty offers the greatest benefit in the sickest patients with Acute Coronary Syndrome and those with ST segment elevation acute myocardial infarction.[4,5]

Jobe et al.[15] have suggested that all new transradial operators should first become facile at angiograms, then gradually move from simpler elective angioplasties with lesions of type A, progressively towards more complex lesions in a graded fashion such as types B1, B2 and C and finally moving to acute coronary syndrome cases and ST segment elevation acute myocardial infarction (emergent) angioplasties as they gain experience.

DIAMETER OF RADIAL ARTERIES AND DEFINITION OF SMALL RADIAL ARTERY

There is a wide variation in radial artery diameters worldwide, with an average size in men in South Asia being 1.8–1.9 mm,[11] and 1.8–2.8 mm in North America. Observational studies on radial and ulnar artery diameters have demonstrated that often both are ≤ 1.5 mm in 8–10% of patients.

Access artery: sheath size mismatch is therefore common and often leads to arterial spasm and subsequent occlusion, especially in those with < 1.7 mm.[16]

The definition of *"Small radial arteries"* remains elusive because of lack of randomized data in the scientific literature on pre-procedure sizing of access arteries; although there is a wealth of registry data[11] on the subject. Small access artery is defined by us as any access artery <1.7 mm in size, and has been shown to be associated with higher cross over rates, procedure failure and access site occlusions on 30 day follow-up.[16]

On comparison with adequate access arteries[16] (defined by us as any artery ≥ 1.7 mm), the crossovers (procedure failure) and access artery occlusions were 3.9% vs 0.9% and 2.8% vs 0.8% respectively (p < 0.0001) in the < 1.7 mm vs ≥ 1.7 mm AAD groups.

Challenge of Transradial Interventions in Patients with Small Radial Arteries

The use of transradial approach is often limited for patients with small radial arteries because of risk of radial artery spasm, with potential for access site cross over, procedure failure and radial artery occlusion preventing its future use as an access site.[6,8]

A recent survey[17] showed that 60% of transradial operators use 6F sheaths, in 75% of all procedures, further, in the RIVAL trial,[7] 77% of the procedure were performed using 6F sheaths.

The outer diameter of radial sheaths varies with manufacturers, with a mean of approximately 2.4 mm for 5F sheaths and 2.7 mm for 6F sheaths.[18]

A Pre-procedure Ultrasound of Assessment of the Access arteries (PPUAA),[11] has been used by us to measure the diameter of forearm arteries (radial and ulnar) bilaterally. This helps minimize difficulties; thus speeding up transradial access and improving overall success.

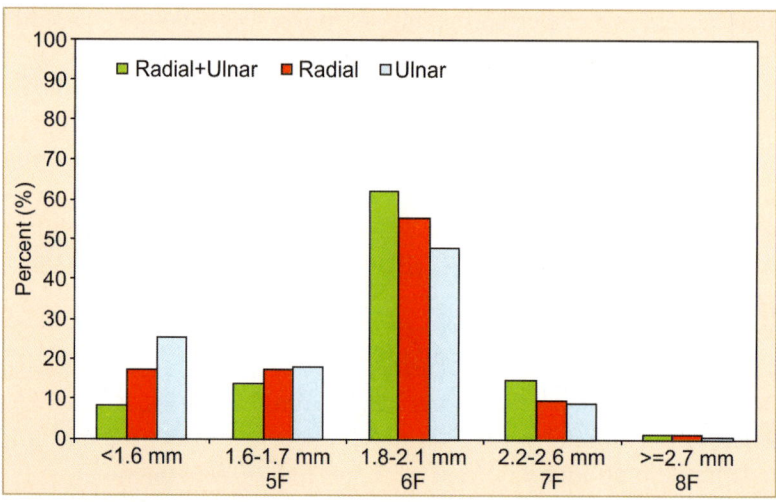

Fig. 1: Sheath-sizing protocol.
Source: SK Chugh et al.

SHEATH-SIZING PROTOCOL BASED ON DIAMETER OF ACCESS ARTERY

Based on a cohort of our patients in India,[11] we created a sheath sizing protocol (Fig. 1).

- For all our interventions, we have commonly used 5F sheath and catheters for access artery diameter (AAD) ≥ 1.6 mm, 6F through AAD ≥ 1.8 mm; 7F sheath for AAD ≥ 2.2 mm.[11]
- Until 2012, transfemoral access was used by us if a patient's bilateral RA and UA diameters did not meet adequate size requirements:
  - AAD ≤ 1.5 mm, inappropriate for 5 F PCIs or coronary angiogram (CA)
  - AAD < 1.7 mm, inappropriate for 6F PCIs (where the use of 6F was indicated)
  - AAD < 2.1 mm, inappropriate for 7F PCIs (where the use of 7F was indicated)

As per our working protocol, until 2012, for percutaneous coronary interventions, the minimum arterial diameter used for angiography was 5F in ≥ 1.6 mm (arterial diameter) and 6F in ≥ 1.8 mm.

Until 2012, it had been our practice that in case this criteria was not met on the right side, the contralateral side (left) was screened for adequate access, failure of which would result in selection of the femoral route. This practice has changed since, with introduction of newer innovative techniques.

Radial artery (RA) was preferred over Ulnar artery (UA), because of a more superficial location, lack of adjacent nerves and easier hemostasis. The preference order that we follow is; right radial artery (RRA) > left radial artery (LRA) > right ulnar artery (RUA) > left ulnar artery (LUA).

Ulnar access was preferred over radial in the following:
1. Anomalous origin of radial artery from the brachial artery
2. Bifurcation of the brachial artery proximal to the antecubital fossa
3. Presence of a radial loop
4. Bilaterally small radial arteries.

New Techniques for Overcoming the Challenge of Small Access Arteries

There are 2 ways to overcome the challenge, as described below:
1. *"Compression of the Other Artery"* (COOA)
   After 2012, for RA diameter <1.5 mm, we began to use *"compression of the other artery"* (COOA), a technique to enhance the size of the access artery (Figs. 2A and B).[19] This enabled us to use even 1.4 mm arteries for 5F access with enhanced success thus aiding in reducing puncture failures. Further all small arteries (defined by us as Access Artery Diameter < 1.7 mm) can be augmented with the use of COOA, increasing the overall number of patients meeting selection criteria for transradial interventions, although this technique needs further evaluation in a randomized setting,[16] preliminary assessment of post-procedure radial artery occlusion in these cases suggests occlusion rates of 2.8%.

   Women more commonly[20] only have a single adequate forearm artery out of the 4 available forearm arteries compared to men: 1.5 mm ((17.1% (F) vs 7.8% (M), 1.6 mm (9.6% (F) vs 3.8% (M)) and 1.7 mm groups (10.6% (F) vs 4.5% (M) groups (p<0.001) and 1.8-2.0 mm group (42.8% (F) vs 29.7% (M), p<0.001). Men commonly have more than one adequate forearm access artery.

   This preliminary data supports the need for pre-operative arterial diameter measurement of forearm arteries by ultrasound doppler

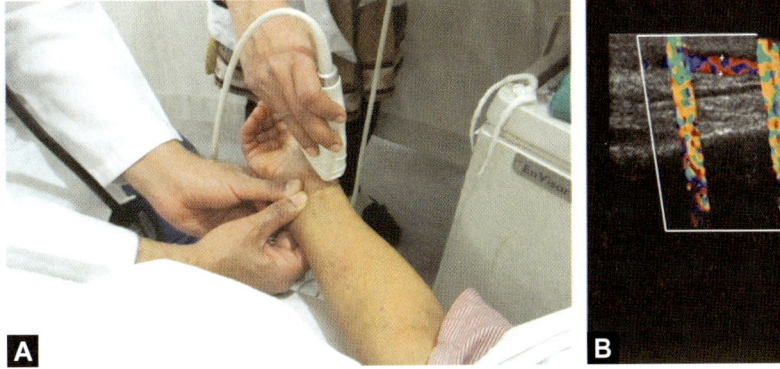

Figs. 2A and B: Compression of the other artery (COOA), a technique to enhance the size of the radial artery by compressing the ulnar.

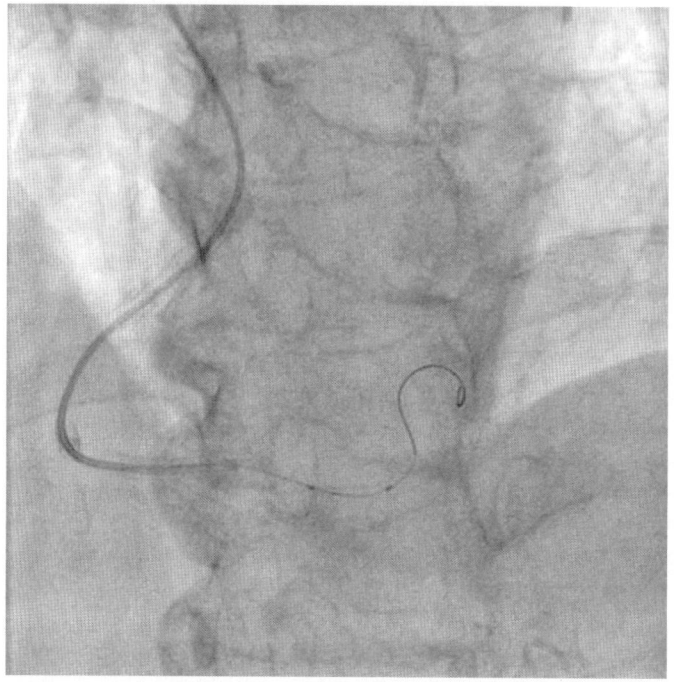

Fig. 3: A 4F angioplasty being done with deep throating of a JR-guiding catheter while the stent is being positioned.

especially in females to find the artery with the biggest diameter for access, in an attempt to prevent unavoidable complications and procedure failures.

2. *Miniaturization of Hardware*: Slender transradial interventions and the GSS slender sheath

   Miniaturization of hardware has led to PCI through 4 French guiding catheters. A 4F PCI was performed for the first time, outside of Japan, 'live' at Gurgaon (now Gurugram), in India on 4th February, 2013 at 'Radial Live' by the author (Fig. 3). It promises to revolutionize transradial interventions especially in patients with small radial artery diameters; but is unavailable in India, at the time of this writing.

   The Miniature hardware (catheters, balloons and wires) are available currently only in Japan where the interventionists use kissing balloons through 5 French guides and trifurcation kissing balloons through 6 French guiding. (Figs. 4A and B, illustrations provided by Dr Matsukage, Pioneer of Slender Radial Club Japan).

   A part of the miniature hardware, the Glidesheath Slender (GSS, Terumo, Japan) is compatible with a 5F guiding catheter and is designed solely for TR access. It has a thinner wall, that reduces its outer diameter to 4F while the diameter of the inner lumen is 5F.

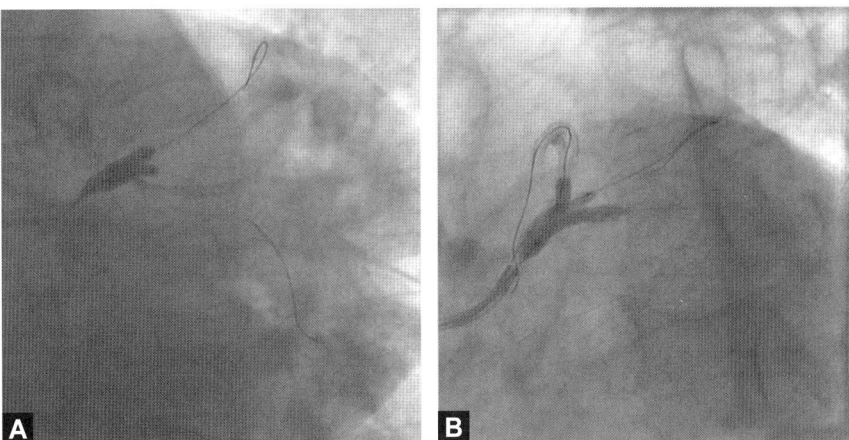

Figs. 4A and B: Bifurcation and trifurcation kissing balloon respectively through a 5F guiding catheter.
Courtesy: Dr Takashi Matsukage, Japan.

MARS PILOT REGISTRY: MINIMIZING ACCESS ARTERY OCCLUSIONS[21]

We performed 9 cases using this GSS as part of a nonrandomized registry, at the Mission hospital at Durgapur in India, and assessed the safety and feasibility of the 5F GSS (4F outer diameter) for complex transradial coronary angioplasty in patients with small radial artery diameters, as part of the MARS Pilot Registry (Minimizing Access Artery Occlusions). The average radial artery diameter in our population was 1.8 ± 0.4 mm. Patients with Coronary Lesions of type B2 or C, AHA/ACC classification, were included. Patients with acute ST elevation myocardial infarction, those with thrombotic lesions requiring thrombo-suction or the presence of known bifurcation lesions with large side branches, those who were unable to consent, or had no indication for a PCI were excluded.

Study Findings

A total of 9 patients were included, of whom 7 were male. The mean (± SD), (range) age was 58.7 (±19.3) years, and the mean body mass index was 21 ± 3.9 kg/m². The mean number of previous punctures of the same radial artery was 0.78 ± 0.44. All patients underwent complex coronary interventions (grade 2B/C, n = 9).

There were no bleeding or vascular complications, one patient had a minor forearm hematoma unrelated to the sheath introducer (Fig. 5). The mean procedure time was 25.1 ± 8.5 min. There were no cross overs, however for one patient the access site was changed to the left radial (diameter

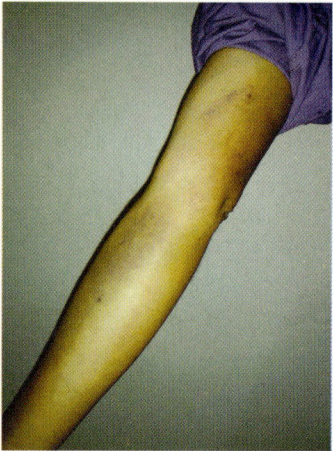

Fig. 5: Minor forearm hematoma from 0.038 terumo guidewire.

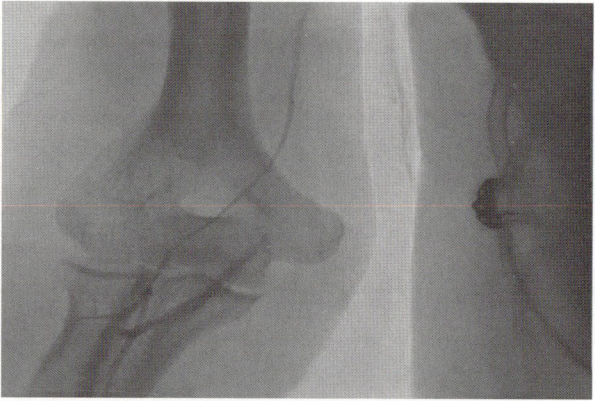

Fig. 6: Complex cubital loop/high origin of the radial artery on the right forearm.

1.5 mm), as a complex cubital loop on the right side could not be negotiated even using an angioplasty wire and balloon (Fig. 6). This patient's right radial artery diameter measured 1.4 mm. One patient who had a anomalously arising radial aretry from axillary artery occluded post-PCI.

In MARS pilot registry: Minimizing Access Artery Occlusions, we demonstrated the safety and feasibility of the new 5 Fr GSS. Pre-procedure determination of radial artery diameter in patients undergoing TRIs, with follow-up Dopplers post PCI, helped us study the impact of interventions with 5F guiding catheters and the GSS sheaths, in patients with small radial artery diameters.

A majority of available stents are compatible with the 5 Fr GSS, additionally this system is compatible with PCIs for chronic total occlusions[19] (Figs. 7A to J) and kissing balloons for bifurcation lesions.[22] Newer low

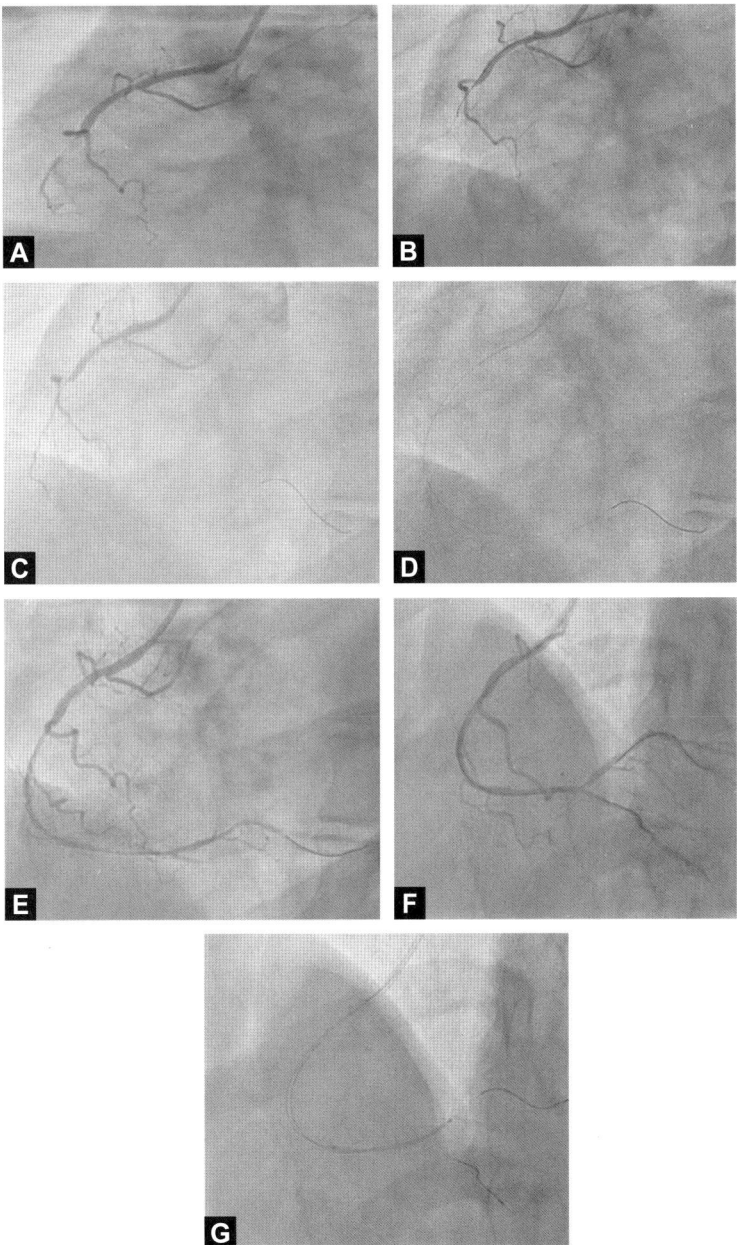

Figs. 7A to G: Successful Transradial Intervention of a right coronary Chronic Total Occlusion (CTO) using the 5Fr GSS sheath and a 5Fr guiding catheter (from left to right). (A) Angiogram shows CTO of proximal right coronary artery (RCA); (B and C) Occlusion crossed with micro-catheter and wizard wire; (D) Wizard wire changed for a BMW wire through the micro-catheter; (E) Angiogram after balloon pre-dilatation in proximal, mid and distal RCA; (F) 2nd BMW wire inserted into posterior descending branch of RCA; (G) Stent being positioned in distal RCA, across the posterior, descending into the posterolateral branch.

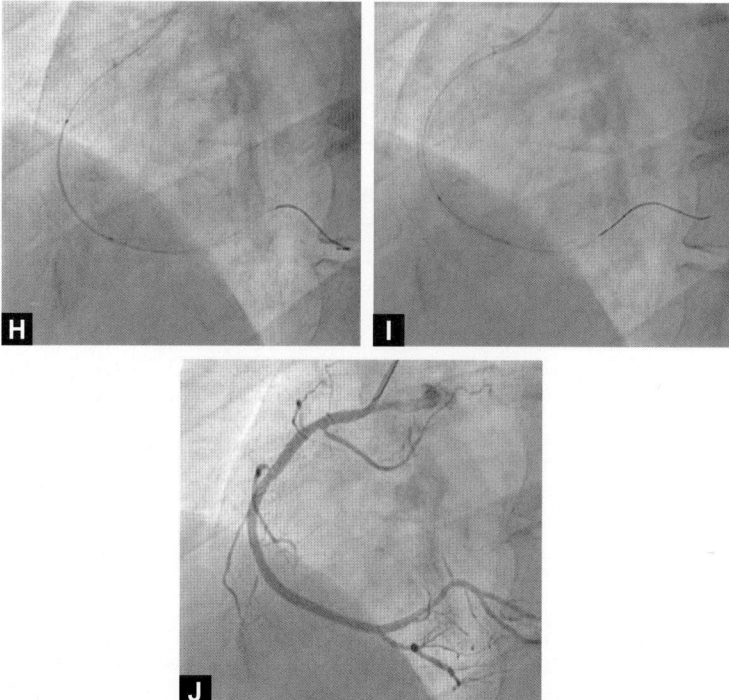

Figs. 7H to J: (H and I) Second and then third stent being positioned in mid and distal RCA respectively; (J) Final angiogram shows successful result.

profile over the wire stents which can go through even diagnostic catheter, are currently under evaluation in Europe and are likely to revolutionize the slender angioplasty field, according to the initial preliminary data.

Prior authors have reported similar procedural success with the utility of 6 Fr GSS[23] and the 5 Fr GSS[24] systems. Our pilot study is the first in a small cohort of Indian patients with small arteries requiring complex PCI. Overall, the use of these sheaths reduced spasm and pain and is a safe alternative for currently available sheaths for angioplasty through 5F guiding catheters. Whether they also reduce incidence of radial artery occlusions needs to be answered by a randomized study.

REFERENCES

1. Hamon M, Pristipino C, Di Mario C, et al. Consensus document on the radial approach in percutaneous cardiovascular interventions: Position paper by the European Association of Percutaneous Cardiovascular Interventions and Working Groups on Acute Cardiac Care and Thrombosis of the European Society of Cardiology. Euro Intervention. 2013;8:1242-51.
2. Rao SV, Tremmel JA, Gilchrist A, et al. Best practices for Transradial Angiography and Intervention: A consensus Statement From the Society for Cardiovascular

Angiography and Intervention's Transradial Working Group. Catheter Cardiovasc Interv 2013.

3. Shah B, Bangalore S, Feit F, Radiation exposure during coronary angiography via transradial or transfemoral approaches when performed by experienced operators. Am Heart J. 2013; 165(3):286-92.
4. Jang JS, Jin HY, Seo JS. The transradial versus the transfemoral approach for primary percutaneous coronary interventions in patients with acute myocardial infarction: a systemic review and meta-analysis. Eurointervention 2012;8(4):501-10.
5. Arzamendi D, Ly HQ, Tanguay JF. Effect on bleeding, time to revascularization, and one year clinical outcomes of the radial approach during primary percutaneous coronary intervention in patients with ST-segment elevation myocardial infarction. Am J Cardiol. 2010;106:148-54.
6. Dehghani P, Mohammad A, Bajaj R. Mechanism and predictors of failed transradial approach for percutaneous coronary interventions. JACC Cardiovasc Interv. 2009;2(11):1057-64.
7. Jolly SS, Yusuf S, Cairns J, et al. Radial versus femoral access for coronary angiography and intervention in patients with acute coronary syndromes (RIVAL): a randomized, parallel group, multicenter trial. Lancet 2011;77:1409-20.
8. Burzotta F, Trani C, Mazzari MA, et al. Vascular complications and access crossovers in 10,676 transradial percutaneous coronary pocedures. Am Heart J. 2012; 163:230-8.
9. Secco GG, Marinucci L, Uguccioni L. Transradial versus transfemoral approach for primary percutaneous coronary interventions in elderly patients. J Invasive Cardiol. 2013;25(5):254-6.
10. Valsecchi O, Vassileva A, Musumeci G, et al. Failure of transradial approach during coronary interventions: anatomic considerations. Catheter Cardiovasc Interv. 2006; 67(6):870-8.
11. Chugh SK, Chugh S, Chugh Y, Rao SV. Feasibility and utility of pre-procedural ultrasound imaging of the arm to facilitate transradial coronary diagnostic and interventional procedures (PRIMAFACIE-TRI). Catheter Cardiovasc Interv. 2013;82:64-73.
12. Romagnoli E, Zoccai GB, Sciahbasi A. et al. Radial versus femoral randomized investigation in ST segment elevation acute coronary syndrome. J Am Coll Cardiol. 2012;60:2481-9.
13. Mehran R, Lansky AJ, Witzenbichler B. Bivalirudin in patients undergoing primary angioplasty for acute myocardial infarction (HORIZONS-AMI): 1-year results of a randomised controlled trial. Lancet. 2009;374:1149–59.
14. Valgimigli M, Gagnor Andrea, Calabro P. et al. Radial versus femoral access in patients with acute coronary syndromes undergoing invasive management: a randomised multicentre trial. Lancet. March 16 2015 published online.
15. Jobe RL, Mann T. Transradial consensus statement: appropriateness ratings for patient selection and physicians' performing procedures. J Indian Med Assoc. 2009;107(9):587-8.
16. Chugh S K, Chugh S, Chugh Y. Addressing the challenges of access of small radial and ulnar arteries in transradial and transulnar interventions: Insights from a color Doppler study. JACC. 2014;63(12):A442.
17. Bertrand OF, Rao SV, Pancholi S, et al. Transradial approach for coronary angiography and interventions. Results of the First International Transradial Practice Survey. J Am Coll Cardiol Intv. 2010;3(10):1022-31.
18. Douglas F, Mamas MA. Mamas. Transradial Sheathless Approach for percutaneous coronary intervention. Cur Cardiol Rep. 2015;14:47.

19. Matsukage T, Masutani M, Yoshimachi F, et al. A prospective multicenter registry of 0.010-inch guidewire and compatible system for chronic total occlusion: the PIKACHU registry. Catheter Cardiovasc Interv. 2010;75:1006-12.
20. Chugh SK, Chugh Y, Chugh S. Overcoming the challenge of transradial interventions in women: insights from a color Doppler study. J Am Coll Cardiol. 2014;64(11):B240.
21. Chugh SK, Chugh Y, Chugh S, et al. Safety and feasibility of the new 5 Fr Glidesheath Slender for complex transradial interventions in patients with small radial artery diameters: a single center initial experience (Insights from the MARS pilot Registry: Minimizing Access Artery Occlusions). Indian Heart J 2016(in Press)
22. Yoshimachi F, Masutani M, Matsukage T. Kissing balloon technique within a 5 Fr guiding catheter using 0.010 inch guidewires and 0.010 inch guidewire-compatible balloons. J Invasive Cardiol. 2007;19:519-24.
23. Aminian A, Dolatabadi D, Lefebvre P, et al. Initial experience with the Glidesheath Slender for transradial coronary angiography and intervention: a feasibility study with prospective radial ultrasound follow-up. Catheter Cardiovasc Interv. 2014;84:436-42.
24. Yoshimachi F, Kiemeneij F, Masutani M, et al. Safety and feasibility of the new 5 Fr Glidesheath Slender. Cardiovase Interv Ther. 2016;31(1):38-41.

4

Left Main Coronary Intervention

Vinay K Bahl, Anunay Gupta

INTRODUCTION

Left main coronary artery (LMCA) involvement is seen in up to 5 % patient in patients undergoing coronary angiography.[1] Inolvement of LMCA is associated with worse prognosis with 50% mortality at three years in patients who are treated medically. LMCA lesion is important clinically as it supplies 100% of myocardium in case of left dominant circulation and around 75% in case of right dominant or balanced circulation.[2] Coronary artery bypass grafting (CABG) has been the standard of care of treatment of LMCA disease. However, recent studies have shown that due to advances in stents technology and use of drug eluting stents, percutaneous coronary intervention (PCI) can be an alternative to CABG. This review highlights the emerging role of PCI in left main disease.

INITIAL EXPERIENCE WITH PCI

Andreas Gruentzig performed first PCI of left main in 1979, however that patient died after four months. Later on it was seen that plain old balloon angioplasty (POBA) alone was associated with poor outcomes in these patients. O Keffe et al. reported 3 years mortality of 64% in patients of LMCA treated with balloon angioplasty. However, later on with development of bare metal stents procedural success rate increased but still over all events rate remain unacceptably high. In a study of 279 patients undergoing left main PCI Tan WA et al reported 1-year incidence of 24.2% for all-cause mortality, 20.2% for cardiac mortality and 9.8% for myocardial infarction.[3]

TRIALS COMPARING PCI WITH CABG

There have been a few randomized control trials which have compared DES with CABG in LMCA disease which are discussed in Table 1.

The Study of Unprotected Left Main Stenting versus Bypass Surgery (LE MANS) was the first randomized controlled trial (RCT) which compared CABG with DES. The primary endpoint of study was change in left

Table 1: Summary of major RCT comparing PCI with CABG in patients with LMCA disease.

Name	Number of patients	Primary outcome	PCI	CABG	P
LEMANS 2008	105	Change in LVEF	3.3%	0.5%	0.04
SYNTAX 2009/2014	705	MACE	36.9%	31.0%	NS
PRECOMBAT 2011	600	MACE	8.7%	6.7%	0.01

(MACE: Major adverse cardiovascular events; LMCA: Left main coronary artery; PCI: Percutaneous coronary intervention; LVEF: Left Ventricular efectige graction; CABG: Coronary artery bypass grafting).

ventricular ejection fraction (LVEF) at 12 months and secondary endpoint were major adverse cardiac and cerebrovascular event (MACCE) at 30 days and 1 year. Trial results showed statistically significant improvement in LVEF with patients treated with PCI versus CABG (58% vs. 54%). PCI was also associated with a lower MACCE rate at 30 days (2% vs. 13%), however MACCE were equal at 1 year in the two groups.

The Synergy between PCI with Taxus and Cardiac Surgery (SYNTAX) trial is the largest RCT which compared PCI to CABG in patients with LMCA disease. PCI with DES (Taxus) was non-inferior to CABG at one year of follow-up. Five-year follow-up of the trial was published recently which also showed non-inferiority of CABG of PCI vs CABG. Rate of MACE at 5 years were 36.9% in PCI versus 31% in CABG which was statistically not significant. It was seen that when patient were subdivided according to there complexity of coronary anatomy, CABG was found to be superior in complex subsets. When stratified by SYNTAX tertiles (0-22, 22-32, >32), the MACE rates were similar between PCI and CABG in the lower two tertiles; in highest tertile, PCI had significantly higher rate of MACCE.[4]

The Premier of Randomized Comparison of Bypass Surgery versus Angioplasty Using Sirolimus-Eluting Stent in Patients with Left Main Coronary Artery Disease (PRECOMBAT) randomized patients with LM disease to first-generation Cypher sirolimus-eluting stents (SES) versus CABG. At 2 years of follow-up rate of MACE were not significantly different between the groups (12.2% for PCI vs. 8.1% for CABG; p = 0.12), however ischemia-driven TVR was significantly more common in the PCI group (9.0% vs. 4.2%; p = 0.02). Similar findings were noted in recently published five-year follow-up.[5]

To summarize, results of above discussed trials conclude that PCI is a possible alternative to CABG in selected subsets of patients. However, these trials have their own limitations such as use of first generation stents and having softer primary end points instead of having harder end points such as mortality.

In a meta-analysis which was published in 2013, MACE rates were not different between PCI and CABG group up to 5 years as discussed above. However, PCI was associated with a lower rate of stroke and CABG was associated with lower rate of target vessel revascularization (TVR).

ROLE OF IMAGING AND FFR

Newer imaging modalities such as intravascular ultrasound (IVUS) and optical coherence topography (OCT) plays a significant role in performing left main intervention. Angiographic assessment of stenosis of left main is challenging. Fractional flow reserve (FFR) and IVUS helps in such situation to take decision regarding revascularization. Minimum lumen area (MLA) of 6 mm^2 has been set as criteria for revascularization in angiographically indeterminate stenosis. However, in Asian population criteria of MLA 4.5 mm^2 has been proposed.

IVUS remains crucial for assessing the degree of lumen compromise and the extent, distribution, and morphology of plaque. IVUS also helps in assessment post PCI of Left main. IVUS can differentiate between plaque versus carinal shift and stent underexpansion versus malapposition. Stent underexpansion has been a predictor of adverse events post LM stenting. It has been seen that long-term mortality in patients who undergo IVUS-guided LM stenting may be lower compared to those who undergo LM stenting under angiographic guidance alone. OCT have higher resolution than IVUS. However, its penetration is poor. Its use is LM intervention developing, importantly in LM Bifurcation PCI.

FFR is the standard method to assess physiological significance of stenosis. In FAME II FFR guided strategy in Non-LM stenosis improved outcomes. Hamilos et al. evaluated the role of FFR in angiographically indeterminate stenosis. Patients with FFR < 0.80 underwent CABG and FFR > 0.80 received optimal medical therapy. There was no significant difference in 5 years survival estimates between two groups. Hence FFR helps in guiding therapy in patients with indeterminate stenosis.

Key Practical Points

- Adjunctive imaging techniques (IVUS and/or FFR) should be used liberally to assess the underlying significance of ambiguous LMCA lesions on angiography
- IVUS guidance should be strongly recommended as the standard of care during LMCA PCI.

OSTIAL LM PCI

Ostial lesions are usually favorable for stenting. However, few points to be kept in mind while performing PCI are summarized in Box 1.

> **Box 1:** Tips and tricks for ostial LM PCI.
> - AO/RAO cranial views are best to visualize ostium of left main.
> - Avoid Amplatz guides
> - Keep guide disengaged after wire has been crossed to avoid damage to ostium
> - Deploy stent 1-2 mm in aorta and flare it with balloon
> - Use IVUS post stenting to ensure optimal results

MANAGEMENT OF LM BIFURCATION

Distal LM lesions are mostly bifurcation lesions involving either Left anterior descending or left circumflex ostium. LM bifurcation can be treated with single or two stent strategy.

Provisional stenting is a single stent strategy which allows placement of second stent if required. In this strategy both the LAD and LCX are wired. LM to LAD is stented. LCX may be or not be treated by final kissing balloon inflation. *Final kissing balloon inflation is must in two stent strategy.* *NORDIC II trial* compared routine final kissing versus no final kissing in patients undergoing provisional stenting. It was seen that there was reduction in angiographic SB restenosis at 8-month follow-up. However, there was no differences in 6-month MACE 2.1% vs. 2.5. But duration of procedure, and contrast use were greater with final kissing balloon inflations.[6] If LCX develops less than TIMI3 flow or patient developed ST/T changes or chest pain or FFR in LCX is less than 0.8, LCX may be stented. After placement of second stent FKBD is must.[4]

Double stent strategy uses either culotte technique, T or the T And Protrusion (TAP) technique, crush stenting or V stenting.

Culotte technique is suitable when angulation of LCX is less than 60° and LCX ostium is diseased. For culotte stenting there should not be more than 1.5 mm difference in vessel diameter between main vessel and side branch. It provides a full coverage of distal LM bifurcation but a significant area of stent overlap.

Crush stenting is preferred when angulation is less than 60 degree and main vessel is larger than side branch. It requires stenting of side branch first with 1-2 mm protrusion in LM which is than crushed by LM to LAD stent. A modification of crush technique is DK crush technique which requires double kissing. In this side branch stent is crushed by balloon instead of stent followed by kissing balloon inflation. First kissing balloon inflation facilitates side branch crossing for final KBI.

V stent technique is used for distal LM bifurcation in which distal LM is not significantly diseased (Medina 0,1,1). Both the stents are simultaneously deployed with minimal protrusion into left main. In *simultaneous kissing*

Flowchart 1: Approach to LM bifurcation stenting in two-stent technique.

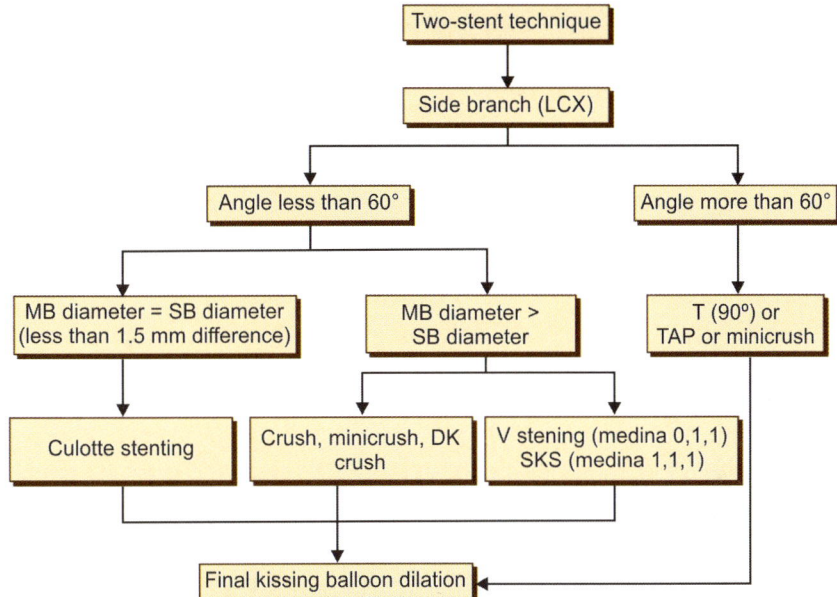

(MB: Main branch; SB: Side branch).

stent (SKS) technique there is 4-5 mm overlap of stents in left main. SKS is used when distal left main is significantly diseased (Medina 1,1,1). SKS is uncommonly used these days. Flowchart 1 summarizes the approach to LM bifurcation disease.

Key Practical Point
• It is important to remember that when there is no significant lesion in the SB (LCX artery), stenting the LM artery with a jailed wire in the SB followed by provisional T-stenting if required is the most reasonable and successful strategy.

WHAT GUIDELINES SAY?

Latest guidelines of European Society of Cardiology were released in 2014.[7] Table 2 summarizes the management of left main coronary artery disease. Heart team approach is recommended when considering LM revascularization.

ACC/AHA guidelines which were updated in 2011 recommends PCI for LM as Class II A in low syntax score versus ESC/EACTS guidelines which recommends PCI as Class I. Ostial or trunk LM is class IIa and LM bifurcation is recommended as II b irrespective of SYNTAX score.

Table 2: 2014 ESC/EACTS guidelines for LM revascularization.

	PCI		CABG	
	Class	LOE	Class	LOE
LMCA disease with syntax score ≤ 22	I	B	I	B
LMCA disease with syntax score 23-32	IIa	B	I	B
LMCA disease with syntax score >32	III	B	I	B

(LOE: Level of evidence, Modified from 2014 ESC/EACTS guidelines on myocardial revascularization).

RECENTLY PUBLISHED TRIALS

Current recommendations of PCI in LM disease solely rely on subgroup analysis of SYNTAX trial. Two major trials EXCEL and NOBLE whose results were published recently had added both clarity and confusion in LM intervention. Table 3 summarizes both the clinical trials.

The Evaluation of XIENCE Prime or XIENCE V vs. CABG for Effectiveness of Left Main Revascularization (EXCEL) was multicenter RCT enrolling patients with a low or intermediate SYNTAX score (<32) with use of the second generation Xience (Abbott Vascular) DES. The composite primary end point of all-cause death, stroke, or MI at 3 years occurred in 15.4% of patients treated with PCI and in 14.7% of patients undergoing CABG. The difference was significant for noninferiority (p = 0.018); but not for superiority (hazard ratio [HR] 1.00, 95% CI 0.79–1.26; p = 0.98). Authors concluded that PCI may be considered an acceptable revascularization modality for selected patients with LM CAD.[8]

Second major trial was The Nordic-Baltic-British Left Main Revascularization Study (NOBLE) trial. It compared PCI using the bioabsorbable polymer biolimus-eluting BIOMATRIX with CABG patients with LM CAD with ≤3 additional noncomplex lesions. Kaplan-Meier 5-year estimates for MACCE at 5 years were 28.9% for the PCI group and 19.1% for the CABG group. The hazard ratio was 1.48, which exceeded the limit for noninferiority and was significant for superiority for CABG compared with PCI (p = 0.006). Major differences between the two trials include a *lower rate of IVUS use post stent deployment in NOBL*E which might have ntributed to the higher stent thrombosis rates and *use of repeat revascularization as one of the end points* which is softer end point as compared to MI or Death and *81 % of patients in NOBLE* had LM bifurcation disease.[9]

To conclude these two landmark trials provide us enough evidence in management of LM disease but they are unlikely to change current guidelines.

Table 3: Salient features of EXCEL and NOBEL trials.

Trial design	Excel	Nobel
	Prospective, multicentre, open label, randomized	
Number of Patients	1905	1200
SYNTAX	<32	Low
Primary end point	Death/MI/CVA	MACE
Follow up	3 years	2 years
IVUS	Recommended	Recommended
FFR	Recommended	Recommended
Stent	EES (Xience)	BES (Biomatrix)
Angiographic follow up	Not recommended	Not recommended
Periprocedural MI	Included	Excluded

CONCLUSION

To summarize left main coronary intervention has evolved from Class III recommendation to Class I recommendation over last one decade. PCI requires careful selection of patients. Heart team approach is must while selecting the patient for LM intervention. Recently published two land mark trials have yielded conflicting results. Still LM PCI should be a suitable alternative to CABG in carefully selected patients. Longer follow-up of these two large trials might add to additional valuable information.

REFERENCES

1. DeMots H, Rösch J, McAnulty JH, et al. Left main coronary artery disease. Cardiovasc Clin. 1977;8:201–11.
2. Kalbfleisch H, Hort W. Quantitative study on the size of coronary artery supplying areas postmortem. Am Heart J. 1977;94:183–8.
3. Tan WA, Tamai H, Park SJ, et al. Long-term clinical outcomes after unprotected left main trunk percutaneous revascularization in 279 patients. Circulation. 2001;104:1609–14.
4. Serruys PW, Morice M-C, Kappetein AP, et al. Percutaneous coronary intervention versus coronary-artery bypass grafting for severe coronary artery disease. N Engl J Med. 2009;360:961–72.
5. Park S-J, Kim Y-H, Park D-W, et al. Randomized trial of stents versus bypass surgery for left main coronary artery disease. N Engl J Med. 2011;364:1718–27.
6. Niemelä M, Kervinen K, Erglis A, et al. Randomized comparison of final kissing balloon dilatation versus no final kissing balloon dilatation in patients with coronary bifurcation lesions treated with main vessel stenting: the Nordic-Baltic Bifurcation Study III. Circulation. 2011 Jan;123:79–86.
7. Kolh P, Windecker S, Alfonso F, et al. 2014 ESC/EACTS Guidelines on myocardial revascularization: the Task Force on Myocardial Revascularization of the European Society of Cardiology (ESC) and the European Association for Cardio-Thoracic Surgery (EACTS). Developed with the special contribution of the

European Association of Percutaneous Cardiovascular Interventions (EAPCI). Eur J Cardio-Thorac Surg 2014 Oct;46(4):517–92.
8. Stone GW, Sabik JF, Serruys PW, et al. Everolimus-Eluting Stents or Bypass Surgery for Left Main Coronary Artery Disease. N Engl J Med. 2016 Oct 31. (Epub ahead of print)
9. Mäkikallio T, Holm NR, Lindsay M, et al. Percutaneous coronary angioplasty versus coronary artery bypass grafting in treatment of unprotected left main stenosis (NOBLE): a prospective, randomised, open-label, non-inferiority trial. Lancet 2016 Oct 28. (Epub ahead of print).

5

Current Approach to Chronic Total Occlusions

Kirti Punamiya

INTRODUCTION

Percutaneous interventions involving chronic total occlusions (CTO), a challenging lesion subset are complex, time and material consuming procedures coupled with a low success rate.[1-4] As our understanding improved with histopathology and intracoronary imaging techniques, newer strategies and techniques evolved along with operator skills to improve success rates.

Although these techniques have been described in various reports the young operator is still at large to compile this into a flowchart for use in his daily practice. The present article is aimed presenting the different techniques and devices with a view to create an algorithm that each operator can then apply to his or her daily practice.

CLINICAL AND LESION-RELATED FACTS

It is important that operators clearly define the benefits of the procedure for every patient and weigh it against the risk and effort required. In carefully chosen patients, successful Percutaneous Coronary Intervention (PCI) of CTOs can potentially relieve angina,[5] improve effort tolerance and left ventricular function[6,7] and achieve complete revascularization.[8] To improve outcomes we must restrict this procedure to patients with a large area of ischemia potentially reversible and exclude those with rather complex distal disease supplying a rather small area of myocardium.

In early 2000, the success rate for CTO PCI was around 50 to 60% and predictors of failure were; age of the occlusion, presence of calcium, non-tapered stump, long occluded segment, bridging collaterals and lack of a visible path.[2] Most approaches then were the conventional antegrade approach using escalating stiffness of wires coupled with lubricity to improve successful wire crossing. By 2005, with introduction of the Fielder family of wires coupled with intravascular ultrasound guidance success rates improved.[9] The concept of wire escalation from soft to stiffer wires was introduced in Japan while the rest of the world used a range of polymeric coated wires.

Ozawa (2006)[10] and Katoh (2006s)[11] described the "retrograde approach" using the septal collateral channels to engage the distal segment and penetrate the distal cap to cross the CTO body successfully in reverse. In the subsequent years, the antegrade and retrograde techniques were used complementing each other in a independent and hybrid fashion. Till date CTO PCI has hinged on these approaches.[12]

The antegrade approach is considered the primary core approach in most CTO lesions and is usually the default first strategy. In certain anatomically challenging subsets where the antegrade approach is likely to have a low success rate like;
1. Aorto-ostial occlusions, long CTO segments more than 20 mm, presence of calcification and ambiguous proximal cap.
2. Previously failed recanalization antegrade attempts by an experienced operator and lesion characteristics like an ambiguous proximal cap with a large straight visible collaterals to a large distal segment would favor a primary retrograde approach.

Setting up for a CTO Case

1. **Angiographic assessment of CTO lesion**: Success in CTO PCI is influenced by the lesion difficulty and the operator skill. Scoring the lesion to grade their complexity and coupling the same to success gives the operator a sense of the likelihood of success. CTO scores developed are to aid operators in this planning. Scoring systems help is assessing the rates of success and thereby in selecting or accepting the appropriate case based on the skill of the operators. By categorizing the lesions a comparison of different techniques to evaluate the comparative success and risks is possible. The first published CTO scoring system was the J-CTO (multicenter CTO registry in Japan) score, created by Morino *et al.* to predict successful guidewire crossing within 30 minutes.[12,13] Newer scores have evolved from other published registries to essentially validate the efficiency of the older scores (Fig. 1A and Fig. 1B).
2. **Collateral circulation assessment**: These are small vascular channels that are recruited to perfuse the myocardium in an occluded territory. Viability is not a pre-requisite for collateral development. Rentrop in 1985 classified collaterals by their effect in filling the occluded arterial segment. While it gave a functional assessment, it was irrelevant by its application in CTO PCI. Werner in 2003 assessed collateral with a view to the retrograde approach, based on continuity and type of connection to the occluded segment.[14] These collaterals regress following a CTO PCI and therefore acute re-occlusion of the re-vascularized CTO vessel can potentially result in an acute coronary syndrome. Further discussion regarding the collaterals will be continued with the retrograde techniques.

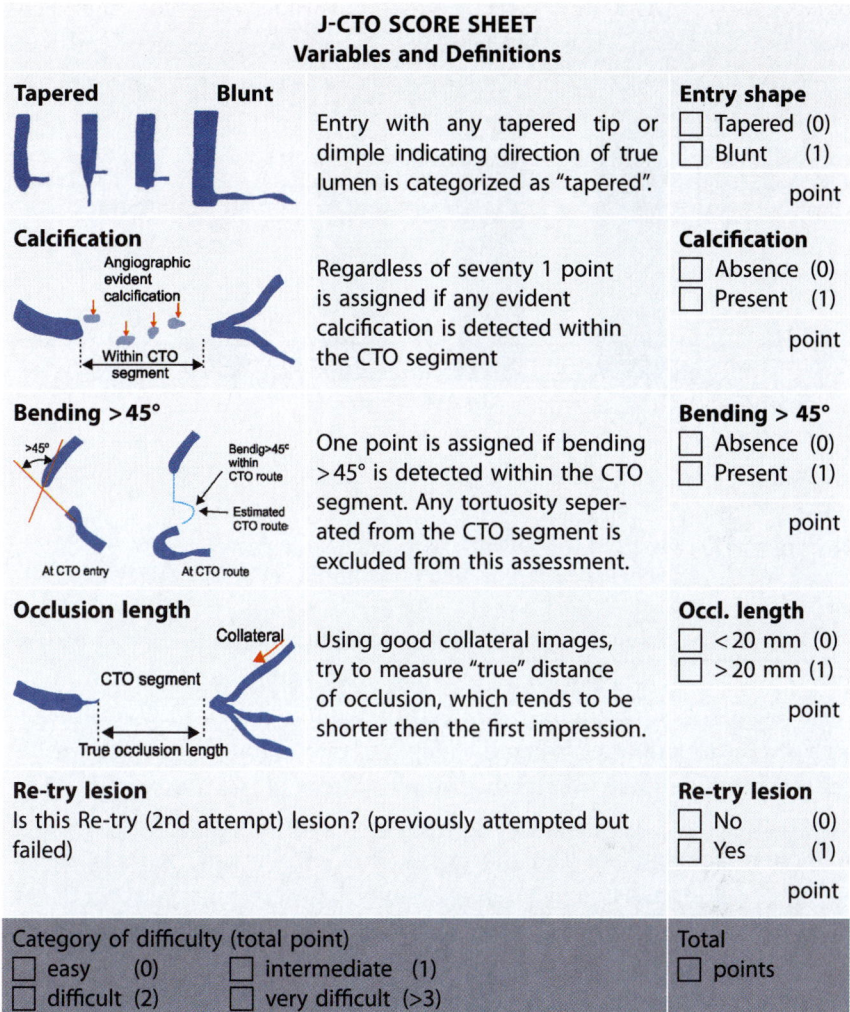

Fig. 1A: J-CTO score sheet to characterize lesion complexity in a standardized way. *Source*: Morino et al.

Access and Dual Angiography

Dual arterial access is recommended and this may be a bilateral femoral, femoral-radial or a bilateral radial approach as well. If intravascular ultrasound (IVUS) guidance is anticipated an 8F access for the occluded vessel and a 7F for the donor vessel is preferred. Long femoral sheaths (45 cm) improve the guide support and are recommended in iliac and aortic tortuosity. Though 7F guides are preferred 6F catheters have been used successfully as well. Guide catheter extensions and branch anchoring techniques can be used to increase support in the selected cases.

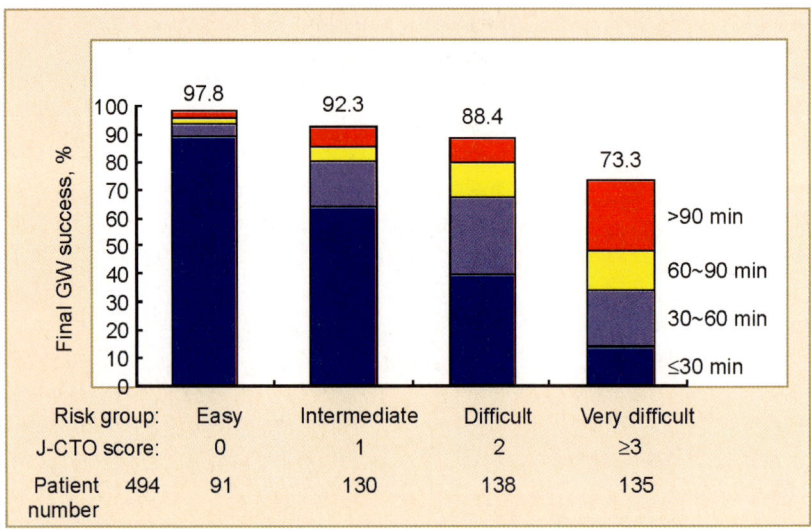

Fig. 1B: Success of wire crossing in 30 minutes based on J-CTO score.

Dual injection angiography or bilateral simultaneous coronary angiography of the occluded vessel and the donor artery supplying collaterals to the distal segment is insightful in strategizing techniques for CTO. It provides relevant information regarding the length of the occluded segment, the distal target by it course, direction, size and extent of disease burden. These observations are collated to choose guide catheters, wires, microcatheters and often the approach. The information on the collateral channels is helpful in retrograde assisted technique. Lesions that were considered CTO were shown to be critical stenosis using simultaneous dual angiography. Though called simultaneous the coronary injections are made in tandem, the donor artery is injected first and as the collaterals fill the occluded distal artery a gentle antegrade injection is made using the antegrade guiding catheter. This staggered injection technique helps capture the entire CTO lesion and distal artery in the same frame while minimizing the radiation exposure as well. In patients with ipsilateral collaterals to the occluded artery dual injections may not be needed, however in case a retrograde approach is contemplated 2 guide catheters into the same coronary origin may still be required.[15]

The author cautions against the use of forceful antegrade injections for visualization as we advance into the procedure for the fear of propagating an intraluminal hematoma and thus a compromising the true lumen that would reduce the chance of a successful recanalization. Following a successful wire crossing IVUS guidance is relied upon to study anatomy and lesion characteristics to complete the PCI.

Rationale of the Approaches

Chronic total occlusion (CTO) lesions studied in cadavers revealed the presence of a proximal and a distal cap.[16] While the proximal cap is densely fibrotic and calcific, the distal cap is less structured therefore making it the favorable end to penetrate and cross the CTO body. Sakakura in an autopsy study showed a negative occlusion remodeling of the occluded segment in chronic CTOs, abundant organized thrombus in short duration CTOs and furthermore the distal cap to be more tapered (78.9%) compared to the proximal cap (48.4%).[17,18] This has been the basis of the retrograde approach to cross the CTO lesion. The findings of neovascular channel (NC) in a CTO body made an exciting concept and operators often used this fact to aid tracking these channels to successful crossing. However, serial sections of the CTO body showed that these channels often traversed the media and into the adventitia. It was actually rare to find a channel communicating the entirely along the length of the CTO body and confined within the intimal space. The CTO body also has islands of calcium and dense fibrous strands that could run horizontally as well as longitudinally to partition the luminal space. These bands are difficult to penetrate and techniques like dissection reentry are thus used to connect the 2 parallel spaces.

Micro-computerized tomography (CT)[19] and IVUS[20] has been used by various groups to study these lesions and this has led a prominent group from Japan to postulate the concept of a path of loose tissue within the CTO body. This loose tissue track or the 'path within the artery' is not usually parallel to the wall of the artery but often tortuous and interrupted by dense fibrous tissue and calcium. To successfully cross these tracks specialized wires are required and the tactile feel of the operator is important. IVUS has helped understand that advancement of wire is not always favorable and may be along a false lumen. This technique of IVUS guidance to track the wire course is amply described in literature.

Antegrade Wire Manipulations and Techniques

Wire Escalation: The Last Decade

This concept was based on the early realization of the hard proximal cap. Experts generally started with a soft tip wire and gradually changed wires with increasing tip force to stiffer tip wires with a view to successful penetration of the fibrocalcific cap. Penetration with increasing tip load was the key and strategy was to increases the stiffness in a stepwise fashion. Even though the penetrative force improved as the stiffness and tip load increased, it was difficult to maneuver these stiff wires around bends and so this approach had its own limitation. Wire handling also included maneuvers like drilling that relied on scouting for an opening in the rigid tissue.[2]

Outside Japan, CTO operators used a philosophy of lubricity-enhanced penetration using polymeric coated wires with increasing stiffness. This approach essentially reduced the frictional force to advance the wire through the CTO body, it took away the tactile feel as the wire passed and this led to penetration of the false lumen more frequently.

Wire Escalation: Current Strategy

The current wire handlings are centered on a point and push technique without the drilling motion using the deflective properties of the wire to deflect off the dense fibrotic and calcified tissue along the CTO body and continue to track the loose tissue. To enable this maneuvering the wires are designed composite core with a 1:1 linear torque, better tip preservation and higher penetrative force with lower tip loads. These wires retain the penetrative force while the reduced stiffness allows them to be deflected successfully to cross the CTO. As these wires (Gaia family) work best within the solid CTO body, any maneuvers like drilling that can potentially create a crescentic false lumen thereby neutralizing the ability of the wire are not recommended.

We recommend, start with a low gram tip load wire like the Fielder XT, XTR or A (Asahi Intecc) using gentle movements to engage into the perceived direction. The microcatheter may be advanced forward to improve penetration and prevent buckling of the wire tip. Sustained resistance to advancement will require escalation to either a moderate tip load wire of 4 to 6 gms or a high penetrative wire of the Gaia family (Fig. 2).

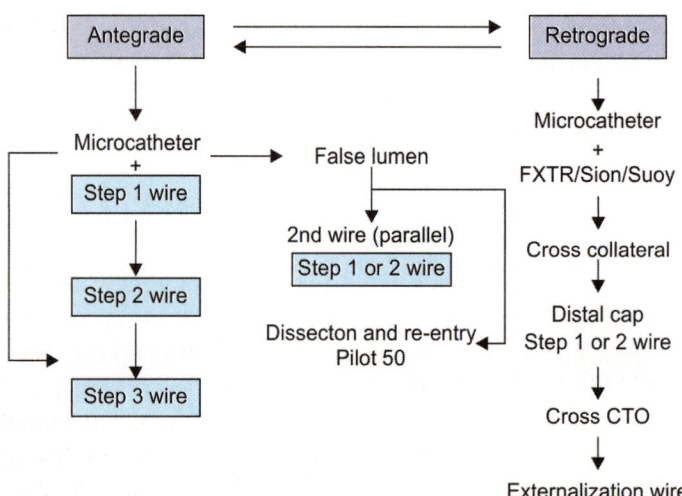

Fig. 2: Strategy based on wire advancement.

Parallel Wire Techniques

If a wire advanced is then visualized to be in a false lumen on the retrograde angiogram, it is best to leave the wire in place and advance a 2nd wire parallel to the first hoping to avoid the path created and explore a new path that may lead to the true lumen. The first wire aids the process by stabilizing and altering the direction, making it feasible for the second wire to advance. The author leaves the choice of this second wire to the operator based on his intuitiveness and tactile perception. Even though this seems like a guided wiring approach it remains a blind approach to track the loose tissue within the vessel space. A good tip to recognize exit from the path is the feeling of fixation of the wire in the dense tissue with a snap like feel on withdrawal. Double barrel microcatheter like the Crusade catheter can be used to facilitate a second wire approach.[21]

In all these wiring techniques it is important to protect the entire length of the wire within a microcatheter. This allows transmission of linear torque to the tip and also allows for easy exchange of wires without loss within the CTO body. Different microcatheters are used interchangeably by various operations (Table 1).

Wires exchanges are done using an extension docking wire, by a trapping balloon in the guide catheter or lubrication push back using the inflation device (Nanto techniques). Care should be taken not to loose wire position as well inadvertent advancement distally into the lesion.

Strategy Based on Wire Advancement

Any antegrade CTO approach has 3 crucial steps:
1. **Penetration of the proximal cap**: A standard workhorse wire is best used to travel the proximal non occluded segment of the occluded artery. Using a microcatheter this wire may then be changed for any of the Step 1 wires (Table 2). Wires are best angled at the distal 1 mm to 45° to 60°. Care should be taken to position the wire in a direction against the proximal cap that is most likely to lead to the true lumen. Any successful advancement should be checked fluoroscopically in at least 2 orthogonal views for early detection of the wire exiting the path. Wire buckling happens when the wire is forced against calcium or dense tissue. This is best avoided because it results in a deformation of the wire creating a extraluminal space. Once such a space is created the wire looses it ability to track the tissue and any forward movement, results in furthering of the false lumen (Fig. 2).
2. **Traversing the CTO body**: Operator should review the anatomy and have some plan of the path to pursue with the CTO segment. Tactile feel with point and push technique helps advance the wire. In chronic CTOs, once

Table 1: CTO toolbox of microcatheters.

Microcatheter	Length	Distal hydrophilic coating	Outer diamater Fr/mm Distal	Outer diamater Fr/mm Proximal	Recommended wire size	Manufacturer
Finecross MG	135/150	70/90 cm	1.8/0.60	2.6/0.87	0.014"	Terumo
Finecross GT	135/150	75/95 cm	1.8/0.60	2.6/0.87	0.014"	Terumo
Corsair	135150	60 cm	2.6/0.87	2.8/0.93	0.014"	Asahi Intecc
Caravel	135/150		1.9/0.62	2.6/0.85	0.014"	Asahi Intecc
Turnpike	135/150	60 cm	0.86 mm	1.02 mm	0.014"	Aquailent Intervensions
Turnpike Spiral	135/150	60 cm	1.02 mm	1.02 mm	0.014"	Aquailent Intervensions
Mogul	130		1.7/0.56	2.5/0.82	0.014"	Goodman
Mizuki Standard	135/150		1.8/0.60	2.5/0.84	0.014"	Kaneka Medix Corp
Mizuki FX	135/150		1.7/0.58	2.5/0.84	0.014"	Kaneka Medix Corp
Specialized microcatheter when balloon fails to cross						
Tornus	135		1.8/0.61	2.1/0.71	0.014"	Asahi Intecc
Tornus 88 Flex	135		2.1/0.70	3/1 mm	0.014"	Asahi Intecc
Turnpike Gold	135	60	1.07 mm	1.02 mm	0.014"	Aquailent Intervensions

Table 2: CTO toolbox of guiding wires.

Wire		Tapering tip	Tip load	Polymer coating	Rope coil	Manufacturer
Step I	Fielder FC	-	0.8 gm	+	-	Asahi Intecc
	Fielder XT	+	0.8 gm	+	-	Asahi Intecc
	Fielder XTR	+	0.6 g	+	+	Asahi Intecc
	Fielder XTA	+	1 g	+	+	Asahi Intecc
	Pilot 50	-	1.5 g	+	+	Abbott Vascular
Step II	Pilot 150/200	-	2.7/4.1 g	+	-	Abbott Vascular
	Cross-it 100 XT	+	1.7 g	-	-	Abbott Vascular
	Progress 40	-	4.8 g	-	-	Abbott Vascular

Contd...

Contd...

	MiracleBros 3*,4,5,6	-	3.0, 4.5, 6.0 g	-	-	Asahi Intecc
	GAIA First (tip 0.010")	+	1.7 g		+	Asahi Intecc
	GAIA Second (tip 0.010")	+	3.5 g		+	Asahi Intecc
	Ultimate Bros 3	-	3 g	-		Asahi Intecc
	Persuader 3 & 6	-	3.0,6.0 g	-	-	Medtronic
Step III	Progress 140T	+	12.5 g	-		Abbott Vascular
	Progress 200T	+	13.3 g	-		Abbott Vascular
	Progress 80, 120	-	9.7,14.9 g	-		Abbott Vascular
	Confianza Pro 9/12/20	+	9/12/20 g	-		Asahi Intecc
	Confianza 9	+	8.6 g	-		Asahi Intecc
	MiracleBros 12	-	12.0 g	-		Asahi Intecc
	GAIA Third (tip 0.012")	+	4.5 g		+	Asahi Intecc
	Persuader 9,12 Hydrophobic	+	9.1 g	-		Medtronic
	ProVia 9,12 Hydrophilic	+	9,13.5 g	-		Medtronic
	ProVia 9,12 Hydrophobic	+				Medtronic
R/G channel crossing wire	Fielder XT/XTR	+	0.8g/0.6 g		+	Asahi Intecc
	SION	-	0.7 g		+	Asahi Intecc
	SION BLUE		0.5 g		+	Asahi Intecc
	SION BLACK		0.8 g		+	Asahi Intecc
	SUOY				+	Asahi Intecc
Externalization wires	Viper		3.6 g			CSI
	RG3		3.0 g			Asahi Intecc
	RotaWire Floppy & extra support					Boston Scientific

into the proximal cap the wire may be difficult to maneuver or advance. This is the time when wire escalation or change may be considered to the Step 2 or 3 wires based on the operator's tactile feel and experience. In event of any deviation from true lumen, parallel wire, wire assisted dissection reentry or a device related dissection reentry might be performed.

3. **Exiting the distal cap**: Orientation of the wire tip in relation to the distal lumen is important. A wire suspected to be in a false lumen should not be advanced without caution and this is best done by a contralateral injection to study collaterals in two orthogonal views. Once crossed the wire movement is characteristic for a luminal location and it is possible to advance the wire at will into several branches with ease. The true lumen position of the wire can be checked by retrograde angiography, advancing the microcatheter and demonstrating a free backflow of blood and wire manipulation in varied branches at will.

Failing to find the true lumen the operator would have one of the three choices to make:

1. **Antegrade wire dissection and reentry**: It was first introduced by Colombo and is a based on the Subintimal Tracking And Reentry (STAR) technique.[22] It involves advancing a knuckled polymeric stiff wire (Pilot 50) into the CTO body, though sub-intimal these wire stay within the vessel framework. When smaller wire loops are used the technique is referred to as a mini-STAR. Once distal to the CTO segment, using a double barrel microcatheter and a stiffer wire one can make an attempt to reenter the distal true lumen by a puncture and reentry method. IVUS can aid an operator in localizing the true lumen in this attempt.

2. **Device-assisted dissection and reentry**: The principle being the same as the antegrade wire dissection reentry. In this technique the CrossBoss coronary catheter (Boston scientific, USA) is used to penetrate the CTO body. A Sting-Ray balloon with lateral ports is used to occupy this subintimal space and pierce into the distal true lumen using a stiff wire.[23]

Across different continents the algorithm are diverging and it is rather difficult to arrive a consensus about application and preferences of these techniques. The antegrade dissection reentry technique though widely accepted in USA is much less accepted in Japan. The author has made an attempt (Fig. 2) put these techniques in perspective, but its applications in daily practice would rely on the devices and individual skills available at the institute concerned.

Retrograde Approach

If the antegrade attempts fail in successful crossing of the CTO segment, retrograde approach is likely to increase the success rate in a few patients. The retrograde approach can be best described in a stepwise fashion to enable the young operator in the strategy.

1. **Collateral assessment**: The assessment of collateral channels made on their favorability of success. Rathore in 2009 graded the type of collaterals from their initial experience in Japan. Collateral channels (CCs) were graded as follows:[23]
   CC0, no continuous connection;
   CC1, continuous thread-like connection; and
   CC2, continuous, small side branch-like connection.

   Collateral channel (CC1), collateral tortuosity < 90°, and angle with recipient vessel < 90° are favorable and were significant predictors of success. Epicardial channel use, CC0, corkscrew[24] channel, angle with recipient vessel > 90°, and non-visibility of connection with recipient vessel were not favorable and found to be significant predictors of procedural failure. The septal collaterals had the advantage because of their multiplicity, straight, intramyocardial course and a reduced chance of a tamponade in case of damage. Epicardial collaterals are frail and not supported by myocardium and only used as a back up option as they risk damage with tamponade. Coronary angiography should be aimed at profiling these collaterals to help plan the procedure.

2. **Collateral channel navigation**: It is important to choose a guide catheter that will ensure a back up and once the septal channel is accessed using a routine wire the microcatheter should be advance into the concerned collateral and a selective angiography performed at low pressure.[25] This angiography serve as a template to negotiate the wires. In case of a straight, non-branching collateral any soft tip polymeric coated wire is acceptable. In tortuous channels the Sion family will have an advantage and in case of invisible channels the Fielder XTR will have a distinct advantage. The Sion black, Suhoy wires have been used recently for effective channel crossing. With every advancement it may be advisable to take angiographic images to chart a path. Following a successful wire navigation the microcatheter (Corsair, Asahi Intecc) should be advanced into the channels using counterclockwise motion. If the microcatheter fails to advance one may use 1.2 to 1.5 mm balloon to gently dilate the channels not beyond 3 atms to facilitate the microcatheter advancement. An important tip is not to leave a wire in the septal or collateral channels without a microcatheter support.

3. **Crossing the occlusion**: Not uncommonly the retrograde wire will directly cross the lesion and pass into the true lumen proximally. More likely though, while the antegrade wire is in the false lumen the retrograde wire ascends parellel to this wire into a secondary false lumen. Here neither wire is in true lumen or the same space but both are likely to be in the intraplaque parallel spaces. The controlled antegrade retrograde subintimal tracking (CART)[26,27] or reverse CART may be attempted. The concept of CART involves balloon dilatation on any one of these wire with

an intention to disrupt the tissue in between and get other wire to enter the dilated space thereby connecting the two lumens. In an attempt to improve long-term results we need to minimize stent placement in the subintimal space and this can be done by using IVUS to determine the level of this connection. The wire choices to enter the CTO body retrogradely are made similar to the antegrade approach with softer wires to start with and escalation based on need and anatomy[28] (Figs. 3A and B).

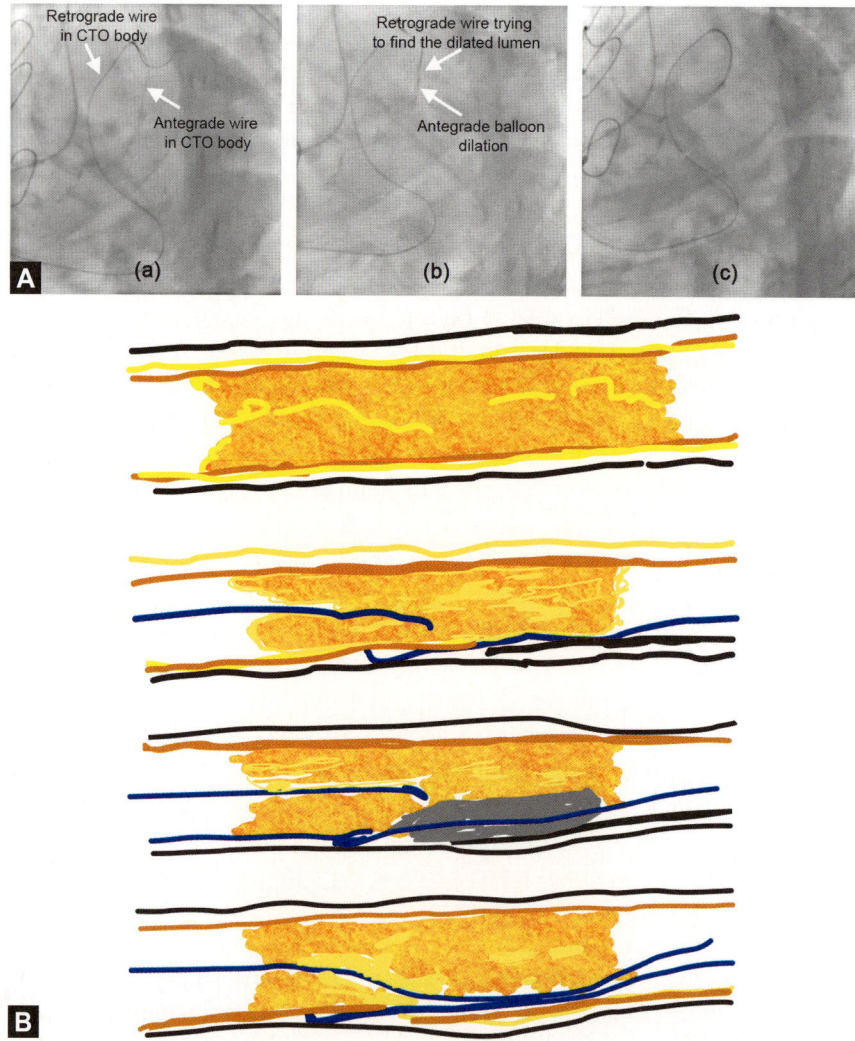

Figs. 3A and B: (A) Depicts the steps of the Reverse CART: (a) Antegrade wire subintimal and retrograde wire intimal space; (b) Balloon on antegrade wire to connect the two spaces, while the retrograde wire attempts to penetrate the antegrade space created; (c) Retrograde wire successfully connects with antegrade lumen. (B) Schematic representation of reverse CART technique.

Intravascular Ultrasound guided reverse CART (Contemporary reverse CART)[29] uses IVUS to:
   a. Optimal sizing of the balloon to enable appropriate tissue disruption within the space for the connection.[30]
   b. Ensure the minimal subintimal course of the connection
   c. In a high plaque burden proximal segment, following a balloon dilation a guideliner can be advanced to keep a protected non-collapsed lumen of the guideliner to enter by the retrograde wire for entry by the retrograde wire.
4. **Securing the retrograde wire in the proximal segment and externalization**.
   a. Retrograde wire that has successfully crossed the CTO body should be further negotiated retrogradely into the antegrade guide catheter (GC).
   b. Once in the antegrade GC, it should be trapped using a balloon inflation in the GC.
   c. On this support trapped wire the retrograde microcatheter should be advanced into the antegrade guide.
   d. The retrograde wire should then be exchanged to an externalization wire as mentioned in Table 2, to pass from the retrograde GC to donor artery through collateral channel into the distal occluded segment beyond the CTO, past the CTO into the antegrade GC, forming a loop.
   e. Once externalized wire is secured at both ends to complete the loop and the PCI may be completed over this wire through the antegrade access.

No wires should be moved in the collateral channel in this fashion without the protection of a microcatheter. It is not common for the wires to cut through the myocardium but on rare occasion can happen with serious or grave consequences.

Cautions specific to the retrograde approach: An important aspect about the CTO retrograde approach is the intubation and instrumentation of both coronary arteries, while one is occluded the other being the donor. Any complication of the donor artery feeding collaterals to the occluded segment can impose an acute and significant ischemia burden.

Donor vessel thrombosis: It is therefore important to maintain Activated Clotting Time (ACT) above 300 secs when doing these procedures. Frequently it is a result of a thrombosis developing in the guide catheter and getting injected into the artery. In case it does occur a rapid response to recanalize the donor artery is most important.

Donor vessel dissection: Typically and most frequently this is a real problem once the loop is established and the guide catheter get drawn into the donor artery inadvertently causing a damage and dissection. The donor artery must be secured before one continues to focus on the occluded artery.

Septal channel rupture and hematoma: Most septal hematomas are small and may be inconsequential. Occasional the hematoma may be massive and result in a tamponade and may be associated with death. It is one of the reason to have a microcatheter over the wire while moving through a collateral channel. It is difficult to detect using echocardiography.

With the newer wires, microcatheters and other devices the need for retrograde procedure has declined and complication rates are low and acceptable.

REFERENCES

1. Puma JA, Sketch MH, Tcheng JE, et al. Percutaneous revascularization of chronic coronary occlusion: an overview. J Am Coll Cardiol. 1995;26:1-11.
2. Tsuchikane E. Complex PCI: PCI for the chronic total occlusion. Coron Interv. 2003;2:8-13.
3. Grantham JA, Marso SP, Spertus J, et al. Chronic total occlusion angioplasty in the United States. J Am Coll Cardiol Intv. 2009;2:479-86.
4. Prasad A, Rihal CS, Lennon RL, et al. Trends in outcome after percutaneous coronary intervention for chronic total occlusions: a 25-year experience from the Mayo clinic. J Am Coll Cardiol. 2007;49:1611-8.
5. Grantham JA, Jones PG, Cannon L, Quantifying the early health status benefits of successful chronic total occlusion recanalization: results from the FlowCardia's Approach to Chronic Total Occlusion Recanalization (FACTOR) trial. Circ Cardiovasc Qual Outcomes. 2010;3:284-90.
6. Finci L, Meier B, Favre J, et al. Long-term result of successful and failed angioplasty for chronic total coronary arterial occlusion. Am J Coardiol. 1990;66:660-2.
7. Bask T, van Geuns RJ, Duncker DJ, et al. Prediction of left ventricular function after drug-eluting stent implantation for chronic total coronary occlusions. J Am Coll Cardiol. 2006;47:721-5.
8. Noguchi T, Miyazaki S, Morii I, Goto Y, Nonogi H. Percutaneous transluminal coronary angioplasty of chronic total occlusions. Determinants of primary success and long-term clinical outcome. Catheter Cardiovasc Interv. 2000;49:258-64.
9. Saito S, Tanaka S, Hiroe Y, et al. Angioplasty for chronic total occlusion by using tapered-tip guidewires. Catheter Cardiovasc Interv. 2003;59:305-11.
10. Ozawa N. A new understanding of chronic total occlusion from a novel PCI technique that involves a retrograde approach to the right coronary artery via a septal branch and passing of the guidewire to a guiding catheter on the other side of the lesion. Catheter Cardiovasc Interv. 2006;68:907-13.
11. Katoh O, Surmely JF, Tsuchikane E, et al. New concept of CTO recanalization using controlled antegrade and retrograde subintimal tracking: the CART technique. J Invasive CArdiol. 2006;18:201-07
12. Morino Y, Abe M, Morimoto T, et al. Predicting successful guidewire crossing through chronic total occlusion of native coronary lesions within 30 minutes: the J-CTO (Multi-center CTO Registry in Japan) score as a difficult grading and time assessment tool. J Am Coll Cardiol. Interv. 2011;4:213-21.
13. Morino Y, Kimura T, Hayashi Y, et al. In-hospital outcomes of temporary percutaneous coronary intervention in patient with chronic total occlusion insights from the J-CTO Registry (Multi-center CTO Registry in Japan). J Am Coll Cardiol Intv. 2010;3:143-51.
14. Werner GS, Ferrari M, Heinke S, et al. Angiographic assessment of collateral function in chronic coronary occlusions. Circulation. 2003;107:1972-77.

15. Singh M, Bell MR, Bergner PB, Holmes DR Jr. Utility of bilateral coronary injection during complex coronary angioplasty. J Invasive Cardiol. 1999;11:291-94.
16. Srivatsa SS, Edwards WD, Boos CM, et al. Histological correlates of angiographic chronic total coronary occlusion: influence of occlusion duration on neovascular channel patterns and intimal composition. J Am Coll Cardiol. 1997;5:955-63.
17. Sumitsuji S, Inoue K, Ochiai M, et al. Fundamental wire technique and current standard strategy of percutaneous intervention for chronic total occlusion with histopathological insights. J Am Coll Cardiol Interv. 2011;4:941-51.
18. Sakakura K, Nakano M, Otsuka F, et al. Comparison of pathology of chronic total occlusion with and without coronary artery bypass graft. Eur Heart J. 2014;35 (25):1683-93.
19. Ehara M, Terashima M, Kawai M, et al. Impact of multislice computed tomography to estimate difficulty in wire crossing in percutaneous coronary intervention for chronic total occlusion. J Invasive Cardiol. 2009;21:575-582.
20. Ito S, Suzuki T, Ito T, et al. Novel technique using intravascular ultrasound-guided guidewire cross in coronary intervention for uncrossable chronic total coronary occlusion. Circ J. 2004;68:1088-92.
21. Rathore S, Katoh O, Tsuchikane E, et al. Mini-focus issue: chronic total occlusion a novel modification of the retrograde approach for the recanalization of chronic total occlusion of the coronary arteries intravascular ultrasound guided reverse controlled antegrade and retrograde tracking. JACC Cardiovasc Interv. 2010;3:155-64.
22. Colombo A, Mikhial GW, Michev I, et al. Treating chronic total occlusion using subintimal tracking and reentry: the STAR technique. Catheter Cardiovasc Inter. 2005;64:407-11, discussion 412.
23. Whitlow PL, Burke MN, Lombardi WL, et al. Use of a novel crossing and re-entry system in coronary chronic total occlusions that have failed standard crossing techniques: results of the FAST-CTO) Facilitated Antegrade Steering technique in Chronic Total Occlusion) trial. JACC Cardiovasc interv. 2015;5:393-401.
24. Galassi A, Grantham A, Kandzari D, et al. Percutaneous treatment of coronary chronic total occlusions: technical approach. Interv Cardiol Rev. 2014;9:201-07.
25. Katoh O, Reifart N. New double wire technique to stent ostial lesions. Cathet Cardiovasc Diagm. 1997;40:400-02.
26 Rathore S, Katoh O, Matsuo H, et al. Retrograde percutaneous recanalization of chronic total occlusion of the coronary arteries: procedural outcomes and predictors of success in contemporary practice. Cir Cardiovasc Interv. 2009; 2(2):124-32.
27. Werner GS, Ferrari M, Heinke S, et al. Angiographic assessment if collateral connections in comparison with invasively determined collateral function in chronic coronary occlusions. Circulation. 2003;107:1972-77.
28. Cohen R, Habbat M, Elhadad S. Retrograde approach reverse CART technique with a single guide for chronic total occlusion of the right coronary via an anomalous left circumflex artery. J invasive Cardiol. 2011;23:E92-E94.
29. Kimura M, Katoh O, Tsuchikane E, et al. The efficacy of a bilateral approach for treating lesion with chronic total occlusions. The CART (Controlled Antegrade and Retrograde subintimal Tracking) registry. JACC, Cardiovasc Interv. 2009; 2:1135-41.
30. Muramatsu T, Tsukahara R, Ito Y, et al. Changing strategies of the retrograde approach for chronic total occlusion during 7 years. Catheter Cardiovasc Interv. 2013;81:E178-E185.

6
Ostial Lesions

Ajit S Mullasari, Srinivasan Narayan

INTRODUCTION

Ostial lesions are defined as lesions occurring within 3 mm of the origin of major epicardial artery or its branches. Ostial lesion present a challenge to the interventional cardiologist due to their peculiar anatomical/pathological features. The results of ostial interventions are also inferior when compared to nonostial lesions in view of the morphology and technicalities involved. Ostial lesions can be classified as below (*see* Fig. 1).

1. Aorto-ostial lesions involving ostia of right coronary artery (RCA), left main stem (LMS) and aortocoronary bypass grafts.
2. Non aorto-ostial lesions involving ostia of major coronary arteries not directly arising from aorta like left anterior descending (LAD), left circumflex (LCX) and ramus intermedius.
3. Branch lesions involving ostia of branches of major coronary vessels, e.g. diagonal branches of LAD, marginal branches of circumflex, posterior descending and poster lateral branches of RCA.

Isolated aorto-ostial disease is more common in women and is seen more commonly in the RCA than LMS.

Common causes of aorto-ostial disease include atherosclerosis, aortitis (takayasu or syphilitic) and mediastinal irradiation.

PECULIARITIES AND CHALLENGES OF OSTIAL LESION INTERVENTIONS[1-3]

1. Higher calcium and fibrous tissue content.
2. Higher tendency to recoil and increased neointimal hyperplasia after ostial stenting resulting in high restenosis rates.
3. Difficulty in engaging the guide and maintaining guide position in aorto-ostial lesions.
4. Different aortic takeoff angles.
5. Difficulty in precise ostial positioning of aorto-ostial stent using conventional fluoroscopic methods due to vessel overlap or foreshortening.

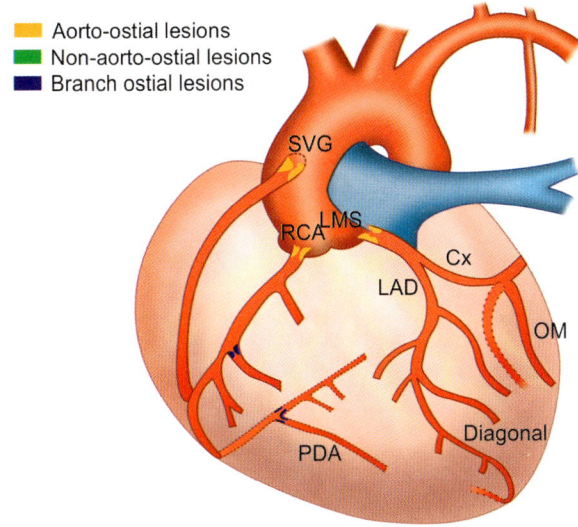

Fig. 1: Various types of ostial lesions and their classification.

Often cardiac contraction makes ostial stent positioning impossible.
6. Pinching of side branch in non aorto-ostial lesions in misplaced stents.
7. "Geographic Miss" in aorto-ostial lesions as high as 54% due to distal migration of ostial stent.[4]
8. More incidence of procedural complications like dissection, abrupt vessel closure and myocardial infarction.

ACCESS

Femoral route is preferred over radial route by many operators in view of better guide stability.

FLUOROSCOPIC VIEWS (SEE FIGS. 2 AND 3)

1. LAO caudal for ostial RCA
2. LAO/AP cranial for ostial left main coronary artery (LMCA)
3. For LAD ostium a combination of caudal views (LAO caudal typically shows least overlap with ramus or LCX but is more foreshortened than the RAO caudal view).
4. For LCX ostium LAO caudal usually best, but if overlap present, LAO cranial may help.
5. For ostial lesions of bypass grafts usually LAO ± caudal for RCA grafts (as for native RCA).
6. For LCA grafts, the ostium is usually least foreshortened in an RAO view.

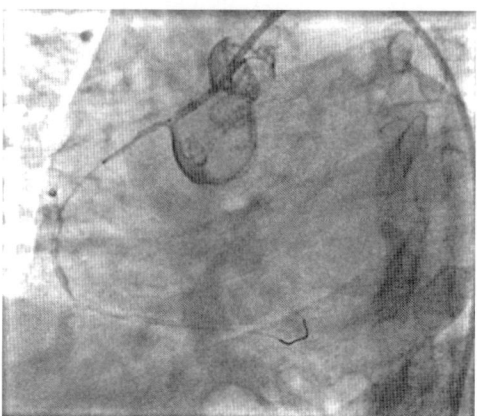

Fig. 2: LAO caudal view for ostial RCA stent positioning.

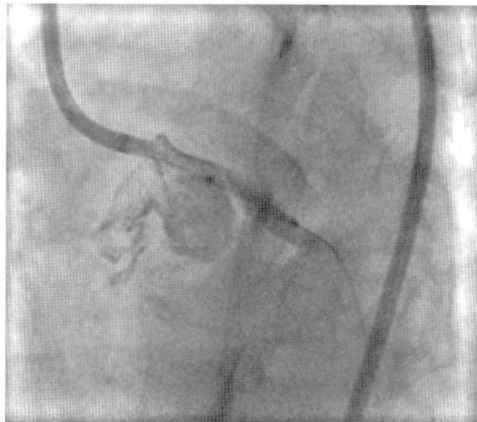

Fig. 3: LAO cranial view for ostial LM stent positioning.

EQUIPMENT GUIDING CATHETERS

For aorto-ostial lesion, less aggressive guide catheters that would provide coaxial alignment without getting sucked/deep seated into the artery should be selected. The guide should not cause trauma to the ostium and should be easily disengageable while positioning the balloon/stent (*See* Fig. 4).

Guides with Side holes would help avoid damping but at the cost of contrast wastage and underestimating the severity of the ostial lesion. Guide selection to be decided based on the vessel take off and various other factors.
- For RCA JR 4 guide with side holes should be used. Avoid using AR or AL guides.
- For LM, JL or FL guides (due to its short tip) with side holes should be used.
- For Bypass grafts, multipurpose or Judkins right guiding with side holes should be used.

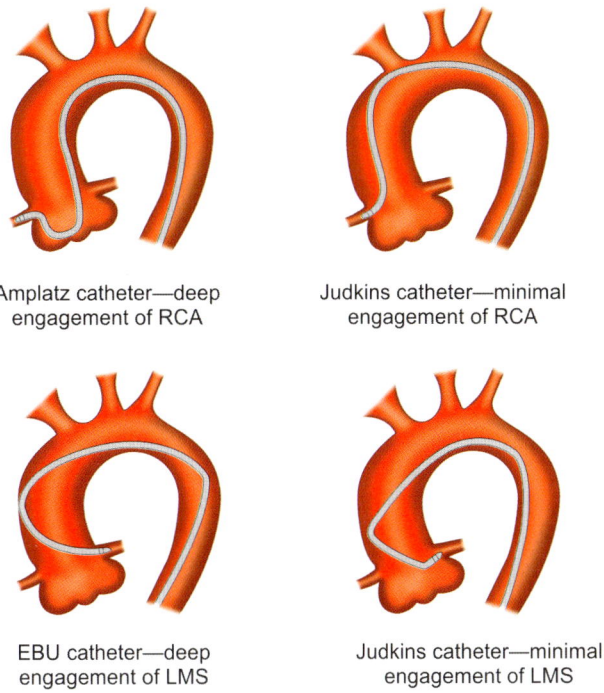

Fig. 4: Various guiding catheters in aorto-ostial lesions.

- For severe ostial disease, pre-load the wire in the guide before vessel intubation. This will facilitate rapid wiring and catheter disengagement after wiring.
- A buddy wire may also be used to provide additional stability or as a marker in the ascending aorta or side branch to assist in positioning the stent.
- Once the device (balloon, stent, etc.) is positioned, the guide is gently withdrawn into the aorta.
  Prior to complete removal of the device from the artery, use the device to "rail in" the guide tip (prevents damage to the deployed stent).

WIRES

Standard 0.014" workhorse wire are sufficient in most cases. Extra support wires can provide additional support in ostial saphenous vein graft (SVG) lesions. Hydrophilic wires are better avoided and the tip of the wire should be monitored throughout the procedure to avoid distal wire perforation during guide manipulation or device positioning.

LESION PREPARATION

Without adequate predilatation it would be a struggle to properly position the stent in aorto-ostial lesions with risk of water-melon seeding. During predilatation the balloon should be inflated slowly 1 atm at a time with guide pulled back in order to properly catch the ostium and avoid balloon migration proximally or distally. A noncompliant balloon can be used with high pressure dilatation initially. Using cutting balloon or scoring balloon-Flextome™ or Angiosculpt™ prior to deployment of the stent is preferable when adequate expansion is not be achieved with high pressure predilatation. Another option is to pass a buddy wire and do force-focused angioplasty.[5] Ostial lesions tend to be more fibrotic with calcium with increased elastic recoil tendency hence adequate preparation of lesion is essential. Intravascular ultrasound (IVUS) and debulking using rotablation is not routinely recommended but is to be used in difficult selected subsets to achieve adequate stent expansion. Some encouraging results have been noted with directional coronary atherectomy (DCA) in ostial lesions in the coronary angioplasty versus excisional atherectomy trial (CAVEAT 1) and balloon angioplasty versus optimal atherectomy trial (BOAT) trials however no clear cut superiority over angioplasty or other debulking techniques have been identified.

STENT POSITIONING

Difficulties in stent positioning in aorto-ostial lesions can occur due to the following reasons:
1. Guide cannot be deeply engaged in the ostium or the lesion and has to be kept in the aorta so only part contrast can enter the vessel and the rest swirls in the aortic sinus.
2. Presence of device (balloon/stent) across the lesion.

One popular method for approaching such aorto-ostial lesions is to engage the catheter and to advance the proximal stent marker just beyond the tip. The entire system is then carefully withdrawn as a unit, with frequent contrast injections to define the true ostium for deployment. This technique is practical only when the stenotic lumen is large enough to allow perfusion around the catheter tip.

How to Properly Position the Aorto-ostial Stent?

1. Use fleck of ostial calcium if present to guide positioning.
2. **Szabo/tail wire technique** (Figs. 5A to C) in aorto-ostial lesions/bifurcation ostial lesions.[6]

First the vessel with the ostial lesion is wired and second wire is placed in the side branch (bifurcation disease) or aorta (in aorto-ostial lesion). The last proximal strut of the stent is lifted up by inflating the stent at 4 atm inside the protective sheath with only the last cell free. The back end of the second wire is introduced through the last stent cell in proximal to distal fashion. The stent is then taken into the guide over the primary wire and the anchor wire and is positioned at the ostium and inflated at low pressures. The anchor wire is then removed and deployment of the stent is done. In the case of an ostial side branch, this technique is used to optimally position the proximal end of a stent at the ostium of the LAD. In case of LCX the anchor wire is placed in the LAD. This technique has been described as a feasible option providing good angiographic and clinical outcome in various larger series.[7]

3. A second wire can be placed and looped in the aorta so that the junction of the coronary artery and the aorta can be better defined (**modified Szabo technique**—Fig. 6). The second wire curving in the aortic sinus will help in preventing deep sucking of the guide as well.
4. **Stent pull-back technique in branch-ostial lesions (Fig. 7)**: A Balloon is inflated at low pressure in the parent vessel (size balloon 1:1), then pull back the stent to the ostium of the SB to create a dent in the balloon that is positioned in the parent vessel.[8]

Stent Deployment

- The stent should be positioned protruding into the aorta by 1-2 mm to prevent recoil of the lesion at the stent edge.
- Confirm proper stent ostial position in different orthogonal views and use stent boost to confirm stent position before deployment.
- In case of too much movement ask patient to hold breath or inflate low pressure 1-3 atm initially and then achieve optimal position before further deployment.
- Avoid using very short (<12 mm) stents to ensure adequate anchoring of the stent and to provide adequate lesion coverage distally.
- Size stent 1:1 ratio and deploy appropriately at high pressures (≥ 12 atm) to ensure optimal apposition. Use stent with high radial strength for optimal stenting.
- Inflation and deflation should be quick in left main lesions (repeat two to three times as needed).
- After stent deployment, pull the stent balloon out partially and do "flaring" of the ostium of the stent (Fig. 8).

SPECIAL SITUATIONS IN OSTIAL LESIONS

1. **Coronary Spasm**
   Excluding spasm as the cause of ostial narrowing during engagement of the coronary catheter is important. This can be done by using NTG as well as by rechecking with a smaller French-guiding catheter.

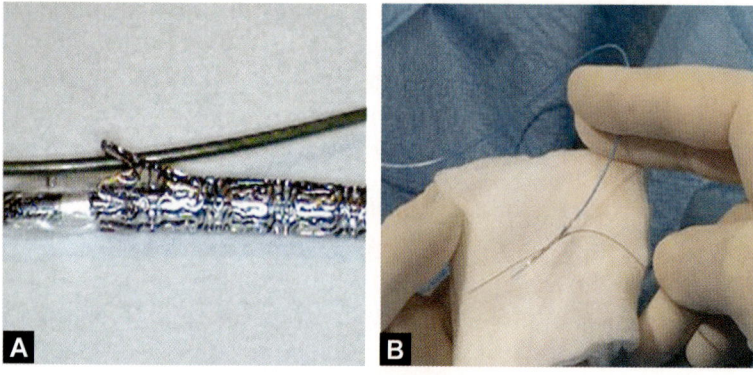

Ostial lesion

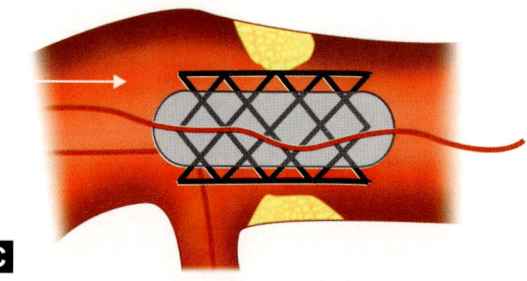

Figs. 5A to C: Szabo technique.

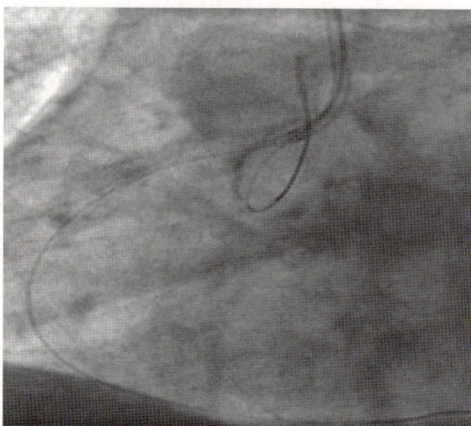

Fig. 6: Looped wire in aortic sinus.

2. Technical Consideration in Ostial LAD Lesions

Issues in ostial LAD stenting include whether to stent from the ostium of LAD or to stent from left main (LM) into LAD across LCX. The presence of significant plaque in the distal LM or at LCX ostium as well as the angle

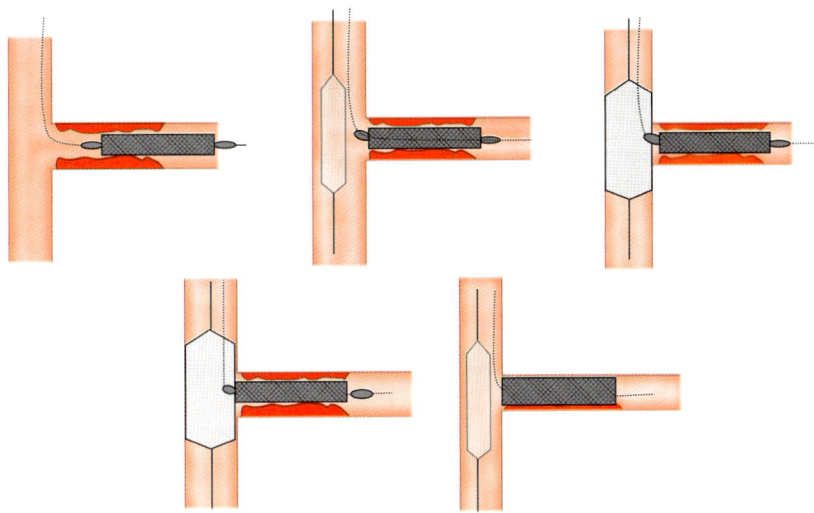

Fig. 7: Stent pull-back technique.

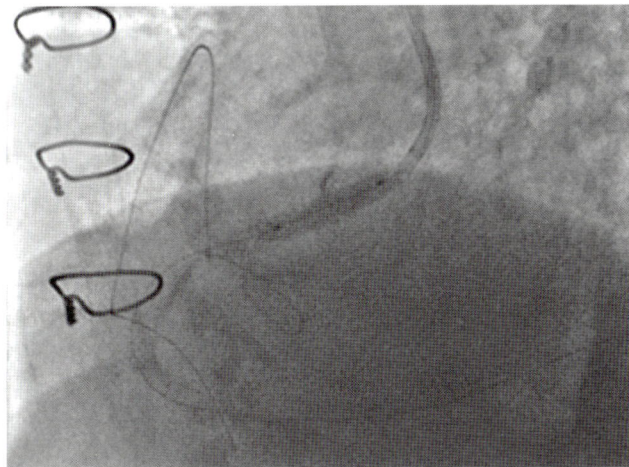

Fig. 8: Ostial RCA flaring with balloon after stent deployment.

of bifurcation between LAD and LCX and the amount of myocardium supplied by the LCX would determine this decision. Bifurcation angle less than 75 degrees is associated with more difficulty in positioning the ostial LAD stent without pinching the LCX as narrow angle is associated with increased incidence of plaque shift.

3. **Side Branch Ostial Stenosis**

   It is neither necessary nor feasible to stent every ostial branch lesion especially in those with small side branch. The balance of risk versus benefit might favor medical therapy in ostial lesions of small side branch.

Before deciding for ostial side branch percutaneous coronary intervention (PCI) we should know.
- What is the size of the side branch and the area of myocardium supplied?
- What is the significance of the degree of stenosis of the ostial lesion and is there evidence of ischemia either based on stress testing or clinical symptoms that warrant treatment?
- Would fractional flow reserve be required since the side-branch procedure may jeopardize the main branch?

4. **Role of Intravascular Ultrasound (IVUS) in Ostial Lesions**
   - Ability to confirm or refute the presence of significant aorto-ostial disease.
   - Assessment of vessel size to guide stent selection
   - Assessment of adequacy of stent expansion
   - Assessment of degree of calcification and need for adjunctive devices
   - Assessment of ostial site restenosis
   - To assess for the presence of proximal or branch vessel disease prior to deciding on a treatment strategy
   - Guide catheter disengagement during pullback risks non-coaxial imaging of the ostium and overestimation of the luminal area.

5. **Role of Fractional Flow Reserve (FFR) in Ostial Lesions**
   Fractional flow reserve (FFR) in aorto-ostial disease may be valuable, with following caveats:
   a. Initial pressure equalization has to be done in the ascending aorta prior to vessel engagement.
   b. Guide catheter needs to be disengaged so as not to occlude flow.
   c. Intravenous adenosine needs to be given rather than an intracoronary bolus, as the latter requires catheter engagement to allow selective injection and flush followed by rapid disengagement to allow FFR measurement.

RECOMMENDED READING

Practical handbook of advanced interventional cardiology/edited by Thach Nguyen, Dayi Hu, Shao Liang Chen, Moo-Hyun Kim, Shigeru Saito, Cindy Grines, C. Michael Gibson, Steven R Bailey. – 4th ed. Chapter 11 Ostial Lesions.

REFERENCES

1. Stewart JT, Ward DE, Davies MJ, Pepper JR. Isolated coronary ostial stenosis observations on the pathology. Eur Heart J. 1987;8:917–20.
2. Rissanen V. Occurrence of coronary ostial stenosis in a necropsy series of myocardial infarction, sudden death, and violent death. Br Heart J. 1975;37:182-91.

3. Popma JJ, Dick RJ, Haudenschild CC, et al. Atherectomy of right coronary ostial stenosis initial and long-term results, technical features and histologic findings. Am J Cardiol. 1991;67:431–3.
4. Dishmon DA, Elhaddi A, Packard K, et al. High incidence of inaccurate stent placement in the treatment of coronary aorto-ostial disease. J Invasive Cardiol 2011;23:322–6.
5. Chetcuti SJ, Moscucci M. Double-wire technique for access into a protruding aorto-ostial stent for treatment of in-stent restenosis. Catheter Cardiovasc Interv. 2004;62:214–17.
6. Szabo S, Abramowits B, Vaitkuts PT. New technique for aorto-ostial stent placement (Abstr). Am J Cardiol. 2005;96:212 H.
7. Wong P. Two years experience of a simple technique of precise ostial coronary stenting. Catheter Cardiovasc Interv. 2008;72:331–4.
8. Kini A, Moreno P, Steinheimer A. Effectiveness of the stent pull-back technique for nonaorto-ostial coronary narrowings. Am J Cardiol. 2005;96(8):1123–8.

7 Coronary Bifurcation Lesions

Nihar Mehta, Ashok Seth

INTRODUCTION

Coronary artery bifurcations are prone to develop atherosclerotic plaque due to turbulent blood flow and high shear stress. Bifurcation lesions are common account for approximately 15–20% of all percutaneous coronary interventions (PCI).[1,2] They pose a complex problem of obtaining an optimal result in the main vessel (MV) while maintaining side branch (SB) patency. With the use of Drug-eluting stents (DES) there has been a reduction in the rate of restenosis and reintervention as compared to Bare metal stents (BMS).[3] While stenting of the MV and stenting of the SB to salvage it if flow was impaired (Provisional Strategy) is preferred, there are instances where upfront elective Two Stent Strategy needs to be employed. The carina and SB ostium are central to the bifurcation anatomy and several strategies can be used to ensure optimal results. Dedicated bifurcation stents are also available and can also be employed but have not been proven to be advantageous.

DEFINITIONS AND CLASSIFICATIONS

A coronary bifurcation lesion is defined as a coronary artery narrowing occurring adjacent to, and/or involving, the origin of a significant SB (Fig. 1). A significant SB is a branch closure which could lead to important adverse sequelae to the patient. Usually there are SB >2.0 mm in diameter.

A bifurcation lesion involves three distinct anatomical segments; the proximal MV, the distal MV and the SB. The bifurcation carina is the transition zone between the MV and the SB and is the core of the bifurcation anatomy.

Each coronary bifurcation is unique because of (a) the conical shape connecting the proximal MV and the distal MV and SB, (b) different diameters of each segment, (c) tapering of the artery from proximal to distal segment, (d) non-uniform geometrical distribution of the plaque, and (e) negative remodeling of the SB ostium.[5]

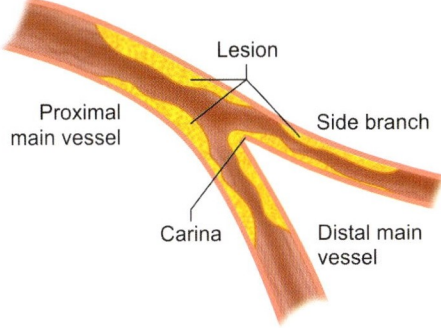

Fig. 1: Anatomy of a coronary bifurcation.

There are various classifications described for bifurcation lesions, the details of which are beyond the scope of this article. They are summarized in Figure 2.

In an attempt to simplify these classifications, Medina et al proposed a classification which divides the bifurcation lesion into three segments: Proximal segment of the main branch, distal segment of the main branch and SB ostium. Any involvement of each segment is assigned suffix 1, otherwise suffix 0. This classification is easier to remember in comparison to older ones. However, the Medina classification has shortcomings. It does not relate to angulation of the distal MB and SB, length of the SB, plaque distribution and the size of the proximal healthy segment which all affect the strategy and decision making (Fig. 3).

A 'True Bifurcation Lesion' is one in which both the MV and the SB have a >50% stenosis (Medina types 1,1,1 or 1,0,1 or 0,1,1). A 'Pseudo bifurcation lesion' is one which does not have significant disease at the ostium of the SB (Medina types 1,1,0 or 1,0,0 or 0,1,0).

ANATOMICAL CONSIDERATIONS

Angle assessment in bifurcation lesions is used to measure two angles: (i) The 'Take – off Angle" or Proximal angle or Angle A (**A**ccess angle)' between the Proximal MV and the SB and (ii) The 'Carina Angle' or Angle B (**B**etween) between the distal MV and the SB (Fig. 4). The angle A gives a measure of difficulty in accessing the SB. The acuteness of Angle B increases the risk of carina displacement and SB occlusion (SBO) after stent placement.[8] The angles between the distal MV and SB (angle B) affect the outcome of PCI pertaining to ease of wire access and stent deliverability, plaque shift or 'snow-ploughing' effect and complete coverage of ostium of SB.[5]

1. Angle B when less than 70 degrees its called a 'Y-angulation' and allows easy wire access to the SB, but plaque shifting is potentially more

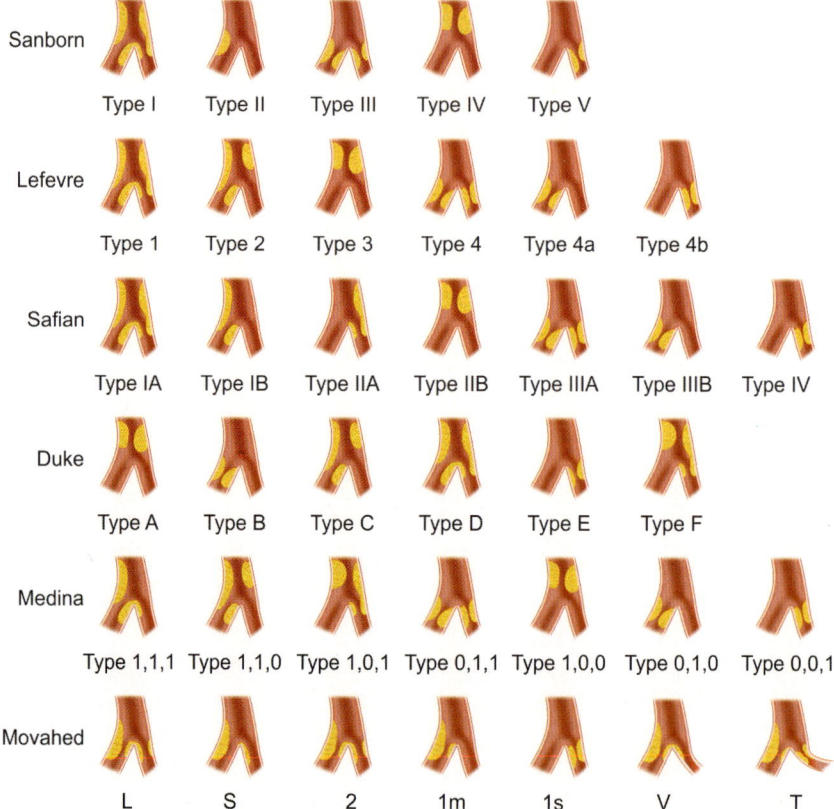

Fig. 2: Summary of the currently known bifurcation classifications.[6]

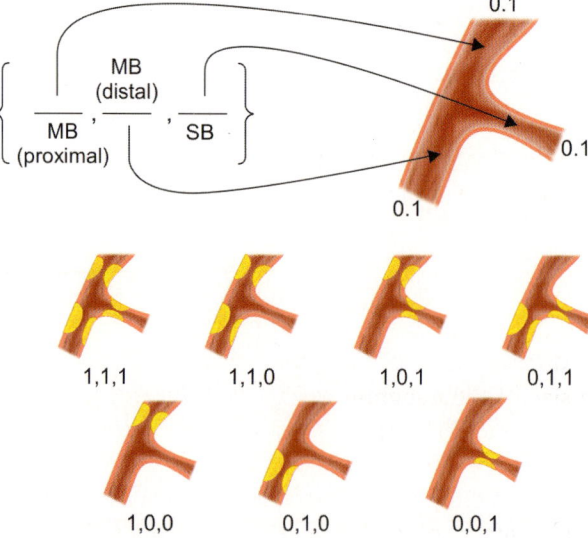

Fig. 3: Medina classification of bifurcation lesions.[7] (MB: Main branch; SB: Side branch).

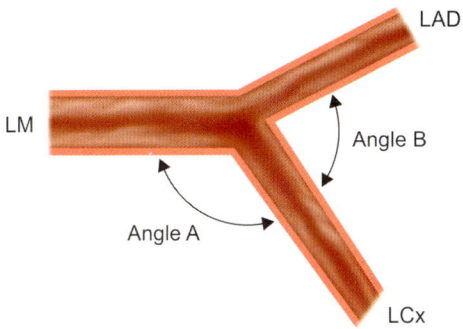

Fig. 4 : Anatomy of the bifurcation angle.
(LM: Left main; LAD: Left anterior descending; LCx: Left circumflex artery).

pronounced and precise stent placement with complete ostial coverage is often difficult or geometrically impossible.

2. Angle B when more than 70 degrees its called a 'T-angulation' and wire access to the SB is usually more difficult. However, plaque shifting is less frequent and precise stent placement with complete ostial coverage is technically easier and more likely.

Analysis of bifurcation angles by multidetector computed tomography revealed that majority of Left main bifurcations [(between left anterior descending (LAD) and left circumflex artery (LCx)] are T-angulations >80 degrees. On the contrary, most non-Left main bifurcations (e.g. Between LAD/Diagonal or LCx/obtuse marginal (OM) artery or posterior descending artery (PDA)/posterior left ventricular artery (PLV)) are Y-angulations with an average angle of 46–53 degrees.[9]

Plaque distribution in bifurcation lesions is localized exclusively to the outer wall of one or both daughter vessels where the wall shear stress (WSS) is low. The term "wall shear stress" refers to the stress on the arterial wall due to the friction associated with the viscous fluid flowing past the arterial wall (Fig. 5). Atherosclerosis occurs early in areas of non-uniform, low WSS. On the other hand, areas of uniform, high WSS are protected. Thus, the carina is usually protected and the plaques develop in both branches opposite to the carina.[10] In studies done using Intravascular Ultrasound (IVUS), this theory has been supported showing sparing of the carina. This has led to a modification in the Medina classification, removing the plaques from the carina.[11]

There is an important mother daughter mathematical relationship first described by Murray. Murray's Law states that the size of the proximal MV (D1) and the size of the daughter vessels (D2 and D3) are represented by the following formula: $D1^3 = D2^3 + D3^3 (+....+...)$.[12] Finet et al modified this to derive the simple formula $D1 = 0.678 (D2 + D3)$.[13] The formula can be used to calculate the size of one vessel if the sizes of the other two vessels in the bifurcation are known; particularly to calculate the proximal vessel diameter when both distal vessel diameters are known.

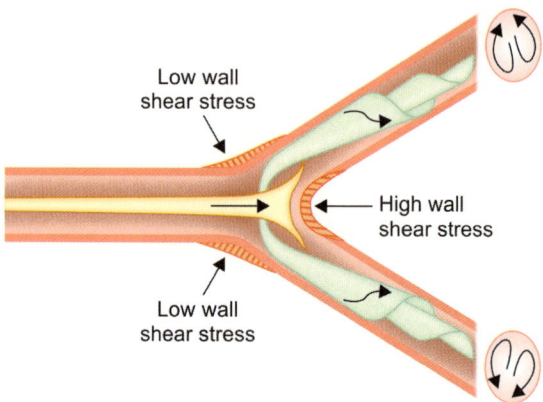

Fig. 5: Illustration of flow patterns and resulting wall shear stress in the region of a bifurcation.
Source: Moore, et al.[10]

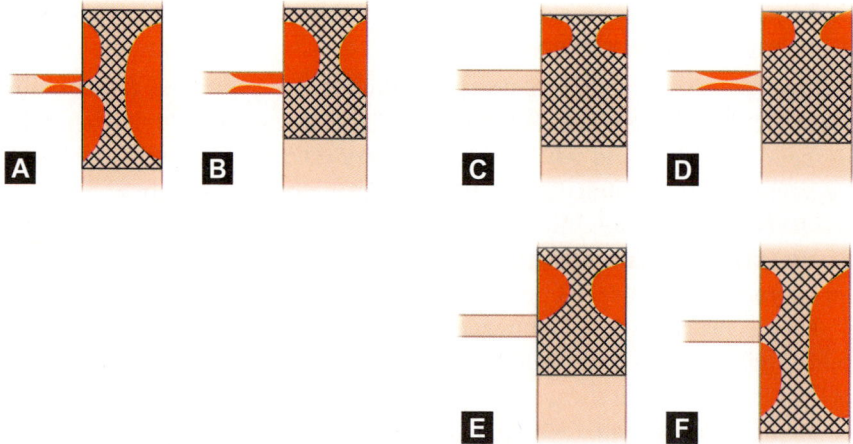

Figs. 6A to F: Threatened side branch morphologies (with permission from Moussa et al.)[4]: (A) SB with >50% ostial narrowing where the origin is completely spanned by either the diseased segment or the index lesion. (B) SB arises adjacent to or is partially contiguous with the diseased index lesion. Non-threatened SB morphologies include: (C) SB without ostial narrowing; (D) SB with ostial involvement; (E) Disease-free SB arising adjacent to diseased segment of the parent vessel; (F) SB without ostial disease arising from parent vessel lesion spanning the entire origin of the SB.

The concept of 'threatened SB morphologies' needs special consideration as regards to the incidence of SBO. In studies done comparing the incidence of SBO based on threatened versus non-threatened SB morphologies, the incidence of SBO was significantly higher in threatened morphologies (80%) as compared to non-threatened morphologies (7.9%)[4] (Figs. 6A to F).

STENTING STRATEGY IN BIFURCATION LESIONS—ONE OR TWO STENTS?

The strategy to use one stent (in the MV) or two stents (one in the MV and one in the SB) for the treatment of bifurcation lesions has been long debated.[14-16] The most important initial questions are whether the SB is large enough (>2.25 mm diameter) and whether the SB supplies a large enough territory to justify its intervention. In the Provisional SB Stenting strategy, the MV is stented first and the SB is stented through the MV stent, only if necessary. Thus the use of the second stent is provisional. Although this is the preferred strategy, the literal adaptation of the conclusions of a given study might be impractical in clinical patient centric decision making. Irrespective of the individual variations in the SB severity and bifurcation anatomy, the provisional stenting hypothesis does not specify lesion specific interventional approach thus creating a caveat in intelligent decision making.

The primary reason why the PCI of bifurcation lesions has been a challenge is the risk of SBO or compromise after treating the MV. Hence understanding the anatomic attributes characterizing the lesion are of importance essence. Multiple classifications of coronary bifurcations including the Medina classification do not characterize the lesion satisfactorily. This includes the bifurcation angle, the size of SB, Myocardial territory supplied by the SB, lesion length in SB and distribution of MV disease. Multiple trials done as mentioned earlier which advocated the preference of a single stent over a double stent strategy assumes the nature of the lesions to be the same without special reference to the "high-risk" bifurcation anatomy. Furthermore, the concept of "threatened" SB morphology is important because of the incidence of SBO varies widely according to varying morphologies that are not reflected in the Medina classification.

Thus, the approach of "one for all" is not practical in all bifurcations. Hence Provisional stenting should not be used as a default strategy in "high risk" bifurcations that involve a large SB. In some patients, elective double stenting (EDS) Strategy is opted for to reduce the risk of large SB compromise.[4]

PROVISIONAL SIDE BRANCH STENTING STRATEGY

This strategy involves stenting the MV first. If necessary, a second stent is delivered to the SB through the MV stent in a classic T, TAP (T and Protrusion), inverted Culotte or Internal Crush technique. Use of the second stent is only provisional.

EVIDENCE

Six randomized studies[19-24] were undertaken in order to compare the provisional SB stenting strategy with one or more dual-stent techniques (Figs. 7A and B).

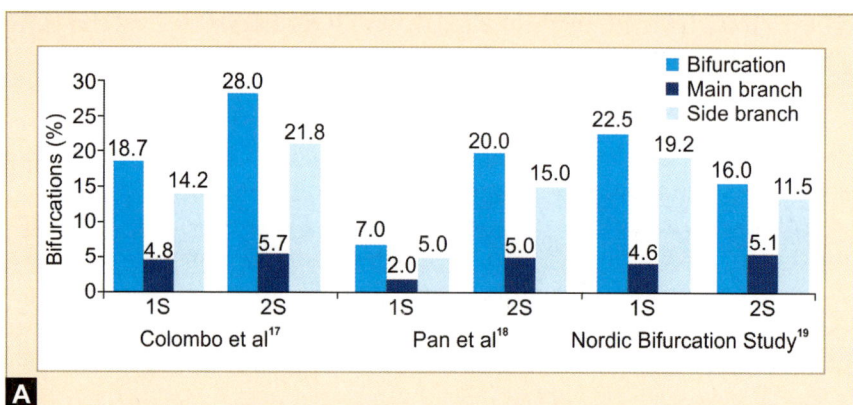

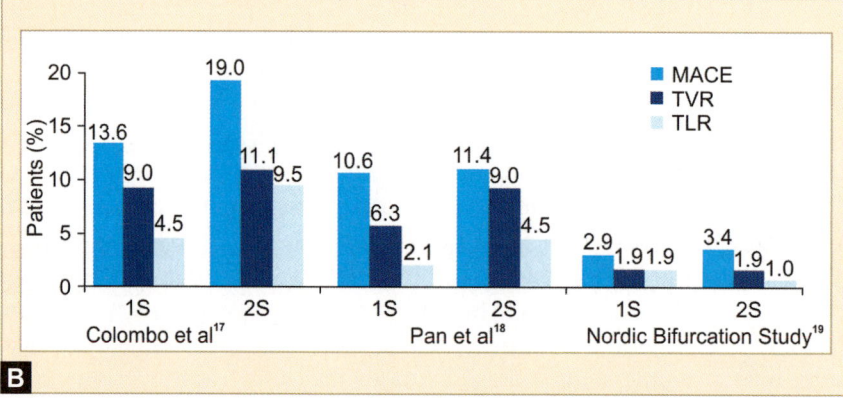

Figs. 7A and B: (A) Angiographic re-stenosis in three randomized trials comparing a one-stent (1S) vs. two-stent (2S) approach in the treatment of coronary bifurcations. (B) Clinical outcomes in three randomized trials comparing a one-stent (1S) vs. two-stent (2S) approach in the treatment of coronary bifurcations. (MACE: Major adverse cardiac events; TLR: Target lesion revascularization; TVR: Target vessel revascularization).

The Nordic Bifurcation Study,[19] a multi-centre, randomized trial designed to compare provisional stenting with routine SB stenting randomized 413 patients to either stenting of the MV (with bailout if necessary) or stenting of the MV and the SB. Six months outcomes did not show any differences in the overall cardiac mortality, target vessel revascularization, myocardial infarction or stent thrombosis. On the other hand, the two-stent strategy was associated with longer procedural times, higher contrast utilization, and unexpectedly, increased post-procedural non-Q wave myocardial infartction (MI).

In the BBC One Study, 500 patients were randomized to a single stent strategy (with bailout if necessary) or a two stent strategy. At 9 months, the composite end-point of death, myocardial infarction or target vessel failure was 8% in the single stent strategy group as compared to 15.2% in the two stent strategy group (p = 0.009). The incidence of myocardial infarction was

3.6% versus 11.2% (p=0.001) in the two groups, respectively. The in-hospital major adverse cardiac events (MACE) rate was 2% in the single stent strategy group as compared to 7.6% in the two stent strategy group (p=0.002).

Similarly, the CACTUS Study, compared provisional SB stenting with the crush technique in 350 patients. The 6 months analysis showed no difference in the clinical or angiographic outcome or stent thrombosis.

The results of these Studies and other relevant prospective registries were pooled in meta-analyses.[24-27] Overall, the meta-analyses did not reveal any differences at 6 to 7 months follow-up in terms of mortality, MACE and target-lesion revascularization (TLR), although there was a significant difference in favor of the single-stent group in the BBC One study.

The Nordic Baltic Bifurcation Study IV randomized 450 patients to compare provisional SB stenting versus two stent strategy in treatment of true bifurcation lesions with a large SB. After 2 years, two-stent techniques for treatment of true bifurcation lesions with a large SB showed no significant difference in MACE rate compared to provisional SB stenting.[27]

Based on these data, current opinion favors provisional SB stenting with placement of DES in the MV. Stenting of the SB is performed only if necessary.

However, one must point out that most of the studies were performed using the first generation thick strut DES in which all two stent strategies resulted in deformed and bulky metal messes into relatively small side SB and adverse sequalae. The present thinner strut DES are more designed for ease and optimization of two stent strategies and hence results have improved. Furthermore, the technical steps of procedure optimization of two stent strategies have also evolved to improve outcomes.

STEPS[28]

- *Wiring both the branches*: Wiring starts with the most difficult branch. The second wire is inserted into the easier branch by limited rotation manoeuvres to avoid wire wrap. The wire inserted in the SB should be without hydrophilic or polymer coating because the coating may get peeled off during removal of the jailed wire. The advantage of securing the SB with a wire is that it serves as a marker to find the SB lumen, if an occlusion occurs.
- *Pre-dilatation*: Pre-dilatation of the MB is left to the operator's discretion. Pre-dilatation of the SB should be avoided if final kissing balloon inflation is planned. It may produce a dissection in the SB. The subsequent step of rewiring the SB through the distal strut of the MB stent may be difficult in presence of dissection.
- *Stenting the MV across the SB*: The selection of the stent is important. The cell area should allow access to the SB ostium. The diameter of the stent

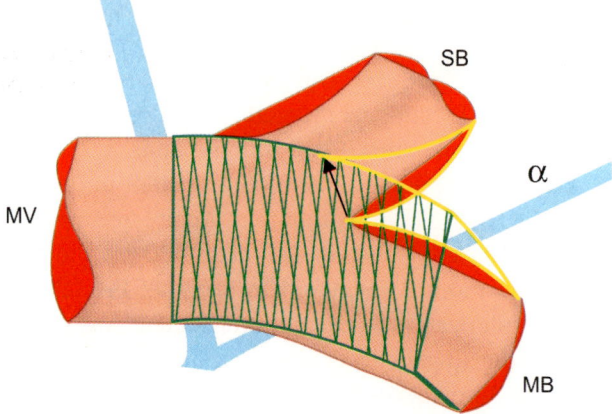

Fig. 8 : Carina shift after MB stenting. (SB: Side branch; MV: Main vessel; MB: Main branch).

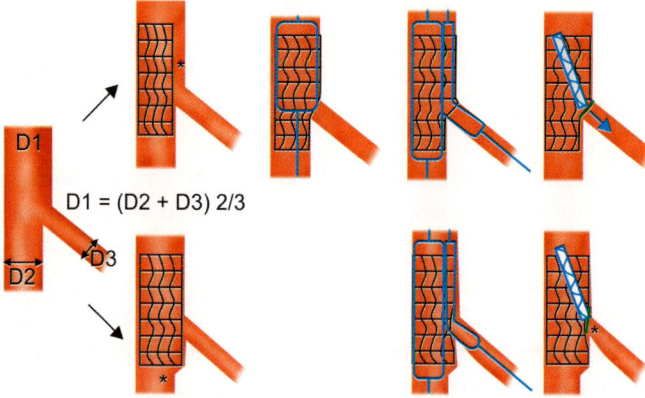

Fig. 9: Consequence of choice of diameter of MV stent: Up – Selection according to the diameter of the distal MV followed by POT technique. Down – Selection according to the diameter of the proximal MV.

should be selected according to the distal MB (not the proximal MB) in order to avoid excess carina shifting (Fig. 8). The proximal part of the stent prior to the bifurcation may be dilated with a short 0.5 mm bigger balloon. This is called proximal optimization technique (POT). This results in optimal diameter of the proximal part of the stent and allows the struts of the stent to face the SB which allows subsequent rewiring of the SB[29] (Fig. 9).

- *SB rewiring or guide wire exchange:* This step starts with removal of the wire in the MB and inserting it into the SB. Alternative a third wire can be used to go through the struts of the MB Stent into the SB so that MB position of the initial wire is not disturbed. The SB jailed wire is then removed or passed into the main branch if MB wire was removed. The manoeuvring of the wire through the MB stent strut should be done

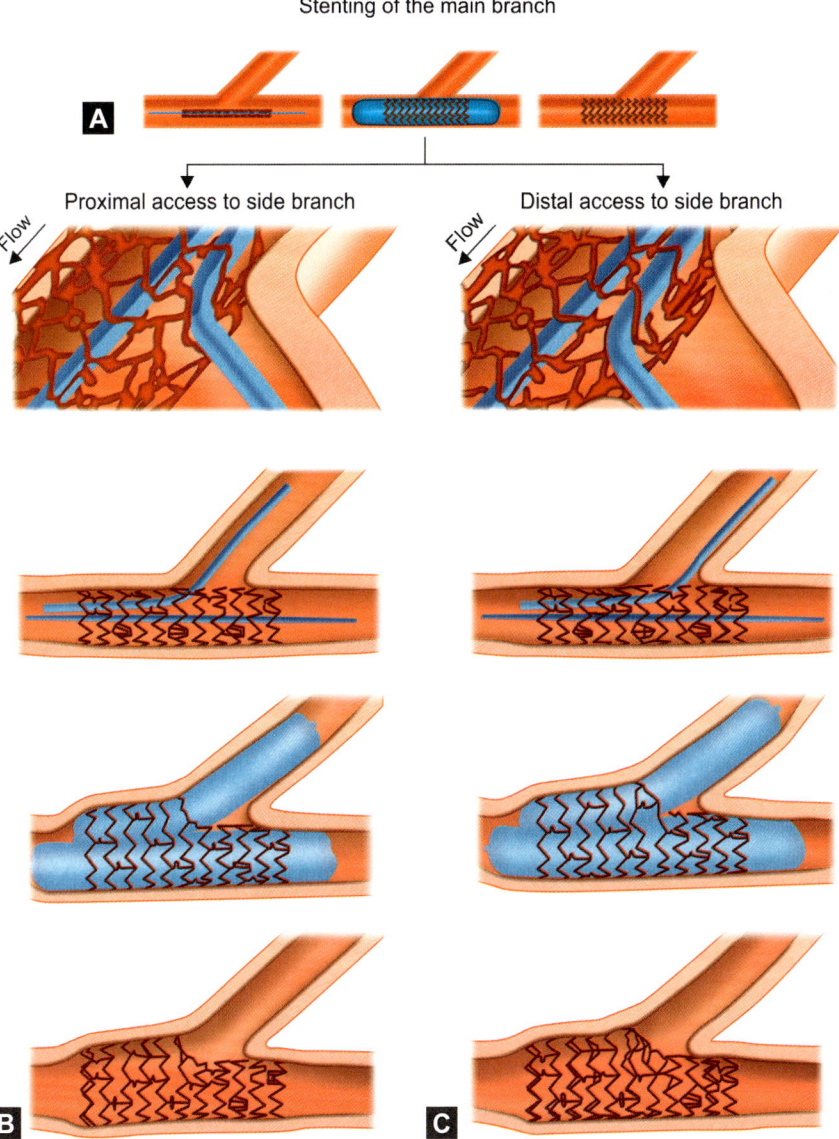

Figs. 10A to C: Proximal versus distal cross during guide wire recrossing and result after final kissing balloon inflation.[31]

carefully, such that the wire enters the distal most strut of the stent. Final kissing balloon inflation performed after this 'distal cross' of the guide wire allows correction of the MV stent deformation, allows a better scaffolding to the SB ostium and facilitates better future access to the SB. On the other hand, final kissing balloon inflation performed after 'proximal cross' of the guide wire results in MV stent deformation and poor SB ostium scaffolding (Figs. 10A to C).

- *Final kissing balloon inflation (FKI)*: Two short balloons are selected based on the diameter of the distal vessels. They are inflated simultaneously to perform the final kissing inflation. For the optimal result of FKI, distal crossing of the wire is preferable.

    A subanalysis of the CACTUS trial showed that FKI was associated with a lower MACE rate and better angiographic result.[19] However, the Nordic Baltic Bifurcation III Study randomized 477 patients to FKI versus no FKI in patients treated with MV stenting. This study showed no difference in the MACE rate or event free survival at 6 months. FKI resulted in better angiographic results, especially in true bifurcation lesions. FKI resulted in longer contrast use, angiography and procedure times.[30] Koo et al. advocated the use of fractional flow reserve (FFR) guided jailed SB intervention. Their study of 110 patients showed no difference in the clinical outcomes at 9 months between the groups with or without FFR guided SB angioplasty.[32]

    The conclusion drawn from these studies does not support routine balloon dilatation of the SB but advocates use of FFR to guide intervention in a jailed SB.
- *Provisional SB Stenting*: In about 70–80% of cases, the procedure ends at the previous step. In about 20% (2–51% in 5 trials)[17-21] results in the SB were unsatisfactory after FKI:
    - \>75% residual stenosis
    - Dissection in SB
    - TIMI Flow grade <3 in a SB >2.5 mm diameter
    - Fractional Flow Reserve <0.75
    - Persistent intra-procedural angina or ECG changes

    In these situations, stenting of the SB is done using

1. *Reverse T technique*: SB stent crosses the struts of the MV stent and is deployed in a T configuration (Fig. 11)
2. *T and Protrusion technique (TAP technique)*: SB stent is implanted with slight protrusion into the MV stent. A balloon is inflated in the MV stent at low pressure (2-3 atmospheres) to help precise positioning of the SB stent.
3. *Internal or reverse crush technique*: The SB stent is deployed, projecting into the proximal part of the MV stent. This is followed by balloon crushing of the proximal part of the SB stent with a balloon in the MV. This is followed by guide wire re-insertion in to the SB and final kissing balloon inflation.
4. *Inverted cullotte technique*: The SB stent is deployed, projecting into the proximal part of the MV stent. The guide wire is then crossed into the MV stent next to the carina. This is followed by final kissing balloon inflation.

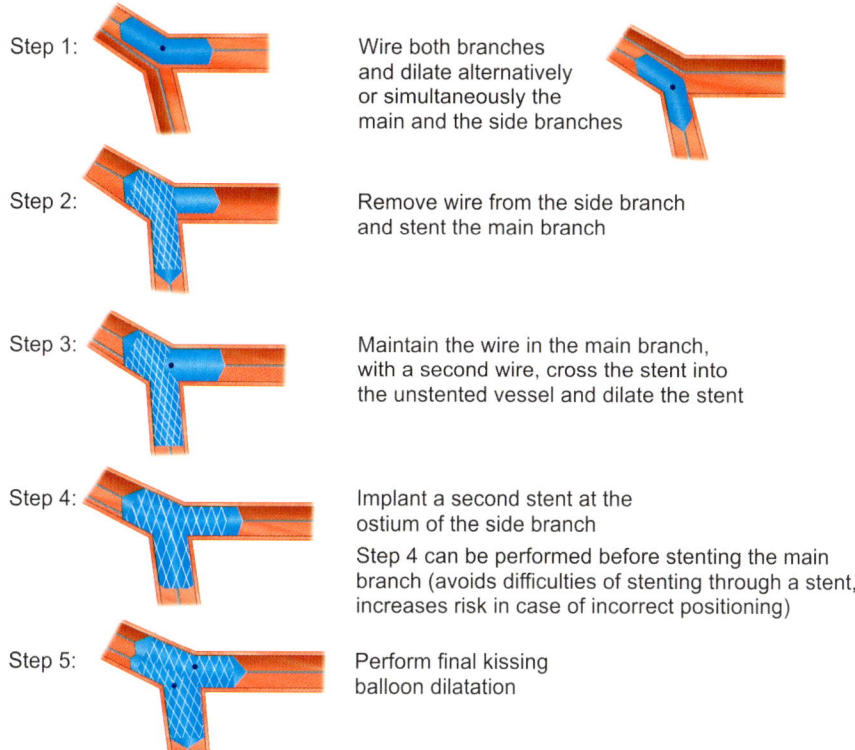

Fig. 11: Classical or reverse T-stenting (Iakovou, et al).[34]

ELECTIVE DOUBLE-STENT STRATEGY

Although provisional stenting has been a preferred option according to many randomized controlled trial,[17-21] in situations where the SB is large or severely diseased, or supplies a large area of myocardium, the two-stent strategy is still often preferred because of its superior acute angiographic result and lower risk of SB compromise.

INDICATIONS

1. True bifurcation lesions – MV and SB have >50% stenosis (Medina classification 1,1,1 or 1,0,1 or 0,1,1).
2. SB supplies a large area of myocardium.
3. SB has a diameter appropriate for stenting; >2.25 mm.
4. SB lesion is severe and/or long.
5. Wide angle between the MV and SB that would lead to difficulty in recrossing the SB after MV stenting.

TECHNIQUES[33]

1. *Classical T-stenting*: The classic T-stenting technique begins with positioning a stent at the ostium of the SB, being careful to avoid stent protrusion into the MV. The stent in the SB is first deployed. The stent balloon and wire in SB are removed. A second stent is deployed in the MV. A wire is then re-advanced into the SB, and final kissing balloon inflations are performed. Reverse T stenting has been described above as a part of provisional SB stenting.
   Indication – Angle between the MV and SB is closer to 90 degrees.
   Advantages – Not technically demanding.
   Disadvantage – Chances of missing the SB ostium in the attempt to prevent protrusion of the stent in the MV (Fig. 11).
2. *Modified T-stenting or Minicrush*:[35,36] is a variation performed by simultaneously positioning stents in the SB and the MV. SB stent is positioned with minimal protrusion into the MV. (In Minicrush technique, the protrusion into the MV is a few millimeters more. It results in increased layers of stents after FKI). This guarantees coverage of the SB ostium. The SB stent is deployed first, and after wire and balloon removal from the SB, the MV stent is deployed. Final kissing balloon inflations are recommended.
   Indications – Preferable if angle is closer to 90 degrees.
   Advantage – Not technically demanding. Ensures complete coverage of the SB ostium.
   Disadvantage – Most bifurcations have a vessel angulation of less than 70 degrees so this technique will lead to incomplete stent coverage at the ostium of the SB (Fig. 12).
3. *Crush technique*:[37] Two stents are placed in the MV and SB, with both the proximal ends in the proximal MV. The MV stent is positioned more proximally than the SB stent. The SB stent is deployed first followed by removal of the stent balloon and guide wire. The MV stent is then deployed at high pressure, crushing the struts of the SB stent which are protruding into the proximal MV. The SB is the recrossed and balloon dilatation in done in the SB at high pressure. This is followed by FKI (Fig. 13A).
   Indication – Can be used for all bifurcation lesions but should be avoided in wide angle bifurcations.
   Advantage – Ensures coverage of SB ostium.
   Disadvantage – Three stent layers in the proximal MV proximal to the origin of the SB and two stent layers in the distal part of SB ostium. This makes rewiring challenging. It also makes the procedure more laborious.

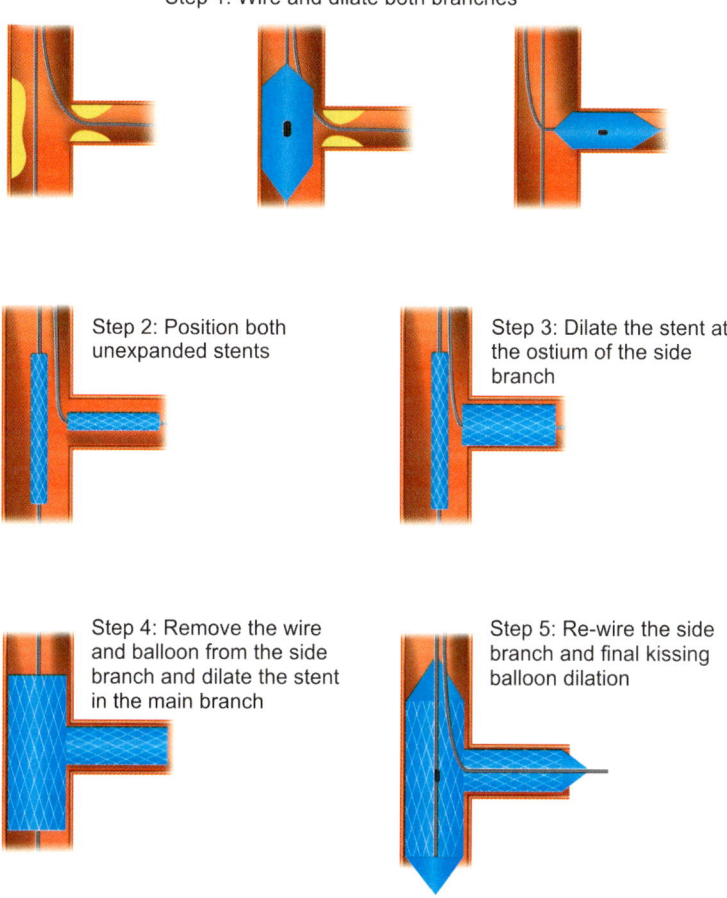

Fig. 12: Modified T-technique (Iakovou, et al)[34]

Variations:
a. *Internal or reverse crush technique*: Described above as a part of provisional SB stenting.
b. *Step crush technique*:[38] In this technique, the SB stent is deployed and first crushed by a balloon. This is followed by advancement and deployment of the MV stent. The other steps remain the same.
c. *Double kiss step crush technique or sleeve technique*:[39] In this technique, the SB stent is deployed and first crushed by a balloon. This is followed recrossing into the SB through crushed SB stent struts and post dilatation with a kissing balloon inflation. This step is then followed by advancement and deployment of the MV stent. The other steps remain the same (Fig. 13B).

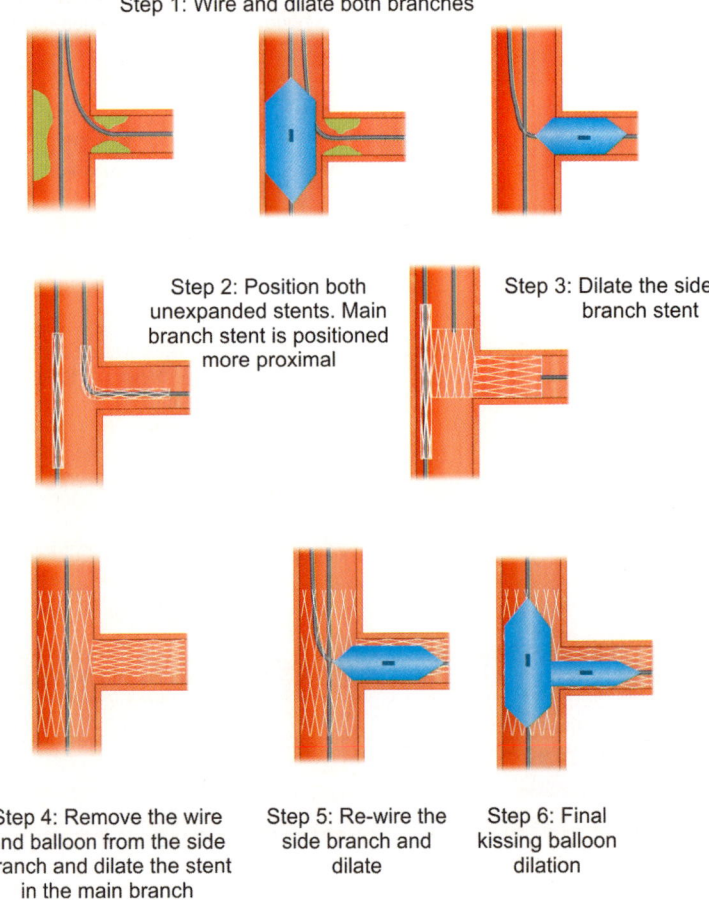

Fig. 13A: Classic crush technique (Iakovou, et al).[34]

d. *'Micro crush' technique*: protruding the SB stent minimally into the MB and then crushing it enables recrossing with wire easily as there are less layers of metal and double kissing (DK) crush to be overall less complex while maintaining the optimal ostial stent coverage of the SB.

The DKCRUSH I bifurcation study by Chen et al showed that the DK Crush technique reduced the incidence of stent thrombosis, target lesion re-vascularization and cumulative MACE rate at 8 months when compared to classical crush technique.[40] The DK CRUSH II study showed that the DK Crush technique reduced the restenosis rate and thus the target lesion revascularization and target vessel revascularization at 12 months as compared to provisional stenting.[41] In the light of these recent studies, this technique has become the technique of choice for two stent strategy in bifurcation stenting when applicable.

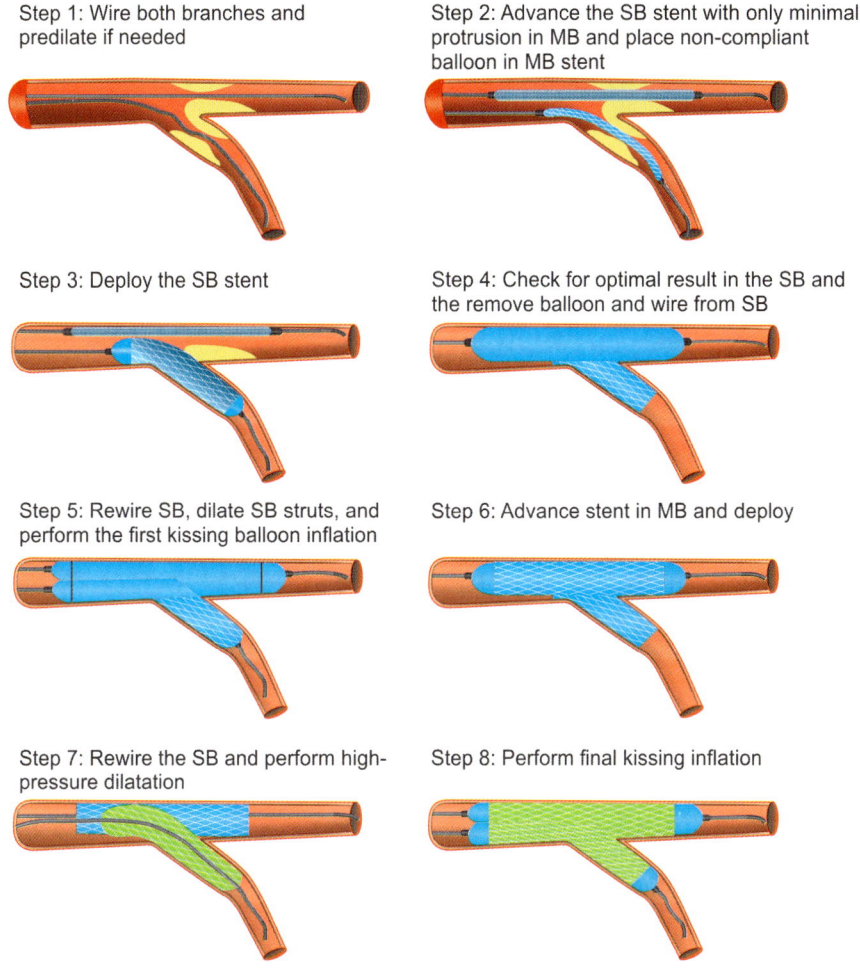

Fig. 13B: Double kissing minicrush technique. (SB: Side branch; MB: Main branch).

4. *Culotte technique*:[42] In this technique, the first stent is deployed in the more angulated branch (usually the SB) with its proximal part protruding into the MV. The wire of the MV which was jailed, is removed and the MV is re-wired through the stent strut. The wire is removed from the SB. The stent struts are dilated with a non-compliant balloon. The second stent is then deployed in the MV. The SB is re-wired through the struts of the second stent. This is followed by FKI (Fig. 14).
 Indication: Any bifurcation lesion, irrespective of the bifurcation angle. It is advisable to use this technique when the MV and the SB have a similar diameter. It can also be used for left main stenting.
 Advantages – Ensures coverage of SB ostium. Can be used for any angle of bifurcation.

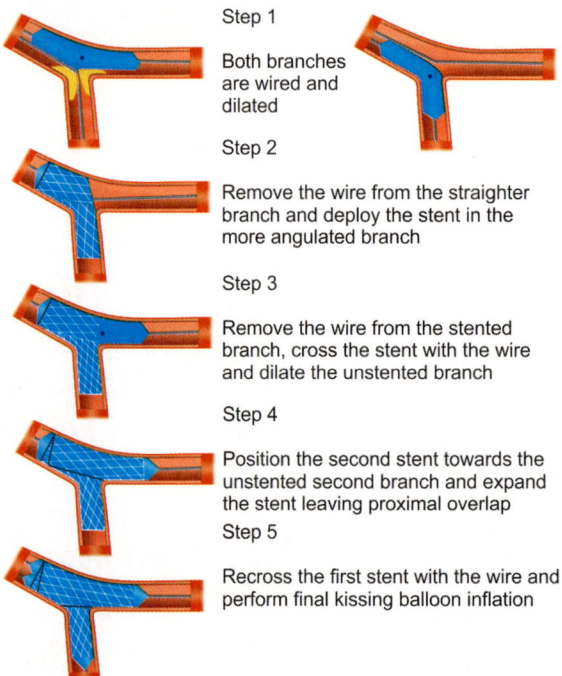

Fig. 14: Culotte technique (Iakovou, et al)[34]

Disadvantage – Double layer of stent in the proximal MV. It requires rewiring of both the branches which can be technically challenging. This is not advisable in case of large discrepancy between the MV and SB due to incomplete apposition of the SB stent in the proximal MV.

Variations – Inverted Culotte: Described above as a part of provisional SB stenting.

5. *The V-stenting technique*:[43] The V-stenting technique consists of implantation of the distal MV and SB stents simultaneously. One stent is advanced in the SB and the other in the distal MV. The proximal edge of both stents touch and forming a small proximal carina (<2 mm). The pre-requisite for this technique is that proximal MV must be free of disease. This is followed by FKI (Fig. 15).

Indication – A 0,1,1 bifurcation lesion as per Medina classification is ideal.

Advantages – Not technically challenging. It does not require rewiring of the vessel through the stent struts.

6. *Simultaneous kissing stents (SKS) technique*:[44] This can be used can be used if there is disease in the proximal MV. The two stents are positioned in the distal MV and SB, but the proximal edge of the stents protrude into the proximal MV to an equal extent. The pre-requisite for this technique is that the Proximal MV should be large enough to accommodate both

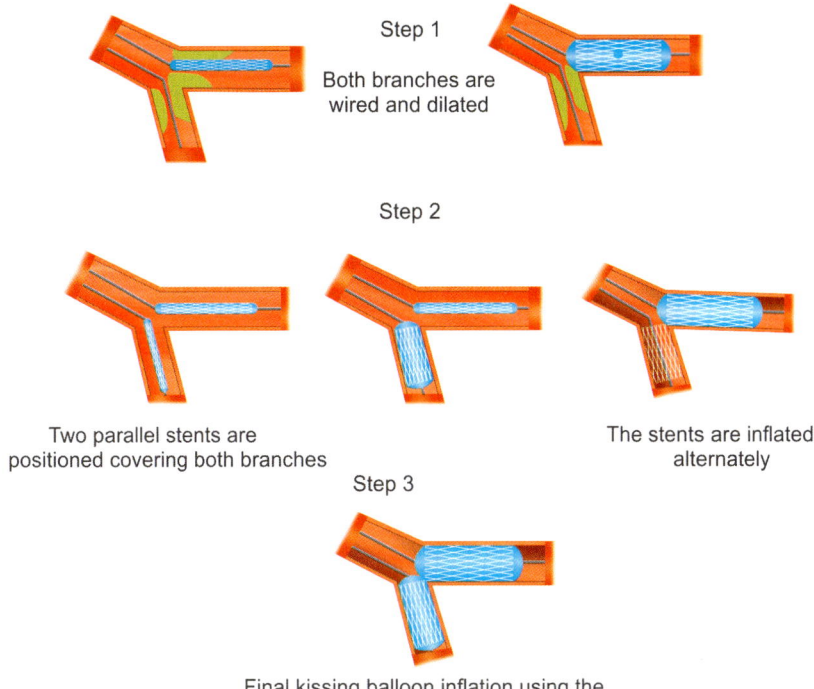

Fig. 15: V-stenting technique (Iakovou, et al).[34]

the stents side by side such as distal left main or proximal LAD/diagonal bifurcations lesions. This is followed by FKI (Fig. 16).

Pre-Requisite – Diameter of Prox MV = 2/3 (Diameter of Distal MV + Diameter of SB).

Indications – Bifurcation lesions with diseased proximal MV, 1,1,1 according to Medina classification. Can be used for left main stenting.

Advantages – Not technically challenging. Does not require rewiring of the vessel through the stent struts.

Disadvantages – In the SKS technique, a metallic neocarina is created in the proximal MV with Stent mal-apposition.

Variation:
a. *Trouser SKS*:[45] Three stents are used in this technique. The first and largest stent is deployed in the proximal MV. This is followed by wiring of the SB through the lumen of the first stent. Two stents are then deployed in the distal MV and SB in a V configuration. This avoids an excessively long double stent carina.
b. *Extended V technique*:[46] Three stents are used in this technique as well. The first and largest stent is deployed in the proximal MV. This is followed by wiring of the SB through the lumen of the first stent. Two stents are

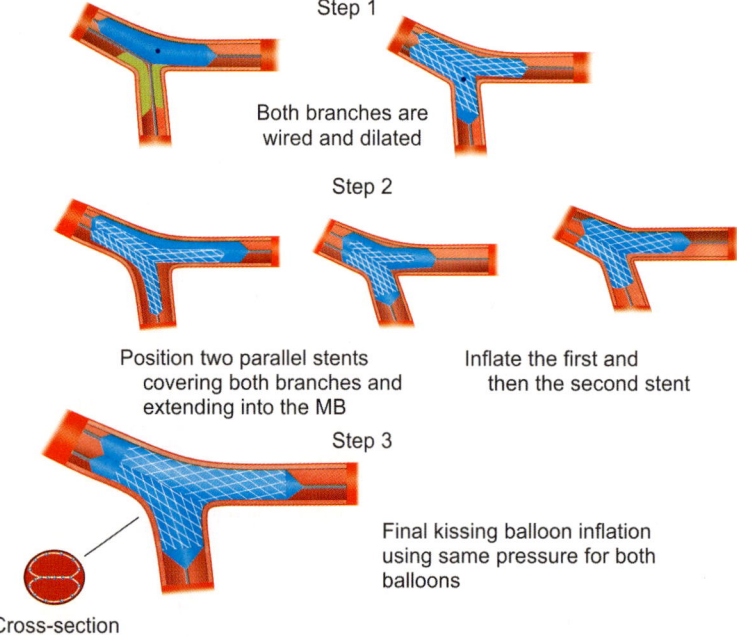

Fig. 16: Simultaneous kissing stents (SKS) technique. (MB: Main branch).

then individually or simultaneously deployed in the distal MV and SB, side by side with slight internal protrusion into the proximal stent.

c. *Y technique*:[47] Three stents are used in this technique as well. Two stents are deployed in the distal MV and SB. This is followed by a third stent deployed in the proximal MV if required. The proximal stent is crimped on two balloons and deployed by inflating both balloons simultaneously (Fig. 17).

Tips and Tricks[32]
1. Guide catheter: 7F or 8F guide catheters are preferred to reduce friction among the hardware and allow easy manipulation. They also provide better support for stent delivery.
2. Wiring the vessel: Wire the branch which seems more difficult first, where manipulation and rotation are expected. This will minimize wire crisscrossing. During insertion of the second wire, minimal rotation should be done. Both wires should be kept separate on the table.
3. Lesion preparation: Lesions in proximal MV, distal MV or SB should be adequately prepared before stent deployment. In case of severely calcified lesions, rotational atherectomy may be used. Cutting balloons may be used in fibrotic lesions. The main problem with aggressive balloon dilatation is dissections.

Contd...

Contd...

4. **Stent selection and deployment:** When using EDS strategy, drug eluting stents have proven to be more effective than BMS.[19-21] Sizing of the stent is also essential for optimal results. Intravascular ultrasound should be used to choose the optimal stent size and to assess the adequate stent deployment or requirement for post dilatation of the stents.
5. **Jailed guide wire:**
   a. When a stenting strategy involves jailing the guide wire, a non-hydrophilic guide wire should be used. This is because the coating on the hydrophilic guide wires may get peeled off when pulling it back.
   b. During deployment of the stent which jails the guide wire (jailing stent), nominal pressure should be used so that retrieval of the jailed wire is easier.
   c. During forceful removal of the jailed wire, the guide catheter may get deep throated. To avoid this, the guide catheter should be pulled back into the aorta before removing the jailed wire. In case the 'jailed wire' cannot be pulled back easily, a balloon can be advanced over the jailed wire.
6. Stents used should have ideal stent strut expansion for optimal SB crossing. Hence stents with 'open cell' design are preferred.
7. **Final kissing balloon inflation (FBKI):** Using noncompliant balloons is an essential step to optimize results.

Contd...

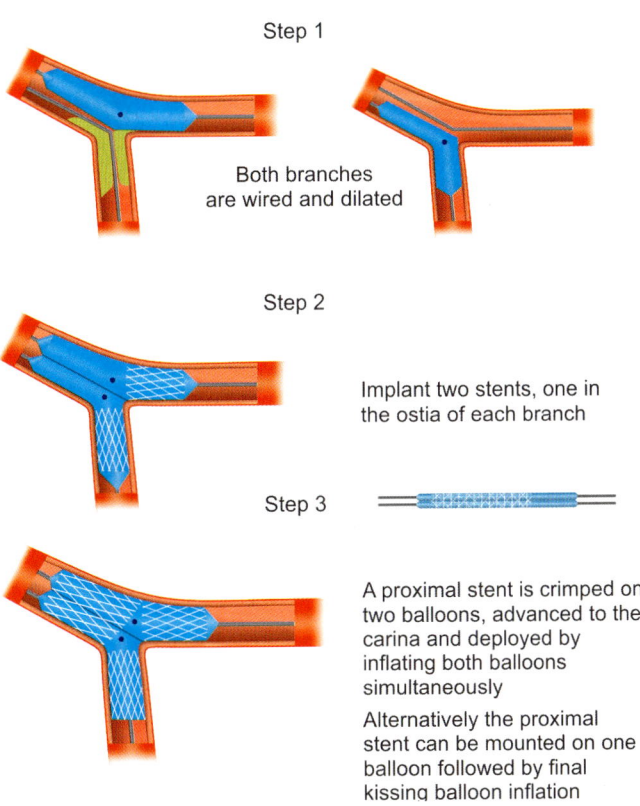

Fig. 17: Y technique.[34]

Contd...

8. Hemodynamic support: May be necessary, especially with left main PCI. Intra aortic balloon pump may be need urgently or may be used electively in some cases. An alternative is the Impella 2.5 device.
9. Dual antiplatelet therapy: Should continue for 12 months after the procedure at least, to reduce the risk of stent thrombosis.

DEDICATED BIFURCATION STENT SYSTEM

On the whole, irrespective of whether a one or two stent strategy is chosen, the results after bifurcation PCI have improved substantially as compared to previous bifurcation studies. Clearly bifurcation PCI is technically challenging and time consuming, especially in order to achieve an optimal long-term result. Dedicated bifurcation stents have been designed to specifically treat coronary bifurcations with the aim of overcoming some of the shortcomings of the conventional approach to bifurcation intervention. Majority of the devices are aimed at facilitating the provisional approach. To understand the need for a dedicated stent technology, one should know about the limitations with current strategies of bifurcation stenting:[48]

1. Maintaining access to SB throughout the procedure.
2. MB stent struts jailing the SB ostium resulting in difficulty in re-wiring SB or passing balloon/stent into SB through the stent struts.
3. Distortion of MB stent by SB dilatation.
4. Multiple layer of stents; Increased rates of stent thrombosis.
5. Inability to fully cover and scaffold ostium of SB.
6. Undue dilatation of the stent in the proximal MV during accommodation of both balloons during FKI.
7. Finally operator skills and technical experience.

As a result, several stents have been specifically designed for bifurcations with the intention of addressing these shortcomings.

WHAT SHOULD AN IDEAL DEDICATED BIFURCATION STENT ACHIEVE?[48]

An ideal dedicated bifurcation stent system should make the PCI of complex coronary bifurcation lesions simpler and should improve short- and long term outcomes. To complete this task the following are necessary:

1. The device should have a low profile and high deliverability even in complex anatomies.
2. It should allow optimal coverage of the carina
3. Allow changing the strategy of approach (e.g. provisional vs. double stent techniques) during the procedure

4. Device should be actively torqueable when alignment of the SB access is needed to accurately place the device.
5. The device should ensure and facilitate rapid SB access and protection during the procedure.

The first generation of dedicated bifurcation stent systems were difficult to deploy, as they were stiff and their accurate positioning was difficult at SB ostium. Many also had larger crossing profiles and less flexibility compared with conventional stents, so that they were difficult to deliver in tortuous or calcified arteries. However, these devices have undergone rapid evolution from their earlier designs along with clinical testing in First-In-Man (FIM) studies. There are now sizeable number of these devices that have a 'CE' mark and are commercially available although none of these are FDA approved.

CATEGORIES OF DEDICATED BIFURCATION STENTS

The currently available (or under investigation) dedicated bifurcation stents can be broadly divided into:
1. Stents that are implanted in both the MB and the SB at the same time; that is, complete bifurcation "Y" stents such as Medtronic Bifurcation Stent.
2. Stents for provisional SB stenting that facilitate or maintain access to the SB after MB stenting and do not require re-crossing of MB stent struts (e.g. Petal™, former AST stent, (Boston Scientific, Natick, MA, USA); Invatec Twin-Rail™ (Invatec S.r.l., Brescia, Italy); Antares™ (Trireme Medical Inc, CA, USA); Y-med Sidekick™ (Y-med Inc, San Diego, CA, USA); Nile CroCo™ (Minvasys, Gennevilliers, France); Multi-link Frontier™ (Abbott Vascular Devices, Redwood City, CA/Guidant Corporation, Santa Clara, CA, USA). These stents allow placement of a second stent on the SB if needed.
3. Stents that usually require another stent implanted in the bifurcation - e.g. Sideguard™ (Cappella Inc, MA, USA); Tryton™ [Tryton Medical, MA, USA); Axxess Plus™ (Devax, Irvine, California)]. The Tryton and Sideguard are designed to treat the SB first and require re-crossing into the SB after MB stenting for FKI. The Axxess Plus is the exception as it is implanted in the proximal MB at the level of the carina and does not require re-crossing into the SB but may require the additional implantation of 2 further stents to completely treat some types of bifurcation lesions.

CHALLENGES OF USING DEDICATED BIFURCATION STENT SYSTEMS[49]

The stent delivery systems (SDS) of these dedicated bifurcation systems have a number of design features which highlight their weaknesses:
1. Double balloon SDS have to be tracked over two wires and thus wire wrap (twisting) is a common problem.

2. These devices still tend to be bulkier than single balloon SDS requiring larger guide catheters
3. Tracking the device over two parallel wires may be limited by wire trap, wire bias and atheroma. This can prevent advancement of the device and subsequent rotation to align with the SB.
4. Although stents with a preformed SB aperture maintain access to the SB during MB stenting, successful implantation of the MV stent is dependent on accurate positioning with a small margin for error.
5. A SDS with a side hole needs to have axial and rotational self-positioning properties, i.e.
   - *Axial*: SDS has a "stopper" to position the side cell at the SB level, closest to the carina.
   - *Rotational*: SDS automatically turns the side hole exactly toward SB.
6. The Nile™, Frontier™, Twin-Rail™, Sidekick™ and Stentys™ SDS have struts that only partially cover the ostium and thus leave the potential for a gap and ostial restenosis.
7. SB specific stents compel the operator to stenting both branches.

ADVANTAGES OF USING DEDICATED BIFURCATION STENT SYSTEMS

1. Stents with a preformed SB aperture maintain access to the SB during MB stenting.
2. Stents that have struts that can be expanded into SB ostium (Petal™, Ariste™) may be clinically advantageous as they provide complete coverage of the SB orifice and offer the possibility of delivering drug to the SB ostium.
3. Reduced layers of stents (as compared to double stenting strategies).
4. Reduced deformation of the stent (as compared to double stenting strategies).
5. Shorter procedure times.

PRELIMINARY CLINICAL RESULTS WITH DEDICATED BIFURCATION STENTS

The first generation bifurcation stents have been tested in FIM studies and multicenter registries only. Although the device success was excellent with most of the devices tested, they suffer from technical problems that may hamper acute clinical results. Restenosis rates with the first generation devices are similar to that reported for BMS in bifurcations[15] with a range varying from 28 to 54% which is in turn coupled with high rates of repeat revascularization and MACE.

Second generation drug-eluting devices have only been very recently introduced and only 1 study has been published. Such experience regards the Axxess Plus™ biolimus-eluting stent which demonstrated a favorable rate of restenosis for the MB and SB, although majority of patients required at least one other stent implanted in the bifurcation.[50] A number of FIM studies and multicenter registries are on-going and the results are eagerly awaited to establish if these new devices will become a good alternative to current bifurcation strategies in different bifurcation scenarios. However, as has been seen with the utilization of two stent techniques in bifurcation PCI, there will be a learning curve in the optimal deployment and utilization of these new devices.

SUMMARY

In the current era of PCI, coronary bifurcations still remain a complex subset. Despite the favorable results shown by multiple trials on coronary bifurcations, achieving success of these interventions requires a learning curve. Understanding of the anatomy of the coronary bifurcation with regards to MV and SB involvement, the carina, angulations and myocardial territory supplied are of crucial importance. As SBO is an important and serious complication with these lesions, anatomical risk stratification is an essential prerequisite.

As per the current evidence, provisional strategy using one stent is the strategy of choice where the risk of the loss of SB by SBO is small or not consequential. In case of a SB narrowing during provisional stenting, FFR guided angioplasty may be performed. In most instances, angiographic SB pinching does not cause ischemia and does not need intervention. It is sensible to resort to the strategy of EDS when the loss of SB is undesirable like in presence of a large SB (>2.25 mm), severe ostial and/or long segment involvement and wide angle (Angle B) with anticipated difficulty in recrossing into SB. Out of all the available techniques for elective double vessel stenting, a choice has to be made on the basis of anatomy, feasibility, operator preference and experience to deliver a good short-term and long-term results. Double Kissing Minicrush technique as a two stent strategy has shown superior results in recent trials. However, in the present era of thin strut open cell design DES, elective TAP with minimal protrusion of SB stent in the MB, especially if MB is large and SB is closer to 60-90º, is a very good and simpler option with favorable results. Various kinds of dedicated stents are aiming at user friendliness but they are far from routine use in the cath lab since the bifurcation anatomy is so variable that 'one stent to fit them all' seems quite elusive.

REFERENCES

1. Dauerman H, Higgins P, Sparano A, et al. Mechanical debulking versus balloon angioplasty for the treatment of true bifurcation lesions. J Am Coll Cardiol. 1998;32:1845-52.
2. Lefevre T, Louvard Y, Morice MC, et al. Stenting of bifurcation lesions: classification, treatments, and results. Cathet Cardiovasc Intervent. 2000;49:274-83.
3. Colombo F, Biondi-Zoccai G, Infantino V, et al., A long-term comparison of drug-eluting versus bare metal stents for the percutaneous treatment of coronary bifurcation lesions, Acta Cardiol. 2009;64(5):583-8.
4. Moussa I, Colombo A. Coronary artery bifurcation interventions; Bridging the gap between research and practice; Tips and Tricks in Interventional Therapy of Coronary Bifurcation Lesions, Issam Moussa, Antonio Colombo (Eds.), 2010; pp. 01-3.
5. Costa R, Kyono H, Costa M, et al. Coronary artery birfucation lesions: Anatomy 101; Tips and Tricks in Interventional Therapy of Coronary Bifurcation Lesions, Issam Moussa, Antonio Colombo (Eds.), 2010; pp. 14-47.
6. Expert review of cardiovascular therapy 2008;6:261-74.
7. Medina et al. Rev. Esp. Cardiol 2006; 59(2):183-4.
8. Louvard Y, Sashikand G, Lefevre T, et al. Angiographic predictors of side branch occlusion during treatment of bifurcation lesions. Cath Cardiovasc Interv. 2005 (Abstr. Supp.).
9. Pflederer T, Ludwig J, Ropers D, et al. Measurement of coronary artery bifurcation angles by multidetector computed tomography. Invest Radiol. 2006;41(11): 793-8.
10. Moore JE Jr., Timmins LH, LaDisa JF Jr. Coronary artery bifurcation biomechanics and implications for interventional strategies; Catheter Cardiovasc Interv. 2010;76:836-43.
11. Oviedo C, Maehara A, Mintz G, et al. A Critical intravascular ultrasound appraisal of the angiographic classification of bifurcation lesions: where is the plaque really located? J Am Coll Cardiol. 2008;51 (Poster 2902-2916): B23-B98.
12. Murray CD. The physiological principle of minimum work: I. The vascular system and the cost of blood volume. Proc Natl Acad Sci USA 1926;12(3):207-14.
13. Finet G, Gilard M, Perrenot B, et al. Fractal geometry of arterial coronary bifurcations, a quantitative coronary angiography and intravascular ultrasound analysis. Euro Interv. 2007;3:490-98.
14. Al Suwaidi J, Berger P, Rihal C, et al. Immediate and long-term outcome of intracoronary stent implantation for true bifurcation lesions. J Am Coll Cardiol. 2000;35:929-36.
15. Yamashita T, Nishida T, Adamian M, et al. Bifurcation lesions: two stents versus one stent - immediate and follow-up results. J Am Coll Cardiol. 2000;35:1145-51.
16. Pan M, de Lezo SJ, Medina A, et al. Simple and complex stent strategies for bifurcated coronary arterial stenosis involving the side-branch origin. Am J Cardiol. 1999;83:1320-25.
17. Colombo A, Moses JW, Morice MC, et al. Randomized study to evaluate sirolimus-eluting stents implanted at coronary bifurcation lesions. Circulation. 2004; 109(10):1244-9.
18. Pan M, de Lezo JS, Medina A, et al. Rapamycin-eluting stents for the treatment of bifurcated coronary lesions: a randomized comparison of a simple versus complex strategy. Am Heart J. 2004;148:857-64.
19. Steigen TK, Maeng M, Wiseth R, et al. Nordic PCI Study Group. Randomized study on simple versus complex stenting of coronary artery bifurcation lesions: the Nordic bifurcation study. Circulation. 2006;114(18):1955-61.

20. Ferenc M, Gick M, Kienzle RP, et al., Randomized trial on routine versus provisional T-stenting in the treatment of de novo coronary bifurcation lesions. Eur Heart J. 2008;29(23):2859-67.
21. Colombo A, Bramucci E, Saccà S, et al. Randomized study of the crush technique versus provisional side-branch stenting in true coronary bifurcations: the CACTUS (Coronary Bifurcations: Application of the Crushing Technique Using Sirolimus-Eluting Stents) Study. Circulation. 2009;119(1):71-8.
22. Hildick-Smith D, de Belder AJ, Cooter N, et al. Randomized trial of simple versus complex drug-eluting stenting for bifurcation lesions: the British Bifurcation Coronary Study: old, new, and evolving strategies Circulation. 2010;121(10): 1235-43.
23. Zhang F, Dong L, Ge J. Simple versus complex stenting strategy for coronary artery bifurcation lesions in the drug-eluting stent era: a meta-analysis of randomisedtrials. Heart. 2009;95(20):1676-81.
24. Brar SS, Gray WA, Dangas G, et al. Bifurcation stenting with drug-eluting stents: a systematic review and meta-analysis of randomised trials. Euro Interv. 2009;5(4):475-84.
25. Katritsis DG, Siontis GC, Ioannidis JP. Double versus single stenting for coronary bifurcation lesions: a metaanalysis. Circ Cardiovasc Interv. 2009;2(5):409-15.
26. Niccoli G, Ferrante G, Porto I, et al. Coronary bifurcation lesions: to stent one branch or both? A meta-analysis of patients treated with drug eluting stents. Int J Cardiol. 2010;139(1):80-91.
27. Lesar MA, Hakeem A, Azarnoush K, et al. Coronary bifurcation lesions: present status and future perspectives. Int J Cardiol. 2015;187:48-57.
28. Albiero R, Boldi E. Provisional Stenting Technique of Non-Left Main Coronary Bifurcation Lesions: Patient selection and Technique; Tips and Tricks in Interventional Therapy of Coronary Bifurcation Lesions, Issam Moussa, Antonio Colombo (Eds.), 2010; pp. 49-66.
29. Darremont O. The POT Technique. European Bifurcation club. Valencia, Sep 2007. http://www.bifurc.net
30. Niemela M, Kervinen K, Erglis A, et al. Randomized comparison of final kissing balloon dilatation versus no final kissing balloon dilatation in patients with coronary bifurcation lesions treated with main vessel stenting. The Nordic Baltic Bifurcation Study III. Circulation. 2011;123:79-86.
31. Chiastraa C, Morlacchia S, Pereirac S, et al. Computational fluid dynamics of stented coronary bifurcations studied with a hybrid discretization method. Europ J Mechanics - B/Fluids; (35) Sep–Oct 2012, p. 76-84.
32. Koo BK, Park KW, Kang HJ, et al. Physiological evaluation of the provisional side branch intervention strategy for bifurcation lesions using fractional flow reserve. Eur Heart J. 2008;29(6):726-32.
33. Favero L, Pacchioni A, Reimers B. Elective Double Stenting of Non-Left Main Coronary Bifurcation Lesions: Patient selection and Technique; Tips and Tricks in Interventional Therapy of Coronary Bifurcation Lesions, Issam Moussa, Antonio Colombo (Eds.), 2010; p. 89-115.
34. Iakovou I, Ge L, Colombo A. Contemporary stent treatment of coronary bifurcations. J Am College Cardiol. 2005;46(8):1446-55.
35. Kobayashi Y, Colombo A, Akiyama T, et al. Modified T stenting. A technique for kissing stents in bifurcation coronary lesions. Catheter Cardiovasc Diagn. 1998; 43:323-26.
36. Colombo A, Stankovic G, Orlic D. et al. Modified T-stenting technique with crushing for bifurcation lesions: immediate results and 30-day outcomes. Catheter Cardiovasc Interv. 2003;60:145-51.

37. Moussa I, Costa R, Lasic Z, et al. A prospective registry to evaluate sirolimus-eluting stents implanted at coronary bifurcation lesions using the 'crush technique'. Am J Cardiol. 2006;97(9):1317-21.
38. Collins N, Drazvik V. A modified balloon crush approach improves side branch access and side branch stent apposition during crush stenting of coronary bifurcation lesions. Cath Cardiovasc Interv 2006;68:365-71.
39. Jim MH, Ho HH, Miu R, et al. Modified crush technique with double dissing balloon inflation (sleeve technique): a novel technique for coronary bifurcation lesions. Cath Cardiovasc Interv. 2006;67(3):403-09.
40. Chen SL. et al. Study comparing the double kissing (DK) crush with classical crush for the treatment of coronary bifurcation lesions: the DKCRUSH-1 Bifurcation Study with drug-eluting stents. Eur J Clin Investig. 2008;38:361-71.
41. Chen SL, et al. A randomized clinical study comparing double kissing crush with provisional stenting for treatment of coronary bifurcation lesions. J Am Coll Cardiol. 2011;57:914-20.
42. Chevalier B, Glatt B, Royer T, et al. Placement of coronary stents in bifurcation lesion by the culotte technique. Am J Cardiol. 1998;82:943-49.
43. Schampaert E, Fort S, Adelman AG, et al. The V-stent: a novel technique for coronary bifurcation stenting. Cath Cardiovasc Diagn. 1996;39:320-26.
44. Sharma SK. Simultaneous kissing drug eluting stent technique for percutaneous treatment of bifurcation lesion in large size vessels. Cath Cardiovasc Interv. 2005:65:10-16.
45. Khoja A, Ozbek C, Bay W, Heisel A. Trouser-like stenting: a technique for bifurcation lesions. Cathet Cardiovasc Diagn. 1997;41:192-6.
46. Helqvist S, Jørgensen E, Kelbæk H, et al. Percutaneous treatment of coronary bifurcation lesions: a novel "extended Y" technique with complete lesion stent coverage. Heart. 2006;92:981-82.
47. Fort S, Lazzam C, Schwartz L. Coronary "Y" stenting: a technique for angioplasty of bifurcation stenosis. Can J Cardiol. 1996;12:678-82.
48. Abizaid A, De Ribamar Costa J, Alfaro VJ, et al. Bifurcated stents: giving to Caesar what is Caesar's. Euro Intervention. 2007;2:518-25.
49. Latib A, Colombo A, Sangiorgi G. Bifurcation stenting: current strategies and new devices; heart published online 23 Sep 2008; doi:10.1136/hrt.2008.150391.
50. Grube E, Buellesfeld L, Neumann FJ, et al. Six-month clinical and angiographic results of a dedicated drug-eluting stent for the treatment of coronary bifurcation narrowings. Am J Cardiol. 2007;99:1691-7.

8

Calcified Lesions

Mathew Samuel Kalarickal, Vijayakumar Subban

INTRODUCTION

Coronary artery calcification (CAC) is a marker of advanced atherosclerosis, and its extent correlates with disease burden and future adverse events. In patients undergoing percutaneous coronary intervention (PCI), the presence of CAC predicts failure of device delivery and optimal lesion dilatation. It has been associated with increased incidence of balloon rupture, coronary artery dissection, vessel perforation, stent underexpansion, malapposition and periprocedural myocardial infarction (MI). Moreover, severe CAC remains an important cause both in-stent restenosis and stent thrombosis.[1-4]

In the recent years, improved understanding of disease process and advancements in device technology have enabled treatment of these complex lesions with high success rate and good long-term outcomes. This article reviews the current status of PCI in calcified coronary lesions including procedure planning, lesion preparation and stent optimization.

PROCEDURE PLANNING

As in any other complex PCI, meticulous procedure planning is very important for successful treatment of calcified coronary lesions. This includes careful assessment of severity of CAC and lumen compromise, estimation of procedure risk and selection appropriate debulking strategy.[5]

ASSESSMENT OF CAC

Assessment of severity and extent of CAC is the cornerstone of treatment of calcified coronary lesions. In the catheterization laboratory, coronary angiography (CAG), intravascular ultrasound (IVUS) and optical coherence tomography (OCT) are used commonly for the assessment of CAC.[6]

CORONARY ANGIOGRAPHY

Fluoroscopy is readily available in catheterization laboratories and remains the most common modality for assessment of CAC. CAC appears as radiopaque densities on fluoroscopy and its intensity depends on the severity of calcification. Fluoroscopically, CAC is classified into 4 grades of severity: None, mild, moderate and severe. Moderate calcification is defined as radiopacities visualized only with cardiac movement prior to contrast administration and severe calcification as densities visualized without cardiac motion, usually involving both sides of the lumen – "tram track" appearance. However, CAG is limited by it poor sensitivity (48%) for the detection of calcification, particularly the milder forms. Further, with fluoroscopy, it is not possible to differentiate superficial calcification from the deeper ones.[1,6]

CORONARY INTRAVASCULAR ULTRASOUND

Intravascular ultrasound (IVUS) detects calcium with a higher accuracy (sensitivity—90 to 100% and specificity—99 to 100%) compared to CAG. On IVUS imaging, fibro-calcific plaques are hyperechoic with a reflectivity more than that of adventitia. Given it the potent reflectively, little ultrasound waves penetrate beyond the surface. This results acoustic shadowing and hence the axial extent of calcium cannot be measured with IVUS. In addition, the strong reflectivity produces various artifacts such as reverberations, and side lobes. IVUS classifies CAC based on it axial (superficial and deep) and circumferential (no of quadrants occupied) and longitudinal extents.[1,6]

OPTICAL COHERENCE TOMOGRAPHY

Optical coherence tomography (OCT) is a light based intravascular imaging modality with 10 times higher resolution than IVUS. With this high resolution, OCT characterize CAC with a very high sensitivity (95 to 100%) and specificity (97 to 100%). On OCT, calcium appears as a heterogeneous, low attenuating, low back scattering structure with well-defined borders. In contrast to IVUS, light penetrates calcium and does not produce artifacts like side lobes, acoustic shadowing, and reverberations. This enables accurate quantification of thickness, depth, arc, area and length of calcification.[1,5,6]

FRACTIONAL FLOW RESERVE

In the presence of CAC, it is very difficult to assess hemodynamic significance of coronary artery lesions by angiography alone. Hence, it is important to evaluate the angiographically ambiguous lesions with fractional flow reserve to appropriately guide revascularization.[7]

RISK ASSESSMENT

Coronary artery calcification (CAC) usually occurs in the setting of complex and multi-vessel coronary artery disease. In addition, most of the patients with CAC are elderly with multiple comorbidities. Hence, it is important to estimate the procedure risk with standard parameters such as EuroScore and SYNTAX score. Patients in the high-risk group should be evaluated by the heart team for the suitable treatment strategy.[7]

TREATMENT OF CALCIFIED SIGNIFICANT NARROWING

Treatment of calcified vessels are essentially different from non calcified narrowings. Direct stenting should be avoided. The lesion/plaque has to be modified to receive the stent/stents.

LESION PREPARATION

Calcified coronary lesions require aggressive preparation before stenting to achieve optimal stent expansion which is a strong predictor of good immediate and long-term outcomes. The choice of lesion preparation strategy depends on the severity and extent of the lesion calcification. Though angiographically moderate to severe calcification predicts the need for some form of debulking, it is very difficult to make the choice of debulking strategy based on angiography alone. Though technically demanding in a significant proportion of patients, some form of intravascular imaging (IVI) has to be used to evaluate the lesion whenever feasible. IVI, particularly OCT, provides valuable additional information on the thickness, depth, area and arc of CAC and lumen area.[5]

In a systematic OCT study, Kubo et al,[8] have shown that a calcium plate thickness of < 505 µ predicted calcium fracture after high pressure balloon angioplasty. In addition, successful calcium fracture was associated with better minimal stent area (5.02 ± 1.43 vs 4.33 ± 1.22 mm^2, p = 0.47), lower binary restenosis (14 vs 41%, p = 0.024) and ischemia driven revascularization (7 vs 28%, p = 0.046). Maejima et al,[9] evaluated the effects of rotational atherectomy (RA) and subsequent balloon angioplasty (BA) on calcified lesions using OCT. Similar to previous study, formation of crack was associated with better minimal stent area (MSA, 7.38 ± 1.92 vs 7.13 ± 1.68 mm^2, p = 0.035) and lumen gain (3.89 ± 1.53 vs 3.40 ± 1.46 mm^2, p < 0.001). The calcium arc and thickness of 227° and 0.67 mm, respectively predicted cracks following RA and BA.

From the above discussion, it is evident that IVI OCT may have an important role to play during calcified lesion PCI. Debulking strategy may be selected based on the thickness and circumferential extent of calcification on OCT. If the calcium is circumferential and the thickness is more than the threshold of 670 µ, the lesion requires pre-treatment with rotational or orbital atherectomy. Post atherectomy OCT reassessment of thickness of the calcium plate at the ablated area determines the need for further ablation (thickness >670 µ). If the calcium thickness in <670 µ, cutting/scoring balloon/noncompliant balloon dilatation alone may achieve optimal lesion preparation. Moreover, OCT confirms adequate lesion preparation (calcium fracture) following balloon dilatation.[9]

In case of eccentric calcium, IVI helps in identifying wire relationship to the plaque components. In case of favorable wire bias (the imaging catheter adherent to the calcified plaque) an atherectomy device may be safely used to modify the lesion. Further, reassessment of the lesion post atherectomy gives information on the adequacy of the plaque removal and the safety of further ablation with a bigger device.[10]

Following DES, IVI helps in identify various abnormalities associated with adverse short and long-term outcomes such as: Underexpansion, malapposition, geographic miss, edge dissection, intramural hematoma, and tissue prolapse.[5]

Figures 1 and 2 provide examples of IVUS and OCT guided treatment of calcified lesions respectively.

DEBULKING DEVICES

Cutting Balloon

Device

Flextome® Cutting balloon (CB, Boston Scientific, Natick, MA) is made up of 3 (2.0 to 3.25 mm) to 4 (3.5 to 4 mm) microsurgical blades mounded longitudinally on a non-compliant nylon balloon. In contrast to the previous generation devices, it incorporates flex points at 5 mm intervals to improve the flexibility and deliverability of the device. The balloon material wraps around the blades and prevents them from being exposed to the vessel wall during device delivery. It is available in diameters ranging between 2.0 and 4.0 mm in 0.25 mm increments and in lengths of 6, 10 and 15 mm.[11]

Mechanism of Action

Cutting balloon angioplasty (CBA) creates longitudinal incisions in the plaque that allows controlled dilatation at lower pressure with less vessel wall injury.[11] OCT assessment of calcified lesion treated with CBA clearly demonstrated localized scoring effect on calcified plaques.[12] Hara et al.[13] compared pre and post intervention IVUS images of patients treated with CBA (n=40) and plain old balloon angioplasty (POBA, n=25) by systematic

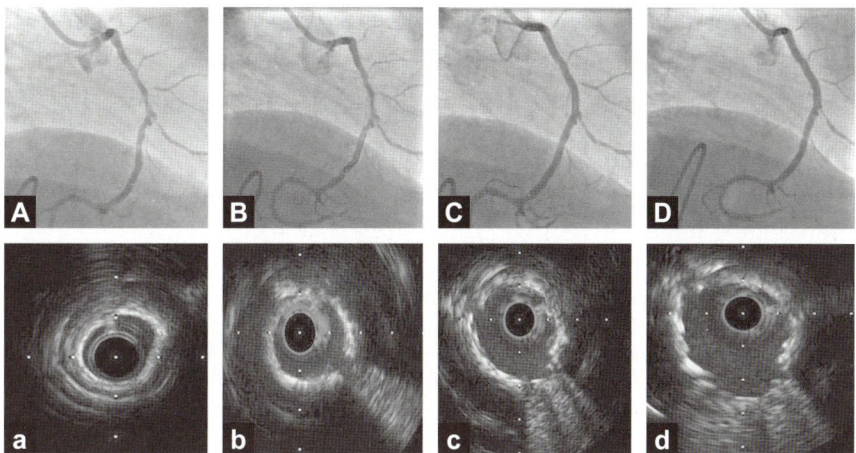

Figs. 1A to D: Intravascular ultrasound (IVUS) guided treatment of severely calcified lesion. (A and a) baseline angiographic and IVUS images. IVUS image showing 360° lesion calcification. (B and b) Post-rotational atherectomy and balloon dilatation IVUS image showing crack at 5 o'clock position. (C and c) Images post stent implantation. (D and d) Final images showing optimally expanded stent.

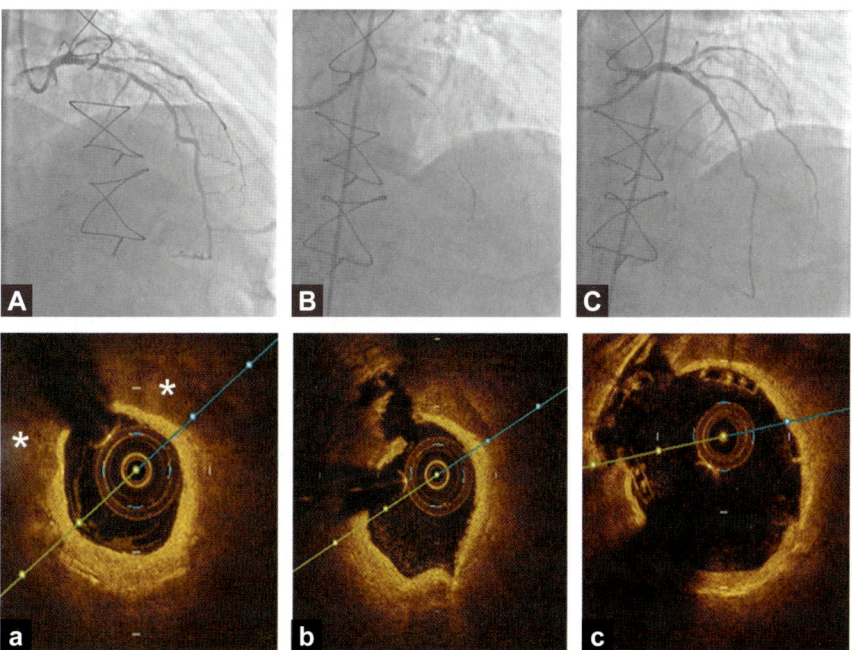

Figs. 2A to C: Optical coherence tomography guided bioresorbable scaffold (BVS) implantation in a severely calcified lesion (stars). (A and a) baseline angiographic and OCT images. OCT image showing 180° lesion calcification. (B and b) Post-cutting balloon dilatation OCT image showing crack (arrow) at 11 o'clock position. (C and c) Final images showing optimally expanded scaffold.

assessment of vessel area, lumen area, plaque area and vessel expansion. All the patients had successful procedure in both the groups. The mean balloon diameter (2.8 mm), balloon-artery ratio and the final minimum lumen diameter (MLD, 2.3 mm) were not different between the groups. However, the maximum balloon inflation pressure was significantly higher in the POBA group (10.1 ± 3.5 vs 8.3 ± 2.3 atm, $p < 0.05$). On IVUS imaging, the minimal lumen area (MLA) was comparable between CBA and POBA groups (5.5 ± 1.2 vs 5.7 ± 1.2 mm), but CBA was associated with smaller increase in vessel size (13.9 ± 3.2 vs 14.8 ± 3.2 mm^2, $p < 0.01$), smaller plaque area (8.5 ± 2.7 vs 9.1 ± 2.2 mm^2, $p < 0.05$) and smaller vessel expansion ratio (1.05 vs 1.22, $p < 0.05$). Lumen enlargement with CBA resulted mainly from plaque compression (55 vs 33%) than vessel stretch (45 vs 67%).

Tips and Tricks[11,14,15]
1. 6 Fr or bigger guiding catheter with optimal back up support
2. Support guide wire
3. Balloon to artery ratio not exceeding 1.1:1
4. Shorter lengths for tortuous vessels
5. Double wet negative preparation
6. Slow inflation and deflation (1 atm every 5 seconds)
7. Angiography before each inflation
8. Avoid torqueing catheters between inflations.

Clinical Evidence

In the pre- stent era CBA had been compared with POBA in a number of studies with conflicting results. Though smaller studies showed promising results, the same was not replicated in the large randomized studies. The Global Randomized Trial (GRT) randomly assigned 1,238 patients between CBA (n = 617) and POBA (n = 621). The primary end point of 6-month angiographic binary restenosis was not different between the CBA and POBA groups (31.4 vs 30.4%, $p = 0.75$). At 9 months follow-up, CBA was associated with higher incidence of MI (4.7 vs 2.4%, $p = 0.03$) and mortality (1.3 vs 0.3%, $p = 0.06$).[16] Similarly, in a meta-analysis of 4 randomized trials of CBA vs POBA in calcified and non-calcified lesions, there was no difference in the rate of restenosis and major adverse cardiovascular events between the two strategies. However, CBA was associated higher incidence of perforations and MI.[17]

There were no major studies that specifically evaluated CBA + bare metal stent (BMS) implantation vs balloon angioplasty (BA) + BMS in calcified lesions. In the restenosis reduction by cutting balloon evaluation III (REDUCE III) trial, 521 patients were randomized to either CBA followed by BMS (CBA-BMS, n = 260) implantation or BA followed by BMS (BA-BMS, n=261). IVUS was used to guide procedure in 279 (54%) patients. At 7 months follow-up, CBA-BMS group was associated with lower incidence of binary restenosis (11.8 vs 19.6%, p<0.05). At 12 months, CBA-BMS group had better target lesion revascularization (TLR, 9.6 vs 15.3%, p<0.05). Lowest incidence of restenosis was observed in IVUS-CBA-BMS arm (6.6%) when compared to Anglo-CBA-BMS (17.9%), IVUS-BA-BMS (19.8%) and Anglo-BA-BMS (18.2%) arms (p<0.05).[18]

Similarly, there were no randomized studies that evaluated CBA + drug eluting stent (DES) vs balloon BA + DES in calcified lesions. Vaquerizo et al,[19] have reported outcomes of 145 patients with 164 moderate to severe calcified lesions modified with CBA (56.7%) or RA (15.9%) or combination of RA and CBA (27.4%) and followed by DES implantation. Procedure was successful in all the patients. At 15±11 months follow-up, major adverse cardiovascular events (MACE) occurred in 9.6% of the patients (3.4% cardiac death, 2.3% MI, and 3.4% TLR). The outcomes were not different between plaque modification strategies.

Scoring Balloon

Device

AngioSculpt® scoring balloon (ASB, Angioscore, Fremont, California) consists of three rectangular spiral nitinol scoring elements wrapped on a semi-compliant nylon balloon. The balloon in the folded position covers the scoring elements from the vessel wall. It is available in diameters ranging between 2.0 and 5.0 mm and in lengths of 10, 15 and 20 mm. The balloon has a larger working range ranging between 2 and 18 atm. The smaller crossing profile (2.7 Fr) and enhanced flexibility facilitates deliverability of the catheter in tortuous anatomies.[11]

Mechanism of Action

During dilatation, the rectangular scoring elements lock the device in place and prevent watermelon seeding. The dilatation force is concentrated over a small area of the scoring elements and exerts a force equal to 15–25 times that of conventional balloon. This allows large initial lumen expansion with limited vessel wall injury.[11] OCT examination of the calcified lesions treated with AngioSculpt® scoring balloon showed evidence of plaque scoring and lumen expansion independent of severity of calcification.[20]

Clinical Evidence

There have been no major randomized trials comparing plaque modification with AngioSculpt® scoring balloon vs BA before DES. de Ribamar Costa et al,[21] evaluated the impact of three difference modes of vessel preparation (no preparation, semi-compliant balloon predilatation, and ASB predilatation) on DES expansion by IVUS. ASB predilatation was associated with larger minimum stent diameter (2.6±0.4 vs 2.5±0.4 vs 2.8±0.4 mm, p=0.048) and minimum stent cross-sectional area (MSA, 6.0±1.7 vs 5.9±1.6 vs 6.8±1.5 mm^2, p=0.02). In addition, final stent areas were <5 mm^2 only in 11% of patients in ASB group comparing to 26% each in other two groups (p<0.001).

Grenadier et al,[22] have recently reported 30 days and 3 years outcomes of a large cohort of patients treated with ASB in two Israeli centers. Over all 521 patients and 745 lesions were included in the study. The procedure was successful in 97.9% of the patients. The 30 day and 3-year MACE rates were 2.9% (Cardiac death – 0.2%, MI – 1.9%, stent thrombosis, ST – 0.4% and TLR – 1.2%) and 7.1% (Cardiac death – 0.4%, MI – 3.8%, stent thrombosis, ST – 0.9% and TLR – 5.9%) respectively. Angiosculpt scoring balloon (ASB) has a higher rated burst pressure (RBP) compared to cutting balloon (CB). This is a significant advantage over CB.

Complications[11,23]

The potential complications of CBA/ASB are coronary spasm, dissection, perforation and entrapment. **Coronary spasm** is not uncommon with CBA and responds well to intracoronary nitroglycerine. **Coronary dissections** occur in about 10% of the patients, but most of them are minor and non-flow limiting. As CBA is followed by stent implantation in most instances, dissections are rarely a problem with these devices in current practice. **Perforations** are rare with CBA and occur commonly with balloon oversizing (>1.1 vs 1.0 balloon – artery ratio). Perforations are managed in the usual way with reversal of anticoagulants, prolonged balloon inflation or covered stent implantation. **Late aneurysms** have been reported in perforations managed with prolonged balloon inflation and also in patients without obvious perforation. **Device entrapment** is a serious complication with these devices that occurs during the treatment of in-stent restenosis when the wire inadvertently passes through an unopposed stent strut. Various maneuvers have described to remove the entrapped device: (1) advancing the device forward and rotating it to unhook the trapped strut or atherotome, (2) inflating a second balloon alongside the entrapped device, (3) deep seating of the guiding catheter and controlled retraction of the device, or (4) surgical removal if the other maneuvers are unsuccessful.

Rotational Atherectomy

Device

Rotational atherectomy (RA, Boston Scientific) equipment consists of five components – cylinder, console, foot pedal, advancer and guidewire. The cylinder provides continuous supply of compressed air/nitrogen to the console. The tank pressure should be at least 500 PSI and the pressure delivered to the console should be between 90 and 110 PSI. The console regulates the amount of air delivered to the advancer and in turn controls the rotational speed of the burr. In addition, it displays the rotational speed and event and procedure durations. Foot pedal activates the advancer air turbine and also switches the rotational speed between ablation and Dynaglide modes. Advancer houses the air turbine that generates high speed rotation using compressed air, an in built wire break, a break defeat button, and an advancer knob. Burr has a long drive shaft with a brass burr coated with diamond chips at the end. The rota guide wire is 325 cm long and has a 0.009" body and 0.014" tip. The burr is available in sizes from 1.25 to 2.5 mm.[24]

Mechanism of Action

The basic principles of rotational atherectomy are *differential cutting* and *orthogonal displacement of friction*. By differential cutting, the rapidly rotating burr selectively ablates rigid inelastic tissue components (calcium and fibrous tissue) while the elastic normal vessel wall components deflect away from the cutting edge. In addition, high speed rotation changes the longitudinal friction vector between the wire and burr to circumferential direction which facilitates burr advancement through tortuous anatomies. The particles generated during ablation are about 5 μ in size and cleared by the reticuloendothelial system.[24]

Tips and Tricks[24,25]

1. Hold beta blockers 24 hours prior to procedure.
2. Adequately hydrate the patient preprocedure.
3. Temporary pacing for right coronary and dominant left circumflex lesions.
4. Guide catheters with simple curves and co-axial alignment to reduce wire bias.
5. Avoid spring type Y connectors.
6. Wire the lesion directly with Rota wire using torque device.
7. Check DRAW (D [Drip] - Check drip from catheter sheath tip and beneath advancer, R [Rotation] - set the RPM at 180000, A [Advancer]—Check free movement of advancer knob, W [Wire]—Check wire clip is attached and tug on wire while rotating to ensure break is activated).
8. Avoid activated burr advancement within the guiding catheter.
9. Beware of wire looping at the guide catheter tip.
10. Platform the burr in a disease free zone proximal to the lesion. Ensure free flow of contrast beyond the burr.

Contd...

Contd...

11. Relieve any forward tension on the drive shaft and guidewire.
12. Ablate the lesion with a gentle pecking motion and moving forward only when there is light resistance.
13. Do not allow the RPM to drop more than 5000 from the platform speed.
14. Limit runs to less than 20 seconds.
15. Give enough time for the artery to perfuse in between the ablation runs.
16. Watch for slow flow, ECG changes, and hypotension (Keep atropine, vasopressors and dilators on the table).
17. Never advance the burr to the point of contact with the spring tip (radiopaque point which is 0.014").
18. Do not keep the rotating burr in the same position for long time.
19. Always withdraw the burr to the platform segment before stopping it.
20. Finish with polishing run (no rpm drop, no resistance).

Clinical Evidence

The recent major studies with RA are summarized in Table 1. The ROTAXUS (Rotational Atherectomy Prior to TAXUS Stent Treatment for Complex Native Coronary Artery Disease) was a prospective, randomized study designed to evaluate the impact of RA on the effectiveness of DES. Overall the study enrolled 240 patients: 120 in the RA arm and 120 in the control arm. There were significantly more cross overs from the control arm to the RA arm (12.5 vs 4.2%, p=0.02). The RA arm was associated with better strategy success rate (92.5 vs 83.3%, p=0.03) and higher acute lumen gain (1.56 ± 0.43 vs. 1.44 ± 0.49 mm, p = 0.01). However, the primary end point of in-stent late lumen loss at 9 months was significantly higher in the RA arm (0.44 ± 0.58 vs 0.31 ± 0.52, p = 0.04). In addition, there was no significant difference in in-stent binary restenosis (11.4 vs. 10.6%, p = 0.71), TLR (11.7 vs. 12.5%, p = 0.84), definite ST (0.8 vs. 0%, p = 1.0), and MACE rates (24.2 vs. 28.3%, p = 0.46) between the two groups.[26] Similarly, there was no difference in 2 years outcomes of MACE (29.4 vs. 34.3%, p = 0.47), death (8.3 vs. 7.4%, p = 1.00), MI (8.3 vs. 6.5%, p = 0.80), TLR (13.8 vs. 16.7%, p = 0.58), and target vessel revascularization (TVR) (19.3 vs. 22.2%, p = 0.62) between the groups.[27]

Complications[25]

Complications during RA are common and occur even in experienced hands. The common complications and their management are summarized in Table 2.

Table 1: Rotational atherectomy—Relevant recent clinical evidence.

Publication	Study design	Treatment	No. of patients	Duration of follow-up	End-points
ROTAXUS Trial (2016)[27]	Randomized	RA+DES vs BA+DES	240	2 years	No difference in MACE events between groups
Couper LT et al (2015)[28]	Multicenter registry	RA+BMS/DES	167	12 months	MACE 15.6%. This was not different from patients not received RA during this period
Jinnouchi et al (2015)[29]	Single center registry	RA+newer generation DES	252	2 years	MACE 20.3%. Predictors of MACE were ACS, hemodialysis, previous CABG
Yabushita et al (2014)[30]	Single center registry	RA in de novo LM disease	64	1 year	Rota is associated with high procedural success and low complication rates
Abdel-Wahab et al (2013)[31]	Single center registry	RA+DES	205	15 months	High procedural success (98%) and MACE 17.7%
Naito et al (2012)[32]	Single center registry	RA+SES vs RA+PES	223	630 days	No difference in MACE events
Mangiacapra et al (2012)[33]	Single center registry	RA+DES vs RA+BMS	187	1 year	Lower MACE with DES

(ROTAXUS: Rotational Atherectomy Prior to Taxus Stent Treatment for Complex Native Coronary Artery Disease, RA: Rotational atherectomy, DES: Drug eluting stent, BA: Balloon angioplasty, BMS: Bare metal stent, SES: Sirolimus eluting stent, PES: Paclitaxel eluting stent, MACE: Major adverse cardiovascular events).

Table 2: Major complications of rotational atherectomy.		
Complication	*Causes*	*Management*
Slow-flow/ no-reflow	• Large burrs and higher speeds • Shorter time interval between ablation runs	• Retraction of the burr • Optimization of perfusion pressure • Intracoronary vasodilators (nitrates, adenosine, verapamil, nicorandil) • Intra-aortic balloon pump support
Perforation	• Oversized burr • Angulated lesions	• Reversal of anti-coagulation • Prolonged low pressure balloon dilatation • Covered stent implantation • Surgical closure and distal grafting

Burr entrapment	• Burr crossing the lesion without adequate ablation (Excessive tension on the burr – jumps forward when activated)	• Gentle controlled traction with
		  – Guide catheter deep intubation
		  – Mother and child catheter
		• Balloon inflation besides the burr
		• Snare assisted traction
		• Surgical removal

Orbital Atherectomy

Device

The Diamondback 360° coronary orbital atherectomy system (OAS; Cardiovascular Systems, Inc., St. Paul, Minnesota) contains an electric motor powered handle with a power switch, speed controller and an advancer knob. The ablating component is a diamond encrusted crown that is mounted eccentrically at the distal end of a drive shaft. The crown tracks over a dedicated 0.12"/0.14" Viper guidewire. ViperSlide® lubricant solution reduces friction and heat generation, and facilitates clearing of microdebris during procedure. The system is simple to set up and easy to control from the operating field.[34]

Mechanism of Action

Orbital atherectomy system (OAS) works on a principle of *differential sanding* and *centrifugal force*. In contrast to rotational movement with RA, the eccentric crown orbits over the guidewire at two different speeds (80,000 and 120,000 rpm). Each pass of device sands off a thin layer of the plaque.

As with RA, OAS selectively ablates the rigid plaque components while the elastic tissue flexes away from the crown. The diameter of the orbit is proportional to the rotational speed (centrifugal force) which can be controlled by the operator. Thus, a single 1.25 mm crown can be used to ablate a diameter up to 3.5 mm without changing the crown size. The crown possesses diamond chips on both front and back that enables ablation in both antegrade and retrograde directions. This decreases the risk of crown entrapment, a feared complication with rotational atherectomy. The orbital motion allows continuous flow of blood, saline and particulate debris distally that reduces potential ischemia, heat generation and consequent thermal injury and restenosis. The particles generated are approximately 2 μ in size, much smaller than that of RA which in turn lessens the incidence of slow flow or no reflow with OAS.[7,34]

Clinical Evidence

ORBIT I trial evaluated the safety and feasibility OAS in an open label, prospective, observational study of 50 patients with severely calcified de novo coronary lesions. Device success (≤50% residual stenosis after OAS before stenting) and procedural success (≤20% residual stenosis after stenting) were achieved in 98 and 94% of patients respectively. Procedural complications occurred in seven patients (6 dissections and one perforation). The in hospital, 30 days, and 6-month MACE (death, MI, and TLR) rates were 4% (two non Q - MI), 6% (one additional non Q- MI resulted in TLR), and 8% (one additional cardiac death) respectively.[35] 33 of these patients from one of the centers participated in the study were followed up over a period of 5 years. The 2, 3 and 5-year MACE rates were 15.2, 18.2 and 21.2% respectively.[36]

The ORBIT II trial was a prospective, single arm, multi-center registry designed to further assess the safety and efficacy of OAS in preparing severely calcified lesions for stent placement. The study enrolled 443 patients across 49 centers in US between May 2010 and November 2012. The primary safety end point of freedom from MACE (MI, TVR and cardiac death) at 30 days occurred in 89.6% of patients against a performance goal of 82%. Similarly, the trial also met the primary efficacy end point of < 50% post-stent residual stenosis without in-hospital MACE (88.9% vs performance goal of 82%). Stent delivery was successful in 97.7% of cases.[37] The 1 - year MACE, TLR and ST rates were 16.4% (cardiac death - 3%, MI - 9.7%, and TLR - 5.9%), 4.7 and 0.2%. The outcomes were maintained at 2 years follow-up with a MACE, and TLR rates of 19.4% (cardiac death - 4.3% and TVR - 8.1%) and 6.2% respectively.[38]

In a large, real world registry of 458 patients including those with very high surgical risk and complex anatomy, OAS was associated very low

30-day major adverse cardio-cerebrovascular event rate (1.7%). The 30-day all-cause mortality, MI, TVR, stroke, and ST rates were 1.3, 1.1, 0, 0.2 and 0.9% respectively. Angiographic complications occurred in 2.3% (perforation 0.7%, dissection 0.9%, and no-reflow 0.7%) and emergency coronary artery bypass graft surgery in 0.2% of the patients.[39]

Rotational Atherectomy vs Orbital Atherectomy

Comparing to RA, the new comer OAS has been proposed to have multiple advantages such as lower incidence of no reflow, crown entrapment and less thermal injury. In a small OCT study, OAS was associated with deeper dissections, improved stent expansion and lower incidence of stent strut malapposition.[40] However, there has been no published head to head comparison between these devices till date. An ongoing observational study (Moderate to Severe Calcified Coronary Lesions, MACE) is expected to provide some comparative data in future.[7]

Laser Atherectomy

Device

The CVX-300® cardiovascular Excimer laser system (Spectranetics Inc., Colorado Springs, CO, USA), consists of a console, laser catheter and a foot pedal. The laser catheter uses Xenon Chloride (XeCl) as active medium to generate pulsed gas laser. The laser catheter is available in both over the wire and monorail designs and four sizes: 0.9, 1.4, 1.7 and 2.0 mm. It is compatible with 0.014" guide wire. The 0.9 mm catheter is compatible with 5 F guiding catheter, 1.4 and 1.7 mm with 7 Fr catheter and 2 mm is with 8 F catheter. The catheter needs calibration before insertion into the guiding catheter. The laser unit need to undergo a warm up period of about 5 minutes. The lasing procedure requires continuous saline infusion to reduce temperature and uncontrolled photoablation of the coronary artery.[41]

Mechanism of Action

Electrical activation of XeCl medium emits light rays in UV spectrum (308 nm) with a tissue penetration capacity of 50 μ. It causes tissue removal by photoablation (vaporization). The process of photoablation occurs in 3 stages: Photochemical, photo thermal and photomechanical. UV light is absorbed by tissue and results in breakdown of carbon – carbon molecular bands (photochemical). It causes high frequency molecular vibration that results in cellular breakdown and formation of vapor bubbles at the tip of the catheter (photothermal). These vapor bubbles expand and implode to cause further tissue distruption (photomechanical).[41]

Clinical Evidence

Excimer laser assisted angioplasty was compared with plain ordinary balloon angioplasty in the randomized Amsterdam-Rotterdam (AMRO) trial. The trial randomly assigned 308 patients into ELCA followed POBA (151 patients/157 lesions) or POBA (157 patients/167 lesions). There was no difference in the procedural success rate between ELCA and POBA groups (92 vs 91%, p = 0.69). Though, ELCA group was associated with larger lumen post procedure (1.69 vs 1.59 mm, p = 0.05), there was no significant difference in the lumen diameters (1.17 vs 1.25 mm, p = 0.34) or restenosis at 6 months follow-up (51.6 vs 41.3%, p = 0.13).[42]

The Excimer Laser, Rotational Atherectomy, and Balloon Angioplasty Comparison (EBARC) study compared the atherectomy strategies with POBA in a population of 685 patients (POBA = 222, ELCA = 232 and RA = 231). RA was associated with higher procedural success rate (diameter stenosis < 50%, absence of death, Q-wave myocardial infarction, or coronary artery bypass surgery) than ELCA and POBA (89 vs 77 and 80%, p = 0.0019). ELCA failed to cross the lesion in 18.5% patients and required cross over to either POBA (12.9%) or RA (2.6%). However, there was no difference in major in-hospital complications (3.2 vs 4.3% versus 3.1%, p = 0.71). During follow up, ELCA group was associated with higher late loss (0.77 ± 0.73 vs 0.55 ± 0.68 and 0.62 ± 0.77 mm; $p = 0.052$; ELCA vs PTCA group, p < 0.05) and increased incidence of restenosis compared to POBA and RA (59 vs 47 and 57%, p = 0.14 for the three-group comparison; $p = 0.039$ for PTCA vs ELCA). ELCA and RA groups underwent more revascularization during follow-up (46.0 and 42.4 vs 31.9%, p = 0.013). Similarly, the MACE (death, Q-wave myocardial infarction, coronary bypass surgery, or repeated angioplasty) rate was higher with ELCA and RA groups (47.9 and 45.9 vs 36.6%, $p = 0.057$ for the three-group comparison; p = 0.015 for PTCA vs ELCA; p = 0.04 for PTCA versus PTRA)[43]

In a single center study, Badr S, et al.[44] reported outcomes of excimer laser in 25 patients with de novo calcified lesions. Fourteen of these lesions were balloon non-crossable. The device success rate was 80% (the laser catheter successfully crossing the stenotic lesion) and 24% of the lesions required additional debulking with RA. Two (8%) patients underwent emergency bypass graft surgery and one procedure (4%) was complicated by coronary perforation.

The early outcome of high energy Laser (Excimer) facilitated coronary angioplasty ON hARD and complex calcified and balloon-resistant coronary lesions (LEONARDO) study enrolled 80 patients (calcified lesions - 45 patients [56.3%], balloon failure - 25 patients [31.2%], and chronic total occlusion - 10 patients [12.5%]) in 4 centers. Over all there were 100 lesions and 96 of them were treated with laser. Technical success (the laser catheter crossing the entire length of the stenotic lesion), procedural success was defined as (< 50% residual stenosis after laser and adjunctive therapy), clinical success (procedural success with absence of MACE at hospital discharge) were achieved in 93.7, 91.7 and 90.6% of the lesions. Higher laser parameters were used in 49 lesions. There was no major procedure related complications.[45]

One of the major indication of ELCA in current practice is treatment of stent underexpansion that is resistant to high pressure noncompliant balloon dilatation. ELCA can be used to modify the underlying resistant calcific or fibrotic plaque and assists stent expansion with balloon dilatation. This strategy was evaluated in the recent Excimer Laser LEsion Modification to Expand Non-dilatable sTents (ELLEMENT) Registry. Twenty-eight patients with under-expanded stents that were resistant to high pressure non-compliant balloon dilatation were included in the study. High energy laser ablation was performed inside the under-expanded stent with simultaneous injection of contrast instead of saline infusion. Successful laser dilatation was achieved in in 27 cases (96.4%), with an increase in MSD by QCA (1.6 to 2.6 mm, $p<0.001$) and MSA by IVUS (3.5 2 to 7.1 mm^2, $p<0.001$). Periprocedural MI, transient slow-flow, ST-elevation occurred in 7.1, 3.6 and 3.6% of the patients, respectively. Two patients developed MACE at 6 months follow-up (one TLR and one death/MI).[46]

Current Status of Atherectomy Devices

Though data from smaller studies were promising, the results of randomized studies with atherectomy devices are disappointing. However, few important aspects of these studies have to be taken into consideration. First, randomized studies have used angiographically moderate and severe calcification as inclusion criteria. As noted earlier, angiography may not be an ideal modality to quantify CAC and CAG based selection of debulking strategy may not be appropriate in a proportion of patients. Second, majority of the patients included in these studies had only moderate calcification where atherectomy devices would not have made substantial impact on outcomes. Third, significant proportion of patients in BA group were crossed over to the atherectomy group. Thus, atherectomy devices continue to have an important role in the modern PCI era and more so with aging patient population and increasing procedure complexity. However, judicious use in those who derive maximum benefit is at most important.[47]

CONCLUSION

Calcified coronary lesions are often complex and pose challenges to interventional cardiologist. Careful patient selection and procedure planning are essential. Intravascular imaging guidance and appropriate use of atherectomy devices are cornerstones of procedure success and good long-term outcomes.

REFERENCES

1. Madhavan MV, Tarigopula M, Mintz GS, et al. Coronary artery calcification: pathogenesis and prognostic implications. J Am Coll Cardiol. 2014;63:1703-14.
2. Lee MS, Shah N. The impact and pathophysiologic consequences of coronary artery calcium deposition in percutaneous coronary interventions. J Invasive Cardiol. 2015;28:160-7.
3. Liu W, Zhang Y, Yu C-M, et al. Current understanding of coronary artery calcification. J Geriatr Cardiol. 2015;12:668-75.
4. Chambers JW, Behrens AN, Martinsen BJ. Atherectomy devices for the treatment of calcified coronary lesions. Intervent Cardiol Clin. 2016;5:143-51.
5. Shimamura K, Guagliumi G. Optical coherence tomography for online guidance of complex coronary interventions. Circ J. 2016;80:2063-72.
6. Mintz GS. Intravascular imaging of coronary calcification and its clinical implications. JACC Cardiovasc Imaging. 2015; 8:461-71.
7. Tomey MI, Sharma SK. Interventional Options for Coronary Artery Calcification. Curr Cardiol Rep. 2016;18:12.
8. Kubo T, Shimamura K, Ino Y, et al. Superficial calcium fracture after PCI as assessed by OCT. J Am Coll Cardiol Img. 2015;8:1228-9.
9. Maejima N, Hibi K, Saka K, et al. Relationship between thickness of calcium on optical coherence tomography and crack formation after balloon dilatation in calcified plaque requiring rotational atherectomy. Circ J. 2016;80:1413-9.
10. Attizzani GF, Patrício L, Bezerra HG. Optical coherence tomography assessment of calcified plaque modification after rotational atherectomy. Catheter Cardiovasc Interv. 2013;81:558-61.
11. Seddon M, Curzen N. Cutting balloons and Angiosculpt. In: Redwood S, Curzen N, Thomas M, editors. Oxford textbook of interventional cardiology. New York: Oxford university press; 2010. p. 586-600.
12. Martín-Reyes R, Jiménez-Valero S, Moreno R. Effectiveness of cutting balloon angioplasty for a calcified coronary lesion. Evaluation by optical coherence tomography and intravascular ultrasound. Rev Port Cardiol. 2010;29:1889-90.
13. Hara H, Nakamura M, Asahara T, et al. Intravascular ultrasonic comparisons of mechanisms of vasodilatation of cutting balloon angioplasty versus conventional balloon angioplasty. Am J Cardiol. 2002;89:1253-6.
14. Bittl JA. The Role of Adjunct Devices: Atherectomy, Cutting Balloon, and Laser. In: Topol EJ, Teirstein PS, editors. Text book of interventional cardiology. Philadelphia, PA: Elsevier, Inc; 2016. p. 564-75.
15. Krishnaswamy A, Whitlow PL. Calcified Lesions. In: Bhatt DL, editors. Cardiovascular intervention. Philadelphia, PA: Elsevier, Inc; 2016. p. 199-208.
16. Mauri L, Bonan R, Weiner BH, et al. Cutting balloon angioplasty for the prevention of restenosis: results of the Cutting Balloon Global Randomized Trial. Am J Cardiol 2002;90:1079-83.
17. Bittl JA, Chew DP, Topol EJ, et al. Meta-analysis of randomized trials of percutaneous transluminal coronary angioplasty versus atherectomy, cutting balloon atherotomy, or laser angioplasty. J Am Coll Cardiol. 2004;43:936-42.
18. Ozaki Y, Yamaguchi T, Suzuki T, et al. Impact of cutting balloon angioplasty (CBA) prior to bare metal stenting on restenosis. Circ J. 2007;71:1-8.
19. Vaquerizo B, Serra A, Miranda F, et al. Aggressive plaque modification with rotational atherectomy and/or cutting balloon before drug-eluting stent implantation for the treatment of calcified coronary lesions. J Interv Cardiol 2010;23:240-8.

20. Kanai T, Hiro T, Takayama T, et al. Three-dimensional visualization of scoring mechanism of "AngioSculpt" balloon for calcified coronary lesions using optical coherence tomography. J Cardiol Cases. 2012;e16–e9.
21. de Ribamar Costa J Jr, Mintz GS, Carlier SG, et al. Nonrandomized comparison of coronary stenting under intravascular ultrasound guidance of direct stenting without predilation versus conventional predilation with a semi-compliant balloon versus predilation with a new scoring balloon. Am J Cardiol. 2007;100:812-7.
22. Grenadier E, Kerner A, Gershony G, et al. Optimizing plaque modification in complex lesions utilizing the angioSculpt device: acute and long term results from a large two-center registry. Am J Cardiol. 2008;102 (Suppl 8A:53i).
23. Chin K. Cutting balloons. In: Ellis SG, Holmes DR, editors. Strategic approaches in coronary intervention. Philadelphia, PA: Lippincott Williams & Wilkins; 2006. p. 125-42.
24. Belder AD, Thomas M. Rotational atherectomy. In: Redwood S, Curzen N, Thomas M, editors. Oxford textbook of interventional cardiology. New York: Oxford university press; 2010. p. 559-68.
25. Barbato E, Carrie D, Dardas P, et al. European expert consensus on rotational atherectomy. EuroIntervention. 2015;11:30-6.
26. Abdel-Wahab M, Richardt G, Joachim Buttner H, et al. High-speed rotational atherectomy before paclitaxel-eluting stent implantation in complex calcified coronary lesions: the randomized ROTAXUS (Rotational Atherectomy Prior to Taxus Stent Treatment for Complex Native Coronary Artery Disease) trial. JACC Cardiovasc Interv. 2013;6:10-9.
27. de Waha S, Allali A, Büttner HJ, et al. Rotational atherectomy before paclitaxel-eluting stent implantation in complex calcified coronary lesions: two-years clinical outcome of the randomized ROTAXUS trial. Catheter Cardiovasc Interv. 2016;87:691-700.
28. Couper LT, Loane P, Andrianopoulos N, et al. Melbourne Interventional Group (MIG) Investigators. Utility of rotational atherectomy and outcomes over an eight-year period. Catheter Cardiovasc Interv. 2015;86:626-31.
29. Jinnouchi H, Kuramitsu S, Shinozaki T, et al. Two year clinical outcomes of newer-generation drug eluting stent implantation following rotational atherectomy for heavily calcified lesions. Circ J. 2015;79:1938-43.
30. Yabushita H, Takagi K, Tahara S, et al. Impact of rotational atherectomy on heavily calcified, unprotected left main disease. Circ J. 2014;78:1867-72.
31. Abdel-Wahab M, Baev R, Dieker P, et al. Long-term clinical outcome of rotational atherectomy followed by drug-eluting stent implantation in complex calcified coronary lesions. Catheter Cardiovasc Interv. 2013;81:285-91.
32. Naito R, Sakakura K, Wada H, et al. Comparison of long-term clinical outcomes between sirolimus eluting stents and paclitaxel-eluting stents following rotational atherectomy. Int Heart J. 2012;53:149-53.
33. Mangiacapra F, Heyndrickx GR, Puymirat E, et al. Comparison of drug-eluting versus bare-metal stents after rotational atherectomy for the treatment of calcified coronary lesions. Int J Cardiol. 2012;154:373-6.
34. Sotomi Y, Shlofmitz RA, Colombo A, et al. Patient selection and procedural considerations for coronary orbital atherectomy system. Interv Cardiol Rev. 2016;11:33-8.
35. Parikh K, Chandra P, Choksi N, et al. Safety and feasibility of orbital atherectomy for the treatment of calcified coronary lesions: the ORBIT I trial. Catheter Cardiovasc Interv. 2013;81:1134–9.

36. Bhatt P, Parikh P, Patel A, et al. Long-term safety and performance of the orbital atherectomy system for treating calcified coronary artery lesions: 5-year follow-up in the ORBIT I trial. Cardiovasc Revasc Med. 2015;16:213-6.
37. Chambers JW, Feldman RL, Himmelstein SI, et al. Pivotal trial to evaluate the safety and efficacy of the orbital atherectomy system in treating de novo, severely calcified coronary lesions (ORBIT II). JACC Cardiovasc Interv. 2014;7:510-8.
38. Genereux P, Lee AC, Kim CY, et al. Orbital atherectomy for treating de novo severely calcified coronary narrowing (1-year results from the pivotal ORBIT II trial). Am J Cardiol. 2015;115:1685-90.
39. Lee MS, Shlofmitz E, Kaplan B, et al. Real-world multicenter registry of patients with severe coronary artery calcification undergoing orbital atherectomy. J Interv Cardiol. 2016;29(4):357-62.
40. Kini AS, Vengrenyuk Y, Pena J. et al. Optical coherence tomography assessment of the mechanistic effects of rotational and orbital atherectomy in severely calcified coronary lesions. Catheter Cardiovasc Interv. 2015;86:1024-32.
41. Rawlins J, Din J, Talwar S, O'Kane P. Coronary intervention with the excimer laser: review of the technology and outcome data. Interv Cardiol Rev. 2016;11:27-32.
42. Appelman YE, Piek JJ, Strikwerda S, et al. Randomised trial of excimer laser angioplasty versus balloon angioplasty for treatment of obstructive coronary artery disease. Lancet. 1996;347:79-84.
43. Reifart N, Vandormael M, Krajcar M, et al. Randomized comparison of angioplasty of complex coronary lesions at a single center. Excimer Laser, Rotational Atherectomy, and Balloon Angioplasty Comparison (ERBAC) Study. Circulation. 1997;96:91-8.
44. Badr S, Ben-Dor I, Dvir D, et al. The state of the excimerlaser for coronary intervention in the drug-eluting stent era. Cardiovasc Revasc Med. 2013;14:93-8.
45. Ambrosini V, Sorropago G, Laurenzano E, et al. Early outcome of high energy Laser (Excimer) facilitated coronary angioplasty ON hARD and complexcalcified and balloOn-resistant coronary lesions: LEONARDO Study. Cardiovasc Revasc Med. 2015;16:141-6.
46. Latib A, Takagi K, Chizzola G, et al. Excimer Laser LEsion modification to expand non-dilatable stents: the ELLEMENT registry. Cardiovasc Revasc Med. 2014;15:8-12.
47. Karatasakis A, Brilakis ES. Atherectomy for calcified coronary lesions: when and how? Catheter Cardiovasc Interv. 2016;87:701-2.

9. PCI in Patients Post Coronary Artery Bypass Grafts

Shirish (MS) Hiremath, Satishkumar S Kolekar

INTRODUCTION

As acute mortality and morbidity in post coronary artery bypass surgery (CABG) is reducing long-term results have increasingly more consideration. Internal mammary artery (IMA), Saphenous vein, radial artery, Gastro-epiploic artery (GEA) are used as conduits in CABG. IMA grafts have best long-term patency rate whereas saphenous vein graft (SVG) has high rate of failure.[1]

The return of myocardial ischemia after CABG is common. The reason is progression of atherosclerosis in native coronary arteries and failure of bypass grafts or proximal subclavian artery stenosis.[2] It has been estimated that by 15 years postoperatively, 62% of patients will have recurrent ischemia, 36% will experience a myocardial infarction.[3]

Repeat revascularization rate among post-CABG patient varies among different study groups driven by atherosclerotic risk factors, graft failure, native coronary disease progression.

The risk factors associated with reintervention are younger age, male gender, more symptomatic, higher serum triglycerides and total cholesterol, better left ventricular function, incomplete revascularization, and less IMA grafting.[2]

National cardiovascular registry (NCDR) analysis between 2004 to 2009 showed percutaneous coronary intervention (PCI) in prior CABG patients contributed 17.5% of all PCI. Target vessel was largely native coronary vessel (62.5%). Bypass graft PCI represented 6.6% of all PCI SVG being the largest (6.1%) contributor, arterial grafts constituted 0.44%, both vein and arterial graft constituted 0.04%.[4]

RECURRENCE OF ISCHEMIA IN POST CABG PATIENTS

Recurrence of ischemia in Post CABG patients is a complex problem selection of intervention must be based on careful analysis. The ischemia can present at various time stages in such patient differs in cause thus the management.

EARLY (IMMEDIATE POSTOPERATIVE PERIOD BEFORE DISCHARGE FROM HOSPITAL)

This is usually attributed to vein graft thrombosis secondary to endothelial damage either due to damage during harvesting or exposure to arterial pressure however other plausible reasons are kinking of graft anastomotic site stenosis, incomplete revascularization, wrong vessel grafting, inaccessible intramyocardial vessel PCI is treatment of choice in this group of patients. American College of Cardiology/American Heart Association (ACC/AHA) 2011 guidelines recommend it as class I indication[5-7] (Figs. 1A to E).

INTERMEDIATE (1 MONTH TO 1 YEAR)

Usually occurs due to perianastomotic site stenosis either in vein or arterial grafts secondary to intimal hyperplasia which is a result of pathophysiologic process causes intimal damage, fibrosis, platelet aggregation, the release of

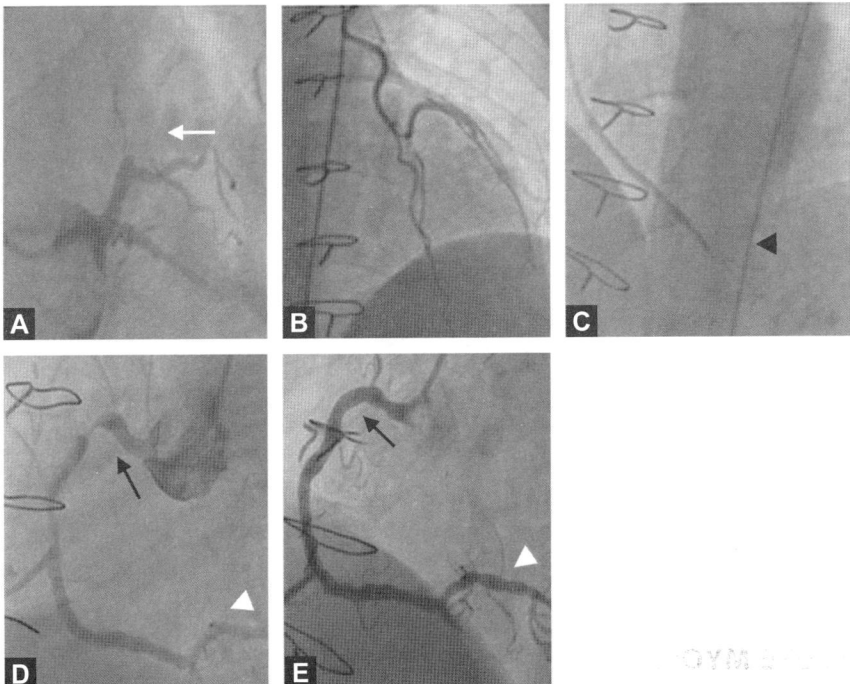

Figs. 1A to E: PCI to native RCA, early recurrence of angina due to graft for wrong vessel (angina through non grafted large vessel). (A) Thrombotic occlusion, ISR of BMS in LAD (white arrow) ISR, CABG: LIMA-RIMA 'Y' graft to LAD, D1, SVG to PDA. (B and C). CAG done for early recurrence of angina, grafts patent but small PD (black arrowhead) grafted ignoring large PLV) circulation cause of recurrence of angina (D and E) Large PLV unaddressed (white arrowheads) PCI to native RCA (black arrows).

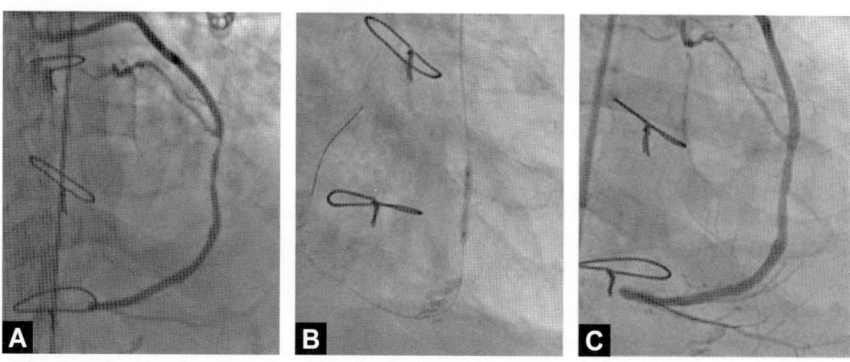

Figs. 2A to C: (A) SVG perianastomotic site stenosis within one year (intermediate) lesion treated (B) PCI without EPD (C) Shows the final result.

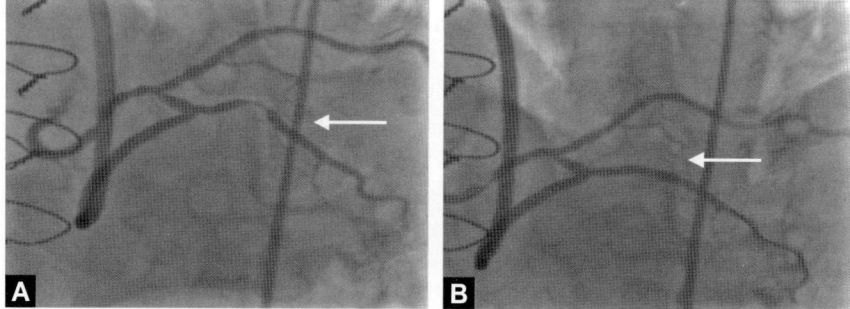

Figs. 3A and B: PCI to native PDA through SVG graft (A) Native RCA CTO, progression of disease (arrow) in PDA distal to graft (LATE). (B) PCI to native PD (arrow) through SVG.

growth factors, and smooth muscle cell proliferation. PCI is safe and recommended option in these patients[5,7] (Figs. 2A to C).

LATE (MORE THAN 1 YEAR)

Obstruction occurs as part of incessant atherosclerotic process in the graft conduits over earlier intimal hyperplasia or native coronary arteries distal to the graft anastomosis. Option of PCI has to be carefully analyzed depending on the site of lesion type of graft and age of the graft especially vein grafts for the reasons discussed later (Figs. 3A and B).

ACUTE MYOCARDIAL INFARCTION

Every year 3% of patients with prior CABG experience acute myocardial infarction (AMI). Therapy in such patient is based on clinical experience. Intravenous thrombolytic therapy is relatively ineffective and not studied by randomized trials in these patient. Nevertheless PCI in such patients have

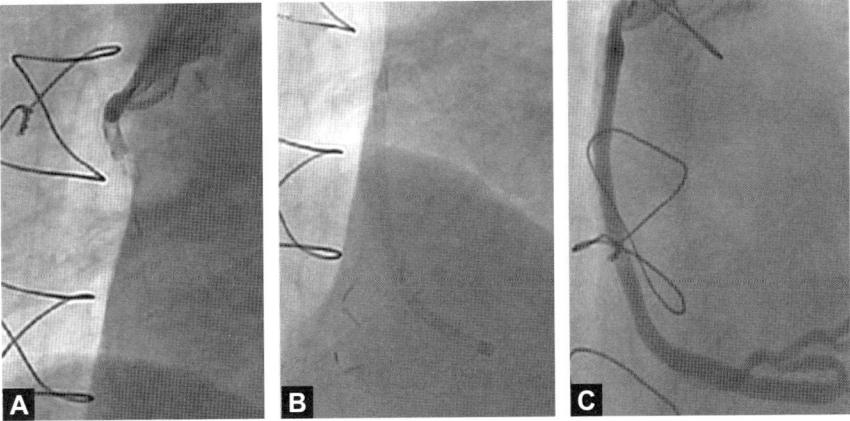

Figs. 4A to C: Post CABG STEMI (a) Thrombolysis, GPIIb/IIIa no effect, (b) aspiration, guide deep in, (c) final result.

inferior short-term and long-term results compared to native vessel PCI in ST elevation myocardial infarction (STEMI). ACC/AHA recommends PCI for recanalization of vein grafts as class IIa intervention[7] (Figs. 4A to C).

TREATING RECURRENT ISCHEMIA

Treatment options for recurrent ischemia include:
- Medical treatment
- PCI of bypass graft or native vessel
- Redo CABG.

Optimization of medical treatment is first step in recurrence of ischemia before advancing to any intervention either percutaneous or surgical as either of two carry higher procedural risk due to complexity of problem. Redo CABG carries high morbidity and mortality and risk of injury to patent grafts. PCI is favored by factors such as, limited areas of ischemia suitable lesions, patent graft to left anterior descending artery (LAD), poor CABG targets and comorbid conditions.[7]

PERCUTANEOUS CORONARY INTERVENTIONS

The results of PCI depend on the types of conduits (native artery, or arterial or saphenous vein grafts) or the locations on the conduits (proximal, mid-, distal, or at the anastomotic sites) and the age of the grafts. Due to advancement in techniques there are very less contraindication for PCI today and most of them are relative in today's date, include unprotected left main disease, heavy calcification, poor distal run-off, long tortuous graft, long diffuse lesion, chronically occluded grafts.

PCI can be done for:
- Native vessel
- Saphenous vein graft
- Arterial graft.

NATIVE VESSEL PCI

In patients with SVG lesions, native vessel PCI carries better short-term and long-term results in comparison to SVG PCI.[4] CI in native vessel encounters unique challenges in view of protected or unprotected LMCA stenosis, ostial stenosis, chronic total occlusions (CTO), limitation associated with native coronary PCI is challenges encountered due to CTO lesions, high burden of calcium, distal vessel lesions especially distal to long or tortuous grafts.[8]

Aorto-ostial Lesions

This particular subset of lesion, i.e. left main coronary artery (LMCA)/right coronary artery (RCA) ostial lesions are rigid, respond poorly to routine balloon dilatations and may require controlled dissection with cutting balloon, scoring balloons or debulking by rotational atherectomy followed by PCI. LMCA stenting proves life-saving especially perioperative graft closure and cardiogenic shock[8] (Figs. 5C and D).

Native Vessel CTO

It is more technically challenging and is associated with lower success rates compared with CTO PCI in non-CABG due to following reason[9] (Figs. 5A and B, Figs. 6A to D).
- Patients tend to be older, have more comorbidities
- Longer duration of the CTOs, diffuse disease, heavy calcification, stenting of the vessels
- Presence of more than one CTO and more than one failed bypass graft, makes visualization of the target vessel and understanding of the anatomic connections between the different vascular territories extremely difficult. This may also limit the available technical approaches (antegrade or retrograde) that can be used.

The technical and procedural success rates of CTO-PCI slightly lower among patients with prior CABG, whereas complication rates were similar to patients without prior PCI.[10]

GRAFT INTERVENTIONS

Vein Graft Interventions

Degeneration and occlusion of SVGs continue to be significant problems in maintaining long-term benefit in patients who have undergone CABG

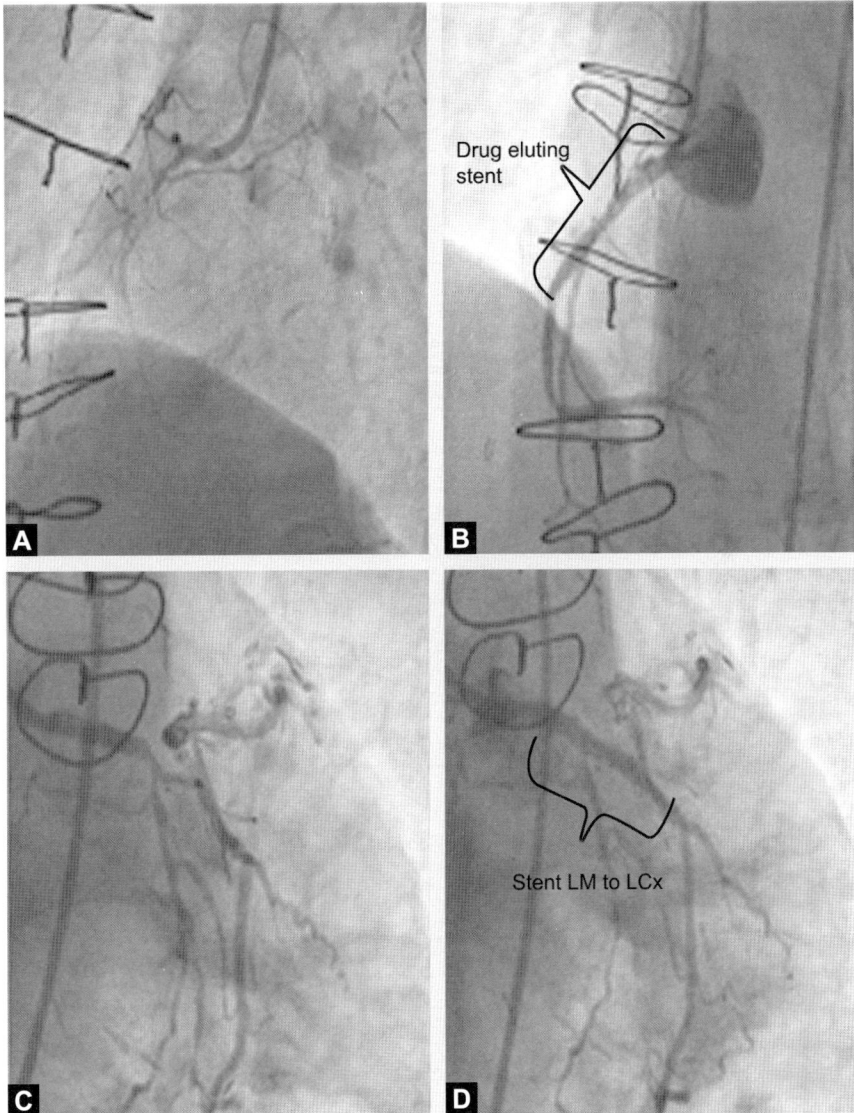

Figs. 5A to D: Intervention in native vessel: CABG 9 years back LIMA to D1 LAD, RIMA 'Y' graft to OM1 OM2 PD exertional angina TMT positive CAG functioning LIMA to D1 and LAD, graft between OM1 and OM2 and. RCA CTO no flowing grafts (A) RCA CTO No flowing grafts (B) PCI to RCA (C) functioning graft between OM1 and OM2 (D) PCI LMCA to LCX.

surgery. SVG occlusion during the first year is high at 15%, and 10-year patency is only 60%.[1]

SVG failure is associated with a significant increase in major adverse cardiovascular events (MACE), including death, myocardial infarction (MI), and the need for repeat revascularization.[11]

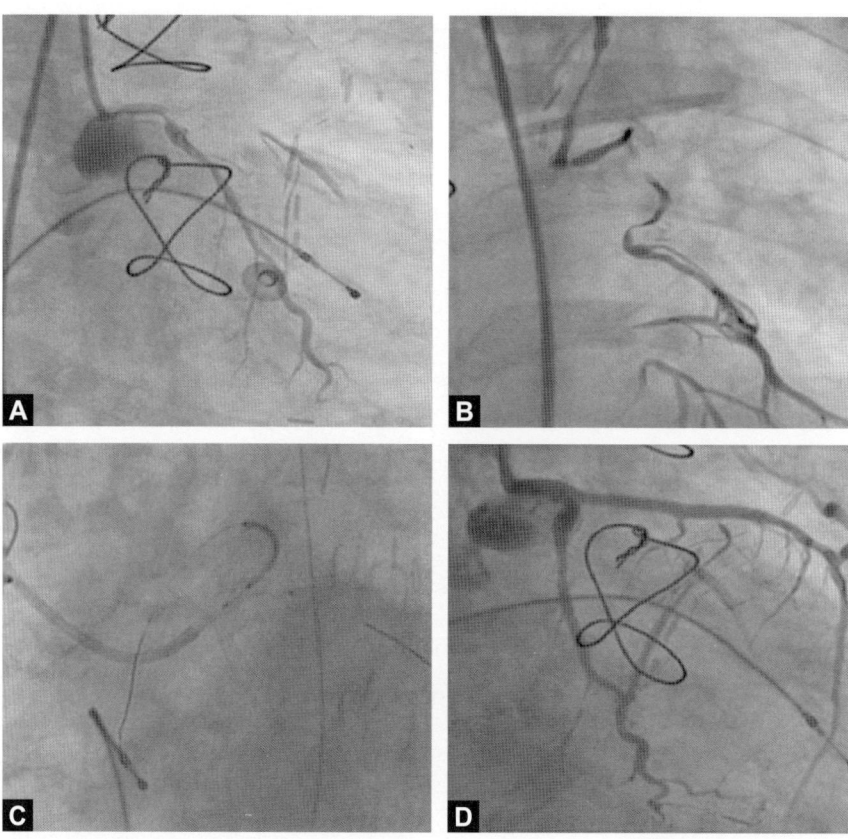

Figs. 6A to D: Native vessel bifurcation stenting in emergency: CTO ISR lesion in LAD prior occlusion of LAD stent, 17-year-old CABG, now, only LIMA functional all other grafts occluded. LIMA: severe disease long and ignored cardiac arrest on ventilator and balloon pump LAD: CTO, wired with cross 200 Bifurcation 2 stents tech (A) Native LAD CTO ISR, ostial LCX critical (B) Severe and long disease in LIMA (C and D) LMCA to LCX and LAD ostial stent bifurcation stenting.

SVG disease occurs in 3 phases as discussed earlier. Atherosclerotic plaques in SVGs are more diffuse, friable, contain more foam and inflammatory cells, have absent or small fibrous caps, and little or no calcification in comparison to native coronary atherosclerosis.[5]

These characteristics predispose SVGs to extensive thrombotic burden and distal embolization during coronary graft interventions, resulting in the '**no-reflow**' phenomenon, and hence, more periprocedural MI. Grafts particularly susceptible to these effects are those of an older age with more ectasia and greater plaque burden.[12]

Use embolic protection devices (EPD), thrombectomy, laser, minimal manipulation of stenotic bed are different strategies used to decrease distal embolization.

Ostial and distal (anastomotic site) lesions are more fibrous and less lipid rich hence less prone for distal embolization compared shaft lesions.[13]

SVG STENTING

The saphenous vein de novo (SAVED) trial was the seminal study that compared balloon angioplasty with bare-metal stents (BMS) in SVG lesions. This demonstrated that the use of BMS had a better composite outcome of freedom from death, MI, repeat CABG, and target lesion revascularization (TLR).[14]

The reduction in restenosis in saphenous vein grafts with cypher (RRISC) trial[15] and the stenting of saphenous vein graft (SOS) trial[16] compared DES to BMS and found a significant reduction in restenosis and TLR, but no difference in mortality. RRISC also found a reduction in TVR. However, at 3-year follow-up from the RRISC trial (delayed RRISC), there were more deaths in the DES compared with the BMS group. In addition, the decrease in TVR seen at 6 months was not noted at follow-up.[17]

Covered Stents

Covered stents were developed as a mechanical strategy to serve as a local filter, trapping plaque against the graft wall to prevent the shower of emboli during stent deployment. In addition, it was hypothesized that neointimal proliferation and the ensuing restenosis would be reduced. Favorable results were initially suggested by a multicenter registry.[18] But randomized trials failed to show any superiority over BMS[19-21] (Figs. 7A to E).

Embolic Protection Devices (Table 1)

Mechanical EPD were developed and proved to be the first treatment modality to reduce MACE during SVG PCI. Currently, there are 3 kinds of this devices available:
1. Distal balloon occlusion/aspiration system
2. Distal filter system
3. Proximal occlusion/aspiration system.

Distal Occlusion/Aspiration System: The PercuSurge GuardWire (Figs. 8A and B)

This was the first EPD to gain Food and Drug Administration (FDA) approval following the results of the saphenous vein graft angioplasty free of emboli randomized (SAFER) trial. This pivotal study showed a remarkable 42% reduction in 30-day MACE and a marked decrease in the no-reflow phenomenon with utilization of EPD.[22]

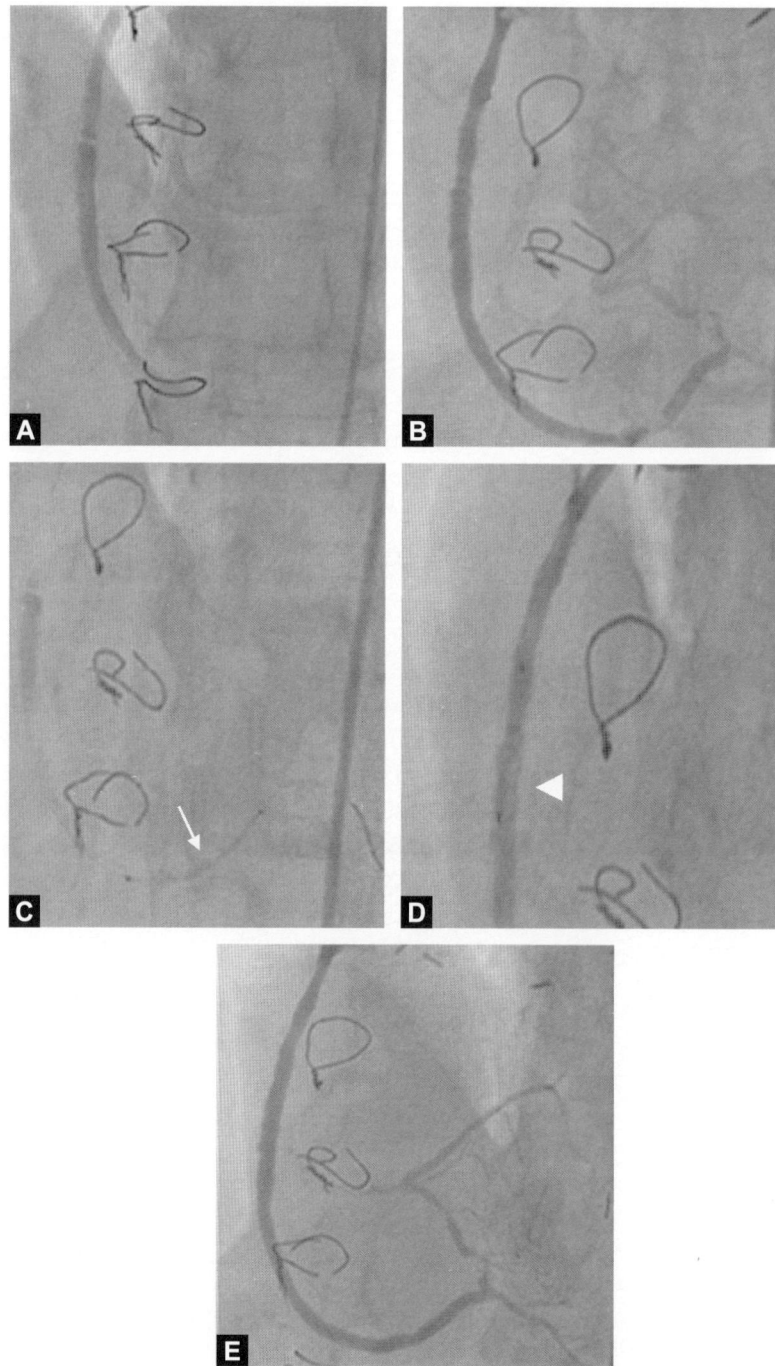

Figs. 7A to E: SVG in stent restenosis (A) Unstable angina symbiot (covered stent) stent 8-year-old ISR mid shaft distal eccentric thrombotic lesion. (B) Mid shaft balloon, thrombus aspiration, no EPD, NO GP blocker, no balloon distally (C) Covered stent distally (arrow) (D) Biomatrix stent (arrowhead) proximally (E) Final result.

Table 1: Embolic protection devices.

Types of EPD	Structure	Mechanism	Disadvantage	Advantage
Filter wire EX, EZ	Windsock shaped filter	Filters large particles	• Large Landing zone 25-50 mm • Incomplete protection • Filters may clog • Delivery catheters may cause embolization before filter deployment • Cannot remove emboli intermittently	• Less Hemodynamic Disturbance • Can be used for ostial lesion • Contrast imaging possible throughout the procedure
Spider	Windsock shaped filter	Filters large particles		
Precusurge Guardwire	0.014"Wire with distal balloon (distal balloon inflation stops complete flow + thrombectomy before deflation)	Filters large particles as well as humoral factors	Cessation of antegrade flow • Possible hemodynamic worsening • Can not be used for ostial lesion (risk of embolization into aorta) • Balloon-induced injury • Not as steerable as PTCA wire • Difficult to image during procedure • Balloon can move during PCI	• Complete protection • small Landing zone 20 mm • Easy to use more tolerable with intermittent occlusion
Proxis	catheter with a protection balloon on its distal tip balloon inflation stops complete flow + thrombectomy before deflation)	Filters large particles as well as humoral factors		

Distal Filtration System (FilterWire EX) (Fig. 9)

This is a guidewire filtration system that uses an oval windsock-shaped filter membrane that is delivered to a "landing zone" distal to the target lesion and then deployed prior to lesion intervention. The intervention is then performed over the wire and a sheath is advanced to retrieve the wire and the filter.[23]

A newer generation of filter devices has since been developed. FilterWire EZ (a second generation of the FilterWire EX) and the Spider Rx filtration device (Figs. 10A to D).

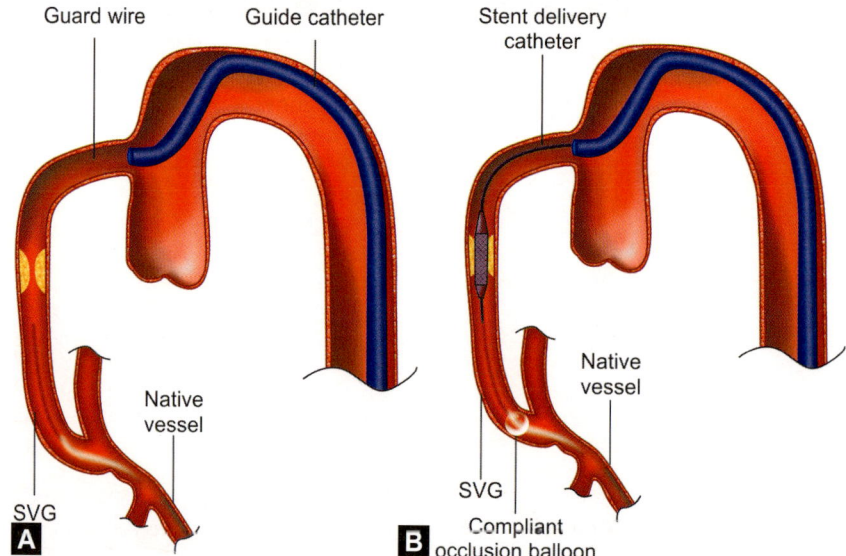

Figs. 8A and B: (A) Distal occlusion/aspiration system. The PercuSurge GuardWire.[22] GuardWire advanced distal to lesion; (B) Distal balloon inflated to occlude flow before stent deployment. Thrombus aspiration catheter used to aspirate stagnant column of blood. Balloon is deflated and retrieved.

Proximal Occlusion/Aspiration System Proxis System (Fig. 11)

These devices occlude the vessel proximal to a target lesion and suspend antegrade flow. As with distal occlusion devices, the stagnant blood and debris are then aspirated. This was based on the proximal protection during saphenous vein graft intervention using the proxis embolic protection system (PROXIMAL) trial that showed the proxis system to be noninferior to distal EPD.[24]

Selection of EPD

- Ostial lesions can be protected by filter type EPD and GuardWire can not be used for as it create stagnant column of blood which can lead to proximal embolization into aorta.
- For shaft lesion any device is suitable.
- Distal lesion can be protected proxis device. For grafts which are less than 2 years duration and lesion due to in stent restenosis (ISR) EPD are not required as embolization risk is less.
- ACC/AHA PCI guidelines give Class I indication for the use of EPD whenever feasible.[7]

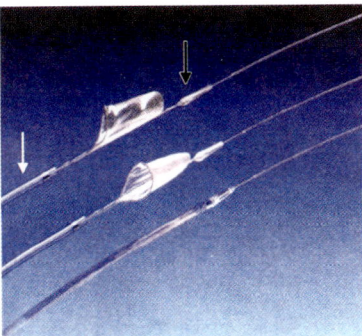

Fig. 9: Distal filtration system (Filter-wire EX). Filter-wire EX consisting of a 0.014" guide wire on which a polyurethane filter is mounted; deployed configuration (top and middle); retracted position (bottom) after being withdrawn into the retrieval sheath (white arrow); a distal nosecone (black arrow) prevents passage of the sheath beyond the wire tip.

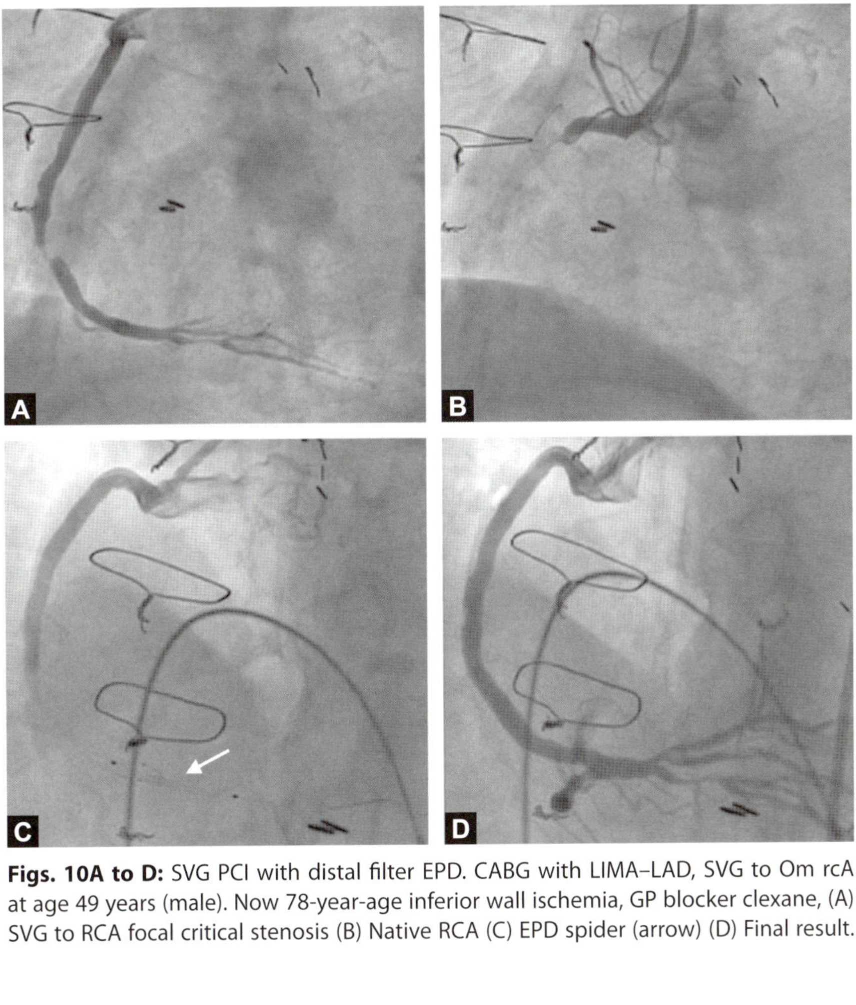

Figs. 10A to D: SVG PCI with distal filter EPD. CABG with LIMA–LAD, SVG to Om rcA at age 49 years (male). Now 78-year-age inferior wall ischemia, GP blocker clexane, (A) SVG to RCA focal critical stenosis (B) Native RCA (C) EPD spider (arrow) (D) Final result.

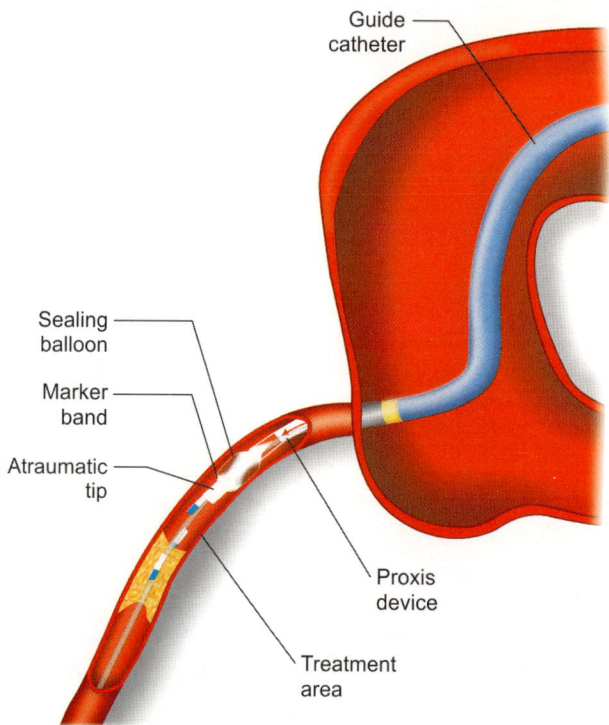

Fig. 11: Proximal occlusion/aspiration system (Proxis system).[24]

Despite benefit in prevention of embolization and MI EPD are underutilized (23%) as per NCDR registry 2004-2009 data.[25] This may be due to anatomic difficulties, such as challenging take-off from the aorta, very large vessel diameter, and the absence of an adequate non-diseased landing zone. EPD use may also be limited due to the higher procedural cost, longer procedural time, and greater radiation exposure.[26]

Other adjunctive modalities such as exciter laser, intragraft vasodilator use or strategies such as undersizing the stent, direct stenting or use of covered stent can be considered for embolic prevention.

Technical Aspects of SVG PCI[27]

- **Adequate guide support**: Important for safe delivery and retrieval of EPDs (Fig. 12).
- Balloon size selection and dilatation:
  - Balloon is sized generally 1:1
  - Oversizing required in case of suboptimal results, or ISR
  - Long balloons (30–40 mm) are used for long and bulky lesions
  - Higher pressures (>12 atm) are required for mature SVG lesions.

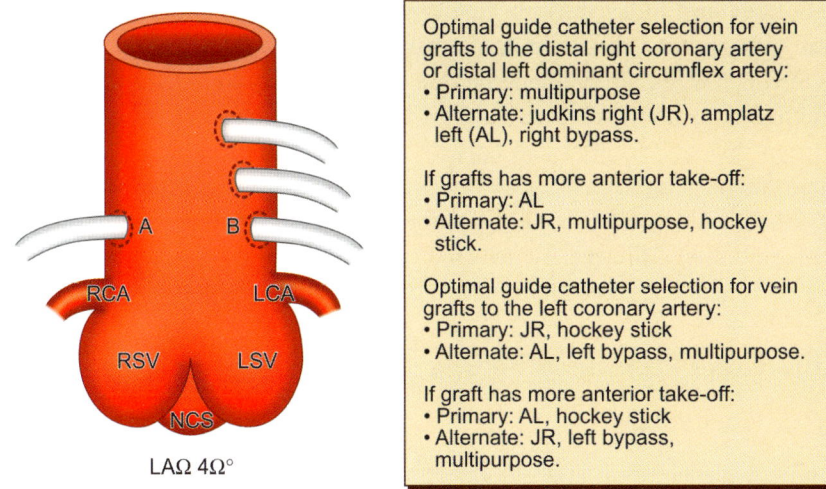

Fig. 12: Adequate guide support: important for safe delivery and retrieval of EPDs.[28]

- Stenting for vein grafts:
  - Rotablation, cutting balloon maybe required for ostial or anastomotic lesions
  - Oversizing, high-pressure inflation is avoided to minimize distal embolization
  - Minimizing post-stent manipulation is also important to prevent embolization.
- Careful EPD retrieval:
  - Balloon and stent must be well enough away from the EPD
  - Guide should be coaxial to prevent filter entrapment in the stent.

Intravascular Ultrasound (IVUS) in SVG PCI

IVUS is not used routinely in SVG PCI as its use increase the risk of distal embolization. SVG lesions are more aggressive compared to native vessel lesions. Conventional angiography underestimates the severity of vein graft remodeling and athermanous plaque development compared to IVUS. Intermediate lesions, better identified by IVUS, might be treated avoiding future recurrence of symptoms attributable to those lesions. It is of help in assessing vessel size. IVUS is performed after stenting to assess results.[28]

SVG CTO

Despite the dramatic reduction in periprocedural morbidity with the use of embolic protection devices during SVG intervention, the MACE rate still remains at 10%, which suggests persistent risk of micro-embolic showers occurring despite embolic protection devices, producing myocardial damage.[22] Plaque burden associated with CTO of SVG is considerably higher with large and bulky thrombi that tend to occupy the entire length of the graft, portending a higher risk of adverse events.[29]

SVG CTOs remain challenging due to an inability to deliver devices, the limitations of poor proximal support and long diffuse lesions, and plaque burden that overwhelms the capacity of current filter devices, prompting the evaluation and need for adjunctive strategies.

This has led to a Class III indication for PCI of SVG CTOs based on current guidelines. However, in selected cases, SVG revascularization is necessitated by the absence of alternative options.[7]

Adjunctive Pharmacotherapy

GP IIb/IIIa Inhibitors

Adjunctive treatment with platelet GP IIb/IIIa inhibitors during SVG intervention do not result in improvement epicardial blood flow and microvascular perfusion or reduction in MACE, plausibly due to excessive atheroembolic and thrombotic burden present during SVG interventions.[30]

Vasodilators

Vasodilators that have been studied in the no-reflow phenomenon include adenosine, verapamil, and nicardipine.

Fischell et al. showed promising results with adenosine in reversing slow-flow and no-reflow phenomenon among patients undergoing SVG PCI.[31]

Michaels et al. showed that there was a significant reduction in no-reflow and a trend toward improvement in TIMI flow grade with prophylactic intragraft administration of verapamil during SVG PCI.[32]

Fugit et al. compared 3 intracoronary vasodilators (nicardipine, diltiazem, and verapamil) on nonsignificant native coronary artery disease and found that nicardipine was the most potent coronary vasodilator with the fewest systemic side effects.[33]

Currently, aspirin, thienopyridine, and anticoagulation with heparin are the only recommended adjuvant pharmacotherapy in SVG interventions.

ARTERIAL GRAFT INTERVENTIONS

Left internal mammary artery (LIMA) is used as most common arterial conduit as a graft others are radial artery and GEA.

LIMA Graft Intervention

Early failure of LIMA graft occurs due to distal anastomosis site stenosis, in Image study was found in 9% of patients[34] (Figs. 13A to C).

Given the increased mortality and morbidity associated with re-do CABG, percutaneous transluminal coronary angioplasty (PTCA) to LIMA stenosis appears to be a viable alternative[35] Gruberg et al. and Ishizaka et al. have reported that IMA grafts underwent PTCA mostly at the distal anastomosis (77-87%).[36,37] Reported success rates of the procedure are between 73% and 97%.[38]

LIMA Graft Restenosis after PTCA

It has been confirmed elsewhere that vessel tortuosity is a significant predictor of angioplasty failure[35,39] which is due to coiling of IMA and preexistent tortuosity in the vessel used as conduit. In other published series of IMA graft angioplasty, angiographic restenosis constituted 8-30% of balloon angioplasties.[35-39] The reported restenosis rates of saphenous vein graft angioplasty (38-52%),[40-42] long-term outcome appears significantly improved using the IMA-based variant. Sharma et al.[43] reported a restenosis rate of 23.5% for stenting in IMA grafts, while Gruberg et al.[36] demonstrated 33% TLR in their stenting group, which was higher than that of balloon angioplasty only. The Gruberg result does not support the proposed benefit of stenting in IMA grafts.

Technical Aspects of LIMA Graft Intervention[27]

Attempting PCI through an LIMA graft is associated with significant technical challenges.

Difficult cannulation of ostium, long and tortuous grafts carry high-risk of ostial dissection jeopardizing entire circulation.

- **Difficult engagement of LIMA ostium**: can be overcome by
  - Dedicated guide use: LIMA or JR-4

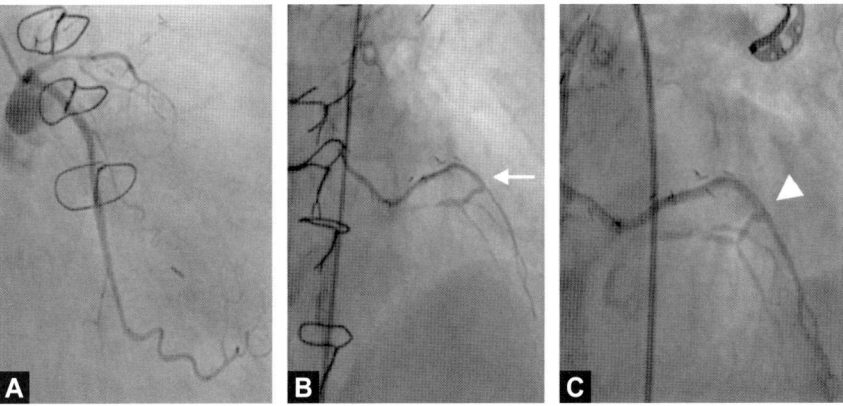

Figs. 13A to C: PCI distal LIMA to D1. Single graft LIMA to D1 and LAD 20 years back now angina. (A) RCA and LCx normal (B) LIMA: normal disease in D1, at and beyond anastomosis (arrow). (C) PCI through LIMA to D1 absorb (arrowhead).

- Use of coronary wire for pulling the guide into the ostium
- Diagnostic catheter may be used to engage followed by exchange to guide
- Alternatively ipsilateral radial or brachial approach can help
- Avoid wedging and too-deep intubation may cause dissection (Figs. 14A to C).
- **Long and tortuous grafts**: can be overcomed by
  - Using shorter guides, longer shaft balloons and stents
  - Using hydrophilic, polymer jacket, wires
  - Microcatheters, deflectable tip catheters (venture).
- **Antegrade IMA flow cessation after wiring**
  - "kinking", pseudo-lesion formation, dissection
  - Antegrade flow is established by removing the wire over a flexible microcatheter
  - "Dual-guide technique."

One guide dedicated for contrast injection and other for delivery of equipment.

TAKE HOME MESSAGE

- Recurrence of ischemia in patients with prior CABG is due to various reasons
- SVG intervention associated with high cardiac event rate especially due to distal embolization
- With the exception of SVG CTO lesion, recurrent ischemia can be managed by percutaneous intervention either graft intervention or native vessel intervention

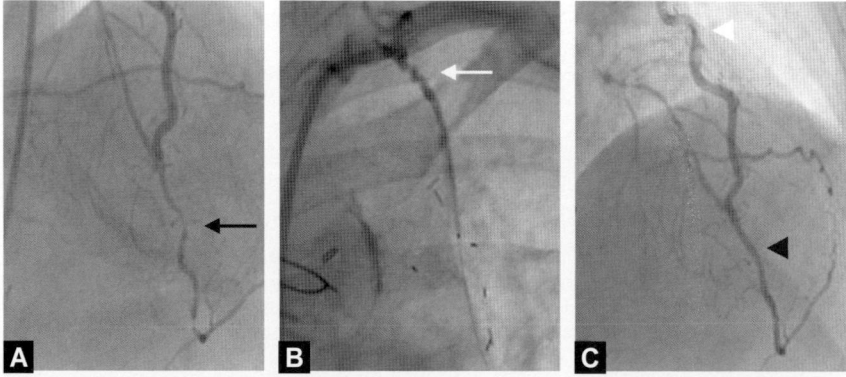

Figs. 14A to C: PCI to diseased native LAD distal to distal anastomotic site through LIMA graft with the help of whisper MS wire, LIMA ostial dissection secondary to deep intubation of catheter. (A) LIMA graft to LAD patent advanced atherosclerosis in distal LAD (black arrow) (B) LIMA dissection due to catheter injury (white arrow) (C) PCI to distal native vessel (black arrowhead) and PCI to osteoproximal LIMA (white arrowhead).

- EPD are strongly recommended in SVG intervention currently they are under utilized
- Stent and balloon oversizing is to be avoided in SVG intervention
- Covered stents and other pharmacological therapy are useful in preventing distal embolization
- Most arterial graft failures are amenable to PCI, role of stent remains controversial
- Arterial graft interventions are prone for dissection of graft due to obstacles in delivery system requires adequate guide and proper wire selection.

REFERENCES

1. Goldman S, Zadina K, Moritz T, et al. Long-term patency of saphenous vein and left internal mammary artery grafts after coronary artery bypass surgery: results from a Department of Veterans Affairs Cooperative Study. J Am Coll Cardiol. 2004 Dec 7;44(11):2149-56
2. Sabik JF 3rd, Blackstone EH, Gillinov AM, et al. Occurrence and risk factors for reintervention after coronary artery bypass grafting. Circulation. 2006 Jul 4;114 (1 Suppl):I454-60.
3. Sergeant P, Lesaffre E, Flameng W, et al. The return of clinically evident ischemia after coronary artery bypass grafting. Eur J Cardiothorac Surg. 1991;5:447–457.
4. Brilakis ES, Rao SV, Banerjee S, et al. Percutaneous coronary intervention in native arteries versus bypass grafts in prior coronary artery bypass grafting patients: a report from the National Cardiovascular Data Registry. JACC Cardiovasc Interv. 2011 Aug;4(8):844-50.
5. Motwani JG, Topol EJ. Aortocoronary saphenous vein graft disease: pathogenesis, predisposition, and prevention. Circulation. 1998;97(9):916-931.
6. Cooper GJ, Underwood MJ, Deverall PB. Arterial and venous conduits for coronary artery bypass. Eur J Cardiothorac Surg. 1996;10(2):129-140.
7. Levine GN, Bates ER, Blankenship JC, et al. 2011 ACCF/AHA/SCAI Guideline for Percutaneous Coronary Intervention. A report of the American College of Cardiology Foundation/American Heart Association Task Force on Practice Guidelines and the Society for Cardiovascular Angiography and Interventions. J Am Coll Cardiol. 2011 Dec 6;58(24):e44-122.
8. Sharma S. Current Management of Saphenous Vein Graft Disease. The Internet Journal of Cardiology. 2003 Volume 2 Number 2.
9. Dimitri Karmpaliotis Does prior coronary artery bypass grafting affect percutaneous chronic total occlusion revascularization ? Interv. Cardiol. (2013) 5(5), 489–492
10. Tanabe, M. Does Percutaneous Coronary Interventions of Coronary Chronic Total Occlusions to Patients with Prior Coronary Artery Bypass Graft Surgery Have Poorer Pocedural Outcome? (2016) J Heart Cardiol 2(4): 1- 8.
11. Halabi AR, Alexander JH, Shaw LK, et al. Relation of early saphenous vein graft failure to outcomes following coronary artery bypass surgery. Am J Cardiol. 2005;96(9):1254-1259.
12. Coolong A, Baim DS, Kuntz RE, et al. Saphenous vein graft stenting and major adverse cardiac events: a predictive model derived from a pooled analysis of 3958 patients. Circulation. 2008;117(6):790-797.

13. Wood FO, Badhey N, Garcia B, et al. Analysis of saphenous vein graft lesion composition using near infrared spectroscopy and intravascular ultrasonography with virtual histology. Atherosclerosis. 2010 Oct;212(2):528-33.
14. Savage MP, Douglas JS Jr, Fischman DL, et al. Stent placement compared with balloon angioplasty for obstructed coronary bypass grafts. Saphenous Vein De Novo Trial Investigators. N Engl J Med. 1997;337(11):740-747.
15. Vermeersch P, Agostoni P, Verheye S, et al. Randomized double-blind comparison of sirolimus-eluting stent versus bare-metal stent implantation in disease saphenous vein grafts: six-month angiographic, intravascular ultrasound, and clinical follow-up of the RRISC Trial. J Am Coll Cardiol. 2006;48(12):2423-2431.
16. Brilakis ES, Lichtenwalter C, de Lemos JA, et al. A randomized controlled trial of a paclitaxel-eluting stent versus a similar bare-metal stent in saphenous vein graft lesions the SOS (Stenting of Saphenous Vein Grafts) trial. J Am Coll Cardiol. 2009;53(11):919-928.
17. Vermeersch P, Agostoni P, Verheye S, et al. Increased late mortality after sirolimus-eluting stents versus bare-metal stents in disease saphenous vein grafts: results from the randomized DELAYED RRISC Trial. J Am Coll Cardiol. 2007;50(3):261-267
18. Baldus S, Koster R, Elsner M, et al. Treatment of aortocoronary vein graft lesions with membrane-covered stents: a multicenter surveillance trial. Circulation. 2000;102(17):2024-2027
19. Schachinger V, Hamm CW, Munzel T, et al; STING (STents IN Grafts) Investigators. A randomized trial of polytetrafluoroethylene-membrane-covered stents compared with conventional stents in aortocoronary saphenous vein grafts. J Am Coll Cardiol. 2003;42(8):1360-1369.
20. Stankovic G, Colombo A, Presbitero P, et al. Randomized Evaluation of polytetrafluoroethylene COVERed stent in Saphenous vein grafts (RECOVERS) Trial. Circulation. 2003;108(1):37-42.
21. Turco MA, Buchbinder M, Popma JJ, et al. Pivotal, randomized U.S. study of the Symbiot (TM) covered stent system in patients with saphenous vein graft disease: eight-month angiographic and clinical results from the Symbiot III trial. Catheter Cardiovasc Interv. 2006;68(3):379-388.
22. Baim DS, Wahr D, George B, et al. Randomized trial of a distal embolic protection device during percutaneous intervention of saphenous vein aortocoronary bypass grafts. Circulation. 2002;105(11):1285-1290.
23. Stone G, Rogers C, Hermiller J, et al. Randomized comparison of distal protection with a filter-based catheter and a balloon occlusion and aspiration system during percutaneous intervention of diseased saphenous vein aorto-coronary bypass grafts. Circulation. 2003;108(5):548-553.
24. Mauri L, Cox DA, Hermiller J, et al. The PROXIMAL trial: proximal protection during saphenous vein graft intervention using the Proxis embolic protection system: a randomized, prospective, multicenter trial. J Am Coll Cardiol. 2007;50(15):1142-1449.
25. Brilakis ES Wang TY, Rao SV, et al, Frequency and predictors of drug-eluting stent use in saphenous vein bypass graft percutaneous coronary interventions: a report from the American College of Cardiology National Cardiovascular Data CathPCI registry. JACC Cardiovasc Interv. 2010 Oct;3(10):1068-73.
26. Mehta SK, Frutkin AD, Milford-Beland S, et al. Utilization of distal embolic protection in saphenous vein graft interventions (an analysis of 19,546 patients in the American College of Cardiology-National Cardiovascular Data Registry). Am J Cardiol. 2007;100:1114-1118.

27. Thach N. Nguyen, Nguyen Quang Tuan, Muhammad Munawar, Interventions in Patients after Coronary Artery Bypass Graft Surgery. In: Thach Nguyen, Dayi Hu, Shao Liang Chen, Moo-Hyun Kim, Shigeru Saito, Cindy Grines,C. Michael Gibson, Steven R Bailey Editors. Practical Handbook of Advanced Interventional Cardiology Tips and tricks, 4th Ed. Chinchester west Sussex: Willey Blackwell; 2012. 293-306
28. Alok Mazumdar Sapheneous vein graft intervention challenges 2014. In: H K Chopra Editor. Cardiology Update 2014 (Cardiological Society Of India) 1st Ed. New Delhi:Jaypee Brothers Medical Publishers; 2015; 474-479
29. Meliga E, Garcia-Garcia HM, Kukreja N, et al. Chronic total occlusion treatment in post-CABG patients: saphenous vein graft versus native vessel recanalization—long-term follow-up in the drug-eluting stent era. Catheter Cardiovasc Interv 2007;70:21-25.
30. Karha J, Gurm HS, Rajagopal V, et al. Use of platelet glycoprotein IIb/IIIa inhibitors in saphenous vein graft percutaneous coronary intervention and clinical outcomes. Am J Cardiol. 2006;98(7):906-910.
31. Fischell TA, Carter AJ, Foster MT, et al. Reversal of "no reflow" during vein graft stenting using high velocity boluses of intracoronary adenosine. Cathet Cardiovasc Diagn. 1998;45(4):360-365
32. Michaels AD, Appleby M, Otten MH, et al. Pretreatment with intragraft verapamil prior to percutaneous coronary intervention of saphenous vein graft lesions: results of the randomized, controlled vasodilator prevention on no-reflow (VAPOR) trial. J Invasive Cardiol. 2002;14(6):299-302.
33. Fugit MD, Rubal BJ, Donovan DJ. Effects of intracoronary nicardipine, diltiazem and verapamil on coronary blood flow. J Invasive Cardiol. 2000;12(2):80-85.
34. Berger PB, Alderman EL, Nadel A, et al, Frequency of early occlusion and stenosis in a left internal mammary artery to left anterior descending artery bypass graft after surgery through a median sternotomy on conventional bypass: benchmark for minimally invasive direct coronary artery bypass. Circulation 1999;100:2353-8.
35. Hearne SE, Davidson CJ, Zidar JP, et al, . Internal mammary artery graft angioplasty: acute and long-term outcome. Cathet Cardiovasc Diagn 1998;44:153-6.
36. Gruberg L, Dangas G, Mehran R, et al, Percutaneous revascularization of the internal mammary artery graft: short- and long-term outcomes. J Am Coll Cardiol 2000;35:944-8.
37. Ishizaka N, Ishizaka Y, Ikari Y, et al, Initial and subsequent angiographic outcome of percutaneous transluminal angioplasty performed on internal mammary artery grafts. Br Heart J 1995;74:615-9.
38. Sketch MH Jr, Quigley PJ, Perez JA, et al. Angiographic follow-up after internal mammary artery graft angioplasty. Am J Cardiol 1992;70:401-3.
39. Dimas AP, Arora RR, Whitlow PL, et al. Percutaneous transluminal angioplasty involving internal mammary artery grafts. Am Heart J 1991;122:423-9.
40. Douglas JS Jr, Gruentzig AR, King SB 3rd, et al. Percutaneous transluminal coronary angioplasty in patients with prior coronary artery bypass surgery. J Am Coll Cardiol 1983;2:745-54.
41. Dorros G, Johnson WD, Tector AJ, et al. Percutaneous transluminal coronary angioplasty in patients with prior coronary artery bypass grafting. J Thorac Cardiovasc Surg 1984;87:17-26.
42. Block PC, Cowley MJ, Kaltenbach M, et al. Percutaneous angioplasty of stenoses of bypass grafts or of bypass graft anastomotic sites. Am J Cardiol 1984;53:666-8.
43. Sharma AK, McGlynn S, Apple S, et al. Clinical outcomes following stent implantation in internal mammary artery grafts. Catheter Cardiovasc Interv 2003;59:436-41.

10
Percutaneous Coronary Intervention in ST Elevation Myocardial Infarction

Hetan C Shah, Ashwin B Mehta

INTRODUCTION

Cardiovascular diseases are leading cause of mortality worldwide. It is estimated that every year 15 million people suffer ST elevation myocardial infarction (STEMI) and 700,000 die as of its consequences. Almost one-third to half of STEMI deaths occur within 1 hour of symptom onset, usually before the first medical contact and this figure has remained constant over the years. The management of STEMI has witnessed enormous change from initial days of its first recognition by James Herrick in 1912.[1] The management of STEMI has evolved over 100 years in four phases (Table 1) and the landmarks *in STEMI thrombolytic therapy* is shown in Table 2.[2]

The use of primary angioplasty as an alternative to thrombolysis was first described in 1983.[3] A meta-analysis comparing these strategies concluded that timely percutaneous coronary intervention (PCI) by an experienced team is superior to in hospital thrombolytic therapy.[4]

PRIMARY ANGIOPLASTY

Primary angioplasty or primary percutaneous coronary intervention (PPCI) is current standard of reperfusion for STEMI.

The greatest benefit gained from reperfusion therapy occurs within the first 2–3 hours of symptom onset however, First "Golden Hour" is the best time window to salvage myocardium.

Table 1: Evolution of management of STEMI.

Phase 1 (1912–1960)	Bed rest	30-day mortality–30%
Phase 2 (1961–1975)	Coronary care unit	30-day mortality–15%
Phase 3 (1976-present)	Myocardial reperfusion	30-day mortality–5%
Phase 4 (Future)	Prevention of reperfusion injury and regeneration	

Table 2: Landmarks in STEMI therapy.

Year	Landmarks
1976	First in man: Intracoronary thrombolysis in STEMI[5]
1980	Unequivocal demonstration of coronary thrombosis as a cause of STEMI[6]
1986	*GISSI trial*: Thrombolysis reduces mortality in STEMI[7]
1993	*GUSTO I trial*: tPA reduces mortality as compared with streptokinase in STEMI[8]
1999	*ASSENT-2 trial*: Single bolus tenecteplase in STEMI[9]
2003	Meta-analysis shows mortality benefits of primary angioplasty over thrombolysis in STEMI[4]

Flowchart 1: Reperfusion therapy for patients with STEMI.

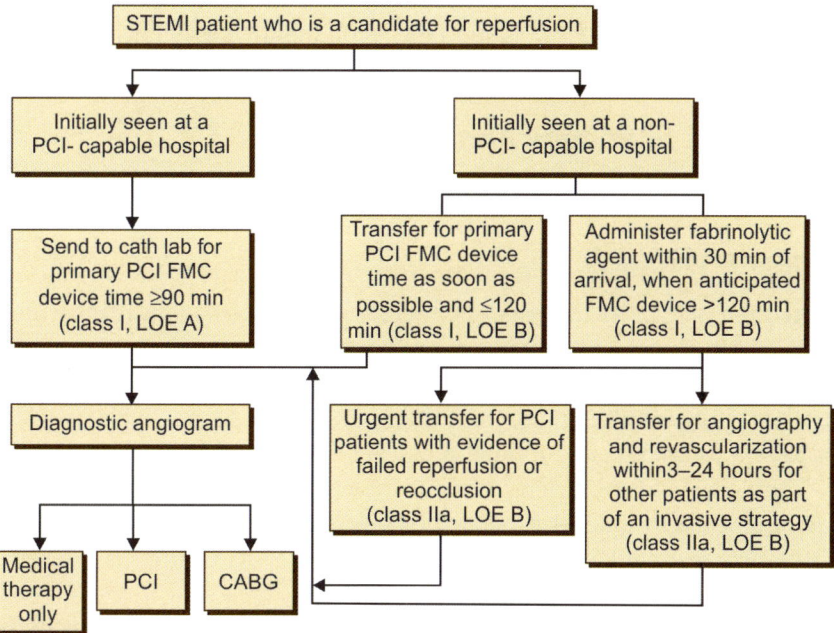

(CABG: Coronary artery bypass grafting; FMC: First medical contact; PCI: Percutaneous coronary intervention; STEMI: ST-elevation myocardial infarction).

The PPCI saves one extra life per 50 treated patients over thrombolysis.[4]

Current recommendations are that if patient after STEMI goes to PCI-capable hospital, then primary PCI is standard of care if it can be performed within 90 minutes.[10] If patient reaches a non-PCI capable hospital then he should be transferred to a PCI-capable center only if PCI could be performed within 120 minutes, otherwise he should receive thrombolysis which should be performed within 30 minutes (Flowchart 1).[10]

Table 3: Recommended indications of primary PCI in STEMI.
Acute STEMI presenting within 12 hours of the onset of symptoms and when primary PCI can be delivered within 120 minutes
Acute STEMI with cardiogenic shock presenting within 36 hours of the onset of symptoms
Active myocardial ischemia presenting >12 hours after the onset of symptoms
Ongoing symptoms of myocardial ischemia OR residual or persistent STEMI elevation 60–90 minutes after fibrinolysis
Clinically stable patients during the same hospital admission after successful fibrinolysis

If patients can be transferred to PCI-capable hospital in reasonable time frame, there is 42% reduction in death, reinfarction and stroke compared to thrombolysis.[11] Primary PCI is specially recommended to following patients as listed in Table 3.

Challenges to Primary Angioplasty

Challenges to primary angioplasty are either logistic or procedure related.

Logistic Challenges

More than 50% of STEMI mortality occurs before the patient reaches hospital in first hour of symptom onset due to ventricular fibrillation caused by ischemia which can be prevented by defibrillation. In low- and middle-income countries like India, there are multiple challenges including lack of patient awareness and trained medical staff, poor emergency services.[10]

There is considerable delay in mean time from symptom onset to presentation in India for STEMI patients which was nearly 360 minutes in largest CREATE (Treatment and Outcomes of Acute Coronary Syndromes in India) registry.[12]

To start successful primary angioplasty requires teamwork at multiple levels from patient education about symptoms, early identification by health personnel and timely referral to capable center and availability of quick transport. Recent white paper discussed challenges and strategies in the management of STEMI with the view of reducing morbidity and mortality specifically addressing management of STEMI in low- and middle-income group.[13]

Challenges to primary angioplasty.
Logistic
• Transport time, trained medical team.
• Pharmacoinvasive therapy—Indian perspective.

Contd...

Contd...

Procedure related
- Choice of adjunct drug therapy regarding thienpyridine.
- Access site complications—femoral versus radial.
- PCI of culprit vessel only vs multivessel PCI in STEMI.
- Crossing the lesion.
- Status of thrombosuction.
- Use of GPIIb/IIIa inhibitors and anticoagulation.
- Status of intra-aortic balloon pumping (IABP).
- Choice of stents: bioabsorbable vascular stents (BVS) versus drug eluting versus bare metal.
- Newer stents.
- Duration of dual antiplatelet therapy (DAPT) after PCI.

Pharmacoinvasive Strategy

Pharmacoinvasive strategy refers to the administration of fibrinolytic therapy either in the prehospital setting or at a non-PCI-capable hospital, followed by immediate transfer to a PCI-capable hospital for early coronary angiography and PCI when appropriate. A meta-analysis of seven trials has shown that death and reinfarction is significantly reduced without increase in stroke by pharmacoinvasive approach. It should be performed within 3–24 hours of thrombolysis.[14] In STREAM trial,[15] the primary end point of all-cause mortality, congestive heart failure (CHF), repeat myocardial infarction (MI) and shock at 30 days occurred in 12.4% patients in the fibrinolysis group and 14.3% patients in the primary PCI group (p = 0.21) without increase in intracranial bleeding (0.5% vs. 0.3%, p = 0.45). STREAM trial reiterates that earlier the reperfusion from symptom onset, lesser the difference between the thrombolysis and primary PCI. STREAM trial for the first time has suggested that in STEMI when PCI cannot be provided in a timely fashion, fibrinolysis followed by rapid transfer to a PCI-capable hospital may provide similar benefits, albeit with some increase in the risk of intracranial bleed.

ANTIPLATELET DRUGS, WHICH TO CHOOSE?

It is recommended that all patients for primary PCI should receive dual antiplatelet therapy (DAPT). All patients should receive 162–325 mg orally as early as possible to ensure rapid bioavailability. High dose of clopidogrel in primary PCI patients (600 mg) significantly reduces cardiac death, MI, stroke and stent thrombosis. Doubling the clopidogrel dose prevents additional six MIs and seven stent thromboses with an excess of three severe bleeds per 1,000 patients treated.[16]

Newer rapid-acting P2Y12 inhibitors, such as ticagrelor and prasugrel offer even greater potential for clinical benefit when administered before primary PCI. In addition to more rapid onset of action, they are also effectively in patients with clopidogrel resistance.

Prasugrel, a novel thienopyridine reduced death, MI and stroke by 19%, stent thrombosis by 46% but at the cost of 32% increase in major bleed in primary PCI setting. Bleed was especially higher in underweight and elderly.

The American College of Cardiology Foundation (ACCF)/American Heart Association (AHA) guidelines (2013) recommend 60 mg loading dose of prasugrel before PCI followed by 10 mg maintenance dose to be continued for 1 year except in patients with high bleeding risk like prior CVA or octogenarians or patients weighing less than 60 kg or other high-risk patients.

Ticagrelor is another newer thienopyridine with rapid onset of action.

The PLATO study compared ticagrelor (180 mg loading dose, 90 mg twice daily thereafter) with clopidogrel (300 or 600 mg loading dose, 75 mg daily thereafter) for the prevention of cardiovascular events in 18,624 patients with acute coronary syndrome (ACS), of whom 35% had STEMI.[17] Significant reductions favoring ticagrelor were seen in the primary PCI subgroup for stent thrombosis (ST) and total deaths, though there were more strokes and episodes of intracerebral hemorrhage (ICH) with ticagrelor. ACC/AHA guidelines recommend 180 mg loading dose of ticagrelor followed by 90 mg twice daily for at least 1 year.

The choice between clopidogrel and newer thienopyridines in patients with STEMI undergoing PCI should be based on the risk of bleeding balanced with the potential clinical benefits. The increased cost and compliance issue (twice a day dosing) are important considerations with ticagrelor in India.

ACC/AHA 2013 recommendation for using P2Y12 inhibitors.
For PCI:
Clopidogrel 600 mg loading dose then 75 mg a day for 1 year, or
Prasugrel 60 mg loading dose then 10 mg a day for 1 year, or
Ticagrelor 180 mg loading dose then 90 mg twice a day for 1 year
Patients should receive DAPT for at least a year regardless of whether they receive a bare metal stent (BMS) or a drug-eluting stent (DES).
For patient undergone fibrinolytic therapy followed by PCI.
Clopidogrel: If loading dose was given with fibrinolytic therapy, continue clopidogrel 75 mg a day for 1 year.
Clopidogrel: If loading dose was not given with fibrinolytic therapy, and PCI is to be performed less than or equal to 24 hours after fibrinolytic therapy, give 300 mg loading dose and continue at 75 mg a day for a year.
Clopidogrel: If loading dose was not given with fibrinolytic therapy, and PCI is to be performed more than 24 hours after fibrinolytic therapy, give 600 mg loading dose and continue at 75 mg a day for a year.
All patients should also receive aspirin 162–325 loading dose, then 81–325 mg a day indefinitely.

Radial versus Femoral Access

Primary PCI still has certain limitations which are access site major bleeding in 7% and vascular complications requiring surgical repair in 0.4–2% of patients.[4,18,19] Radial approach was associated with a significant lower incidence of major bleeding and access site complications and a significant better net clinical benefit as seen in RIVAL STEACS[15] and STEMI-RADIAL[16] trial. We also believe the radial should be the preferred approach in primary angioplasty to reduce bleeding. However, one should follow the approach in which one is more experienced and confident.

Crossing the Lesion

Familiarity and experience should guide the selection of hardware. One should always start with workhorse wire, which is usually "soft-tipped, non-hydrophilic guidewire". Hydrophilic guidewires should not be the first choice, since it increases the risk of perforation or dissection of downstream vessels especially when those vessels cannot be visualized or when encountered with difficult anatomy such as tortuous and calcified vessels.

If one fails to cross the lesion, the next step is to choose floppy hydrophilic wire. One should avoid entering false lumen by careful and gentle wiring, avoiding forceful manipulation. The most important clue suggesting entry into a false channel is the loss of free movement of the wire tip in the distal vessel.

If there is a doubt about the location of the wire in the distal lumen, an over-the-wire balloon or end-hole infusion catheter should be advanced across the lesion, the wire withdrawn, and either by slowly aspirating the blood or injecting diluted contrast gently, it can be confirmed that the distal true lumen has been properly accessed.

Tortuous vessels often limit control of the distal wire tip, wire support with monorail balloon, an over-the-wire balloon or distal end whole infusion catheter may aid in crossing of the lesion.

Percutaneous Coronary Intervention of Nonculprit Vessel

The American College of Cardiology (ACC)/American Heart Association (ACC) 2013 guidelines recommend PCI of culprit vessel only at the time of primary PCI and recommended ***against*** [Class III] the PCI of nonculprit artery stenoses. In hemodynamically stable patients with STEMI, based primarily on the results of nonrandomized studies and meta-analyses and safety concerns.

Four randomized controlled trials (RCTs), such as PRAMI, CvLPRIT, DANAMI 3 PRIMULTI, PRAGUE-13,[20,21] have since suggested that a strategy of multivessel PCI, either at the time of primary PCI or as a planned, staged

Flowchart 2: Algorithm for preferred approach of primary PCI.

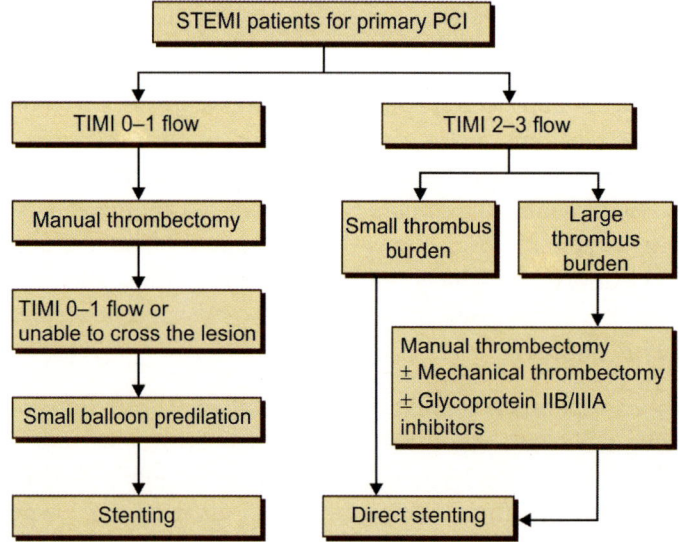

procedure, may be safe and beneficial in selected patients with STEMI. On the basis of these findings, the prior Class III -harm recommendation with regard to multivessel primary PCI in hemodynamically stable patients with STEMI has been upgraded and modified to a Class IIb recommendation to include consideration of multivessel PCI, either at the time of primary PCI or as a planned, staged procedure.[22]

Aspiration Thrombectomy (Flowchart 2)

The 2011 PCI and 2013 AHA/ACC STEMI guidelines' Class IIa recommendation for aspiration thrombectomy before primary PCI was based on the results of 2 RCTs and 1 meta-analysis and was driven in large measure by the results of TAPAS, a single-center study. Since formulation of that recommendation, 3 multicenter trials (INFUSE-AMI, TASTE, TOTAL), 2 of which enrolled significantly more patients than prior aspiration thrombectomy trials, have prompted re-evaluation of this recommendation. These 3 more recent trials, as well as an updated meta-analysis, found no significant reduction in adverse events with routine aspiration thrombectomy. Based on these 3 trials, routine aspiration thrombectomy before primary PCI is now designated as Class III—No benefit. Based on these and other considerations, a Class IIb recommendation was established stating that the usefulness of selective and bailout aspiration thrombectomy in patients undergoing primary PCI is not well-established.[22]

Distal protection devices such as Boston Scientific Filterwire 1 system and the PercuSurge Guardwire system have no role in native vessels primary

PCI since most of the trials failed to show any improvement in microvascular reperfusion, reduction in infarct size as well as clinical outcomes.[23-25]

Glycoprotein (GP) IIb/IIIa Inhibitors

In prethienopyridine era, use of abciximab as adjunctive therapy to PPCI resulted in lesser mortality (2.4% vs 3.4%; p = 0.05) and reinfarction (1.0% vs 1.9%; p = 0.03) without increase in bleeding.[26] In later studies with full dose clopidogrel, none of the three Gp IIb/IIIa inhibitors showed any benefit in death or reinfarction.[27] Benefit of Gp IIb/IIa use appears to be limited to lesions with large thrombus burden and no preloading of antiplatelets. Advent of rapidly acting thienopyridine—prasugrel and ticagrelor, has further restricted the use of Gp IIb/IIIa inhibitors.

CHOICE OF ANTICOAGULANT: BIVALIRUDIN VERSUS UNFRACTIONATED HEPARIN

Bivalirudin has emerged as a new promising agent, which is as effective as unfractionated heparin (UFH) in reducing ischemic complications but has got considerable advantage mainly due to low bleeding risk.[28] Its use during primary PCI has been given class I recommendation by recent ACC guidelines. In situations where bleeding risk is high, it is preferred over UFH (class IIa).

Recently published HORIZONS-AMI trial,[29] EUROMAX trial[30] as well as their pooled analysis[31] reported that primary PCI with bivalirudin improved 30-day net clinical outcomes, with significant reductions in major bleeding, thrombocytopenia and transfusions compared with heparin. In majority of the trials, there was an increased risk of acute stent thrombosis, within first 24 hours after PCI, in the bivalirudin group, which is a cause of concern for the interventional cardiologist. Whether use of novel PCI practices such as more potent newer adenosine diphosphate (ADP) antagonists (i.e. ticagrelor and prasugrel) and post-PCI bivalirudin infusion in conjunction with bivalirudin can lessen acute stent thrombosis is not clearly known and remains an area of further investigation.

Enoxaparin and fondaparinux have been studied less extensively in this setting. The ATOLL trial comparing intravenous enoxaparin with UFH for primary PCI failed to meet its primary, composite endpoint.[32] Fondaparinux is not used since it has been associated with catheter thrombosis in this setting.[33]

Direct Stenting versus Predilation

Pre-stent balloon dilation is associated with distal embolization, no reflow and impaired angiographic outcomes, which have been correlated with

Table 4: Strategies for optimizing outcomes of primary PCI and decreasing risk of no reflow.

Strategy	Mechanism	Disadvantages
M-Guard stent	Thrombus jailing b/w vessel wall and stent	• Little clinical data • Increased target vessel revascularization/restenosis at 1 year follow-up
Manual thrombectomy	Thrombus removal	• Partial thrombus removal • Not always effective • Conflicting data
Direct stenting	Minimizes distal embolization	• Inadequate stent sizing • Suboptimal stent deployment
Delayed stenting	Allow thrombus clearing and optimal stent deployment	• Longer hospital stay • Risk of reocclusion

increased mortality. Observational studies suggest direct stenting might be associated with better angiographic outcomes and less no reflow (Table 4). In a recent meta-analysis,[34] direct stenting was associated with lower mortality, which is likely mediated by reduced microvascular damage, improved myocardial perfusion and low incidence of heart failure.

Balloon versus Stents

Stents do not offer mortality benefit over plain balloon angioplasty but have advantage of lesser restenosis. Drug-eluting stents (DES) are current standard of treatment during PPCI without offering any mortality benefit. Long-term follow-up of 11 trials has shown that with DES there is 47% reduction in target vessel revascularization (TVR) without any change in mortality.[35] Also, stent thrombosis rates were significantly lower in the DES group 4 (0.5%) patients with definite stent thrombosis in the DES group vs 14 (1.9%) in the bare-metal stents (BMS) group in Examination Trial, using second generation everolimus eluting stent, alleviating initial fear of high stent thrombosis in DES.[36]

Periprocedural Thrombotic Complications

Distal embolization is common during primary PCI. Significantly large emboli in distal coronary bed can be managed with manual thrombectomy catheters.

Slow flow and no reflow are one of the most feared complications of primary PCI and occur in 8.8–11.5% of cases. Adequate anticoagulation including glycoprotein IIb/IIIa inhibitors, minimalistic approaches such as direct stenting and minimizing manipulation may reduce the risk of slow/no reflow.

Table 5: Intracoronary drug regimens for slow/no reflow.

Drug	Dose*
Verapamil	100–200 µg up to four doses
Adenosine	24 µg up to four doses
Sodium nitroprusside	100 µg up to total of 1,000 µg
Adrenaline	50–200 µg

*We recommend larger doses as long as patient is hemodynamically stable.

Several pharmaceutical agents such as intracoronary calcium channel blockers, adenosine, nitroprusside, nicorandil and epinephrine can be delivered to distal microvasculature beyond target lesion using either thrombosuction devices or over the wire balloon (Table 5).[37]

Intra-aortic Balloon Pump

A meta-analysis published in 2009 and two more trials published recently have failed to show any benefit for intra-aortic balloon pump (IABP) in the setting of anterior wall STEMI and complex PCI.[38,39] Although, IABP has shown benefit in certain subgroups, its use is primarily limited to individual preferences and clinical judgment.

NONADHERENCE TO P2Y12 INHIBITORS

EDUCATE Study

Any nonadherence (ANA) defined by missing ≥ 1 days of DAPT) is common, with estimated 9.6% of patients demonstrating ANA in the 6 months after DES placement. EDUCATE (Endeavor Drug-Eluting Stenting: Understanding Care Antiplatelet Agents and Thrombotic Events) indicated that ANA within 6 months after DES placement is associated increased all-cause mortality, cardiac mortality, and adverse cardiovascular outcomes.

CONCLUSION

Following are the salient points, which should be taken care while performing PCI in STEMI:
- Successful primary angioplasty requires teamwork at multiple levels from patient education about symptoms, early identification by health personnel, timely referal to capable center and availability of quick transport.
- Pharmacoinvasive approach if performed within 3–24 hours of thrombolysis, results significantly reduction in death and reinfarction without increase in stroke.

- The procedure should be kept as simple and as short as possible.
- All patients should receive dual antiplatelet therapy.
- Choice between clopidogrel, prasugrel and ticagrelor should be based on the risk of bleeding balanced with potential clinical benefit.
- Bivalirudin may be preferred over UFH when bleeding risk is high.
- Adjunctive GP IIb/IIIa inhibitors use at time of PCI can be considered on individual basis for large thrombus burden (as in bail out) or inadequate antiplatelet drug loading.
- Experience should guide the selection of access (radial vs. femoral) as well as selection of hardware.
- Radial access should be preferred over femoral.
- Routine Thromboaspiration in all STEMI cases is not recommended.
- Distal protection devices have no role in native vessel primary PCI.
- DES is standard of care in primary PCI.
- Direct stenting is a feasible option.
- Slow flow and no reflow are dreaded complication but can be easily managed with intracoronary drugs.

REFERENCES

1. Herrick J. An intimate account of my early experience with coronary thrombosis. Am Heart J. 1944;27:1.
2. Braunwald E. The treatment of acute myocardial infarction: the past, the present, and the future. Eur Heart J Acute Cardiovasc Care. 2012;1:9.
3. Hartzler GO, Rutherford BD, McConahay DR, et al. Percutaneous transluminal coronary angioplasty with and without thrombolytic therapy for treatment of acute myocardial infarction. Am Heart J. 1983;106 (5 pt 1):956-73.
4. Keeley EC, Boura JA, Grines CL. Primary angioplasty versus intravenous thrombolytic therapy for acute myocardial infarction: a quantitative review of 23 randomised trials. Lancet. 2003;361(9351):13-20.
5. Chazov EI, Matveeva LS, Mazaev AV, et al. Intracoronary administration of fibrinolysin in acute myocardial infarction (in Russian). Ter Arkh. 1976;48(4):8-19.
6. DeWood MA, Spores J, Notske R, et al. Prevalence of total coronary occlusion during the early hours of transmural myocardial infarction. N Eng J Med. 1980;303(16):897-902.
7. Gruppo Italino per lo Studio della Streptochinasi nell'Infarto Miocardico (GISSI). Effectiveness of intravenous thrombolytic treatment in myocardial infarction. Lancet. 1986;1(8478):397-402.
8. The GUSTO Investigators. An international randomized trial comparing four thrombolytic strategies for acute myocardial infarction. N Engl J Med. 1993;329(10):673-82.
9. Van De Werf F, Adgey J, Ardissino D, et al. Single bolus tenecteblase compared with front loaded alteplase in acute myocardial infarction: the ASSENT-2 double blinded randomized trial. Lancet. 1999;354(9180):716-22.
10. American College of Emergency Physicians; Society for Cardiovascular Angiography and Interventions, O'Gara PT, Kushner FG, Ascheim DD, et al. 2013 ACCF/AHA guideline for the management of ST-elevation myocardial

infarction: a report of the American College of Cardiology Foundation American Heart Association Task Force on Practice Guidelines. J Am Coll Cardiol. 2013;61:e78-140.
11. Dalby M, Bouzamondo A, Lechat P, et al. Transfer for primary angioplasty versus immediate thrombolysis in acute myocardial infarction: a meta-analysis. Circulation. 2003;108:1809-14.
12. Xavier D, Pais P, Devereaux PJ, et al. for the CREATE Registry Investigators. Treatment and outcomes of acute coronary syndromes in India (CREATE): a prospective analysis of registry data. Lancet. 2008;371:1435-42.
13. Baliga RR, Bahl VK, Thomas Alexander et al. Management of STEMI in low- and middle-income Countries Global Heart. 2014;9(4):469-510.
14. Borgia F, Goodman SG, Halvorsen S, et al. Early routine percutaneous coronary intervention after fibrinolysis vs. standard therapy in ST-segment elevation myocardial infarction: a meta-analysis. Eur Heart J. 2010;31(17):2156-69.
15. Armstrong PW, Gershlick AH, Goldstein P, et al. STREAM Investigative Team. Fibrinolysis or primary PCI in ST-segment elevation myocardial infarction. N Engl J Med. 2013;368(15):1379-87.
16. Mehta SR, Tanguay JF, Eikelboom JW, et al. Double-dose versus standard-dose clopidogrel and high-dose versus low-dose aspirin in individuals undergoing percutaneous coronary intervention for acute coronary syndromes (CURRENT-OASIS 7): a randomised factorial trial. Lancet. 2010;376(9748):1233-43
17. Steg PG, James S, Harrington RA, et al. Ticagrelor versus clopidogrel in patients with ST-elevation acute coronary syndromes intended for reperfusion with primary percutaneous coronary intervention: a Platelet Inhibition and Patient Outcomes (PLATO) trial subgroup analysis. Circulation. 2010;122(21):2131-41.
18. Grines CL, Browne KF, Marco J, et al. for the PAMI Study Group. A comparison of immediate angioplasty with thrombolytic therapy for acute myocardial infarction. N Engl J Med. 1993;328:673-9.
19. Aversano T, Aversano LT, Passamani E, et al. for the Atlantic Cardiovascular Patient Outcomes Research Team. Thrombolytic therapy vs primary percutaneous coronary intervention for myocardial infarction in patients presenting to hospitals without on-site cardiac surgery: a randomized controlled trial. JAMA. 2002;287:1943-51.
20. Gershlick AH, Khan JN, Kelly DJ, et al. Randomized trial of complete versus lesion-only revascularization in patients undergoing primary percutaneous coronary intervention for STEMI and multivessel disease The CvLPRIT trial. J Am Coll Cardiol. 2015;65(10):963-72.
21. Wald DS, Morris JK, Wald NJ, et al. Randomized trial of preventive angioplasty in myocardial infarction. N Engl J Med. 2013;369:1115-23.
22. 2015 ACC/AHA/SCAI Focused Update on Primary Percutaneous Coronary Intervention for Patients With ST-Elevation Myocardial Infarction. VOL. 67, NO. 10, 2016. http://dx.doi.org/10.1016/j.jacc.2015.10.005.
23. Stone GW, Webb J, Cox DA, et al. Enhanced Myocardial Efficacy and Recovery by Aspiration of Liberated Debris (EMERALD) investigators. Distal microcirculatory protection during percutaneous coronary intervention in acute ST-segment elevation myocardial infarction. A randomized controlled trial. JAMA. 2005;293:1063-72.
24. Gick M, Jander N, Bestehorn HP, et al. Randomized evaluation of the effects of filterbased distal protection on myocardial perfusion and infarct size after primary percutaneous catheter intervention in myocardial infarction with and without ST-segment elevation. Circulation. 2005;112:1462-9.

25. Silva-Orrego P, Colombo P, Bigi R, et al. Thrombus aspiration before primary angioplasty improves myocardial reperfusion in acute myocardial infarction: the DEARMI (Dethrombosis to Enhance Acute Reperfusion in Myocardial Infarction) study. J Am Coll Cardiol. 2006;48:1552-9.
26. De Luca G, Suryapranata H, Stone GW, et al. Abciximab as adjunctive therapy to reperfusion in acute ST-segment elevation myocardial infarction: a meta-analysis of randomized trials. JAMA. 2005;293:1759-65.
27. Van't Hof AW, Ten Berg J, Heestermans T, et al. Prehospital initiation of tirofiban in patients with ST-elevation myocardial infarction undergoing primary angioplasty (On-TIME 2): a multicentre, double-blind, randomised controlled trial. Lancet. 2008;372:537-46.
28. Wander GS, Gupta NK. Antithrombotics and antiplatelets in acute myocardial infarction. Indian Heart J. 2011;63:58-65.
29. Stone GW, Witzenbichler B, Guagliumi G, et al. HORIZONS-AMI Trial Investigators. Bivalirudin during primary PCI in acute myocardial infarction. N Engl J Med. 2008;358:2218-30.
30. Steg PG, Van't Hof A, Clemmensen P, et al. Design and methods of European Ambulance Acute Coronary Syndrome Angiography Trial (EUROMAX): an international randomized open label ambulance trial of bivalirudin versus standard-of-care anticoagulation in patients with acute ST-segment elevation myocardial infarction transferred for primary percutaneous coronary intervention. Am Heart J. 2013;166:960-7.
31. Stone GW, Mehran R, Goldstein P, et al. Bivalirudin versus heparin with or without glycoprotein iib/iiia inhibitors in patients with STEMI undergoing primary percutaneous coronary intervention pooled patient-level analysis from the HORIZONS-AMI and EUROMAX trials. JACC. 2015;65:27-38.
32. Montalescot G, Zeymer U, Silvain J, et al. Intravenous enoxaparin or unfractionated heparin in primary percutaneous coronary intervention for ST-elevation myocardial infarction: the international randomised open-label ATOLL trial. Lancet. 2011;378:693-703.
33. Yusuf S, Mehta SR, Chrolavicius S, et al. Effects of fondaparinux on mortality and reinfarction in patients with acute ST-segment elevation myocardial infarction: the OASIS-6 randomized trial. JAMA. 2006;295:1519-30.
34. Azzalini L, Millan X, LY HQ, et al. Direct stenting versus pre-dilation in ST-elevation myocardial infarction: a systematic review and meta-analysis. J Interv Cardiol. 2015;28(2):119-31.
35. De Luca G, Dirksen MT, Spaulding C, et al. Drug-eluting vs bare-metal stents in primary angioplasty: a pooled patient-level meta-analysis of randomized trials. Arch Intern Med. 2012;172(8):611-21.
36. Sabate M, Cequier A, Iñiguez A, et al. Everolimus-eluting stent versus bare-metal stent in ST-segment elevation myocardial infarction (EXAMINATION): 1 year results of a randomised controlled trial. Lancet. 2012;380(9852):1482-90.
37. Prasad S, Meredith IT. Current approach to slow flow and no-reflow. Cardiac Interventions Today. 2008:43-51.
38. Sjauw KD, Engström AE, Vis MM, et al. A systematic review and meta-analysis of intra-aortic balloon pump therapy in ST-elevation myocardial infarction: should we change the guidelines? Eur Heart J. 2009;30:459-68.
39. Thiele H, Zeymer U, Neumann FJ, et al. IABP-SHOCK II Trial Investigators. Intraaortic balloon support for myocardial infarction with cardiogenic shock. N Engl J Med. 2012;367:1287-96

11 High-Risk Percutaneous Coronary Interventions

Upendra Kaul, Satyendra Tiwari

DEFINING HIGH-RISK PCI CRITERIA

There is lack of consensus on what defines high-risk percutaneous coronary intervention (PCI) due to diversity of anatomic, procedural and clinical characteristics. Only when these characteristics get combined, it constitutes a high-risk PCI (Table 1). It is the relative inability of the high-risk patient

Table 1: Clinical, anatomic, and hemodynamic criteria used to identify the high-risk percutaneous coronary intervention patients.

Clinical criteria
- Cardiogenic shock occurring within 24 hours or at the start of coronary intervention
- Left ventricular systolic dysfunction on presentation: ejection fraction ≤ 30–40%
- Killip class II–IV on presentation or congestive heart failure
- Coronary intervention after resuscitated cardiac arrest within 24 hours ST-segment elevation myocardial infarction
- Acute coronary syndrome complicated by unstable hemodynamics, dysrhythmia, or refractory angina
- Mechanical complications of acute myocardial infarction age ≥ 70–80 years
- History of cerebrovascular disease, diabetes, renal dysfunction, or chronic lung disease

Anatomic criteria
- PCI to unprotected left main coronary artery or left main equivalent
- Distal left main bifurcation intervention
- Multi-vessel disease
- Previous coronary artery bypass graft surgery including intervention to a graft, particularly a degenerated graft
- Last remaining coronary conduit
- Target vessel providing a collateral supply to an occluded second vessel that supplies > 40% of the left ventricular myocardium
- SYNTAX score ≥ 33

Hemodynamic criteria
- Cardiac index < 2.2 l/min/m^2
- Pulmonary capillary wedge pressure > 15 mm Hg
- Mean pulmonary artery pressure > 50 mm Hg

to withstand the deleterious hemodynamic consequences of dysrhythmia, transient intervals of ischemia-reperfusion injury, or the distal embolization of atherogenic material (i.e., the no-reflow phenomenon) which get associated with PCI. A high-risk patient may have diminished cardiovascular reserve and would be susceptible to post-ischemic stunning of the myocardium. Therefore it becomes important to recognize this subset and anticipate difficulties that might occur during the procedure. The aim being to decide whether mechanical circulatory support (MCS) needs to be instituted. Otherwise, vicious cycle of deleterious events starts, leading to further reduction in cardiac output (CO) and ischemia, which results in cardiogenic shock (CS) or fatal ventricular arrhythmias.

On the other hand patient may be in CS on presentation, a diagnosis based on evidence of hypotension (systolic blood pressure < 90 mm Hg), end-organ hypo-perfusion (cool extremities and urine output < 30 mL/h), a cardiac index (CI) of ≤ 2.2 l/min/m², and a pulmonary capillary wedge pressure of ≥ 15 mm Hg.[1] There is evidence that mixed venous blood oxygen saturation < 65% can also be incorporated.[2]

MECHANICAL CIRCULATORY SUPPORT DEVICES (FIGS. 1 AND 2, TABLES 2 AND 3)

Mechanical circulatory support devices have therapeutic impact on CS by following mechanism:
1. Maintenance of end-organ perfusion
2. Optimization of myocardial perfusion

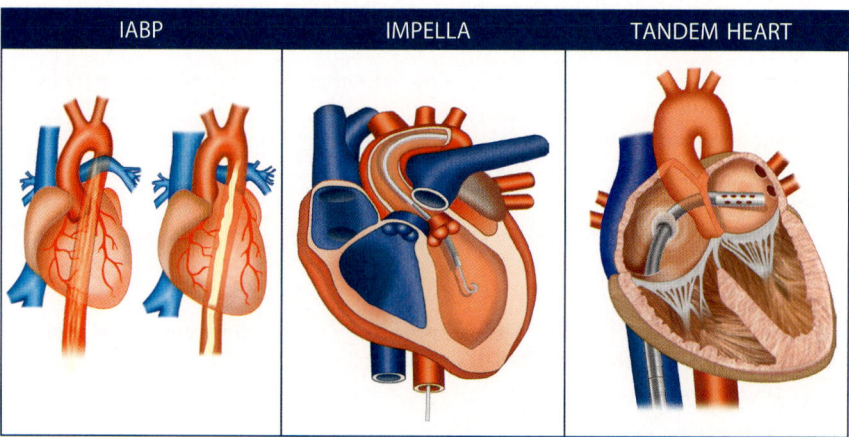

Fig. 1: Mechanical circulatory support devices.

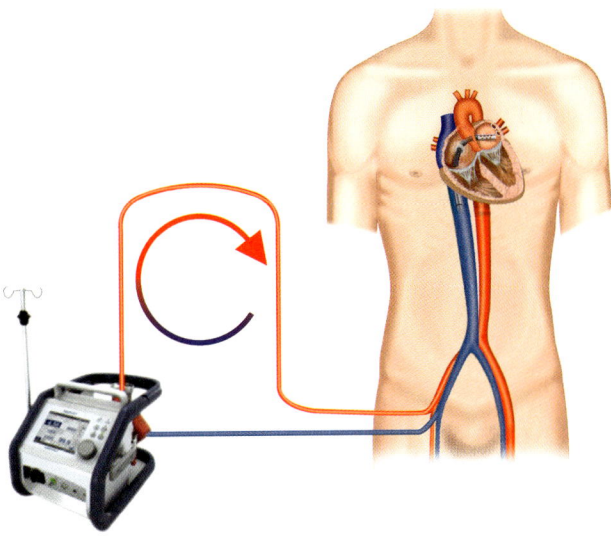

Fig. 2: Percutaneous extracorporeal membrane oxygenation.

Table 2: Percutaneous coronary assist devices.

IABP	Impella	Tandem Heart
Advantages	*Advantages*	*Advantages*
• Available everywhere • Easy implantation • Lower profile so minimizing complications • Newer system calibrate automatically accelerating time to effective diastolic augmentation • Different ranges of balloons available for different heights of patients • Larger volume balloons displace more blood providing enhanced diastolic augmentation	• Can augment CO by • 2.5 l/min (Impella 2.5) to 4.0 l/min (Impella-CP / cVAD) • Can be used to support circulation for up to 7 days • Does not require stable cardiac rhythm or native CO for optimal cardiac function	• Can increase cardiac output by 4–5 l/min • Can be used to support circulation upto 14 days • Does not require stable cardiac rhythm or native CO for optimal cardiac function
Disadvantages	*Disadvantages*	*Disadvantages*
• Can only supplement cardiac output by 0.3 to 0.5 l/min	• Not universally available	• Not universally available

Contd...

Contd...

• Twisting and kinking or clot formation in catheter line/pressure line • Small risk of aortic dissection or rupture • Systemic embolization • Stroke • Infection • Lower limb ischemia • Hemolysis • Bleeding at insertion site	• Requires 12–14 Fr sheath so prone to more vascular complication • Non-pulsatile flow • Risk of displacement of inflow from LV to aorta • Systemic embolism • Stroke • Infection • Lower limb ischemia • Hemolysis	• Require specialized for trans septal technique with 21 Fr cannula • Relatively longer implant time. • Implantation cannot be done during CPR • Complex post implant management • 17 Fr femoral cannula causing more vascular complication • Systemic embolism • Infection • Limb ischemia • Hemolysis

(IABP: Intra-aortic balloon counterpulsation; CO: Cardiac output; CP: Cardiac power; cVAD: Continuous ventricular assist device; LV: Left ventricle; CPR: Cardiopulmonary resuscitation).

Table 3: Percutaneous extracorporeal membrane oxygenation.

Advantages	Disadvantages
• Can augment CO by >4.5 l/min • Can be used to support circulation for several weeks • Does not require a stable cardiac rhythm for optimal function	• Not universally available • Non pulsatile blood flow • Relative lung ischemia • Risk of lung over inflation leading to alkalosis • Possible poor coronary and cerebral perfusion • May require concomitant IABP, inotropes • Stroke • Embolism • Infection • Lower limb ischemia • Hemolysis

(CO: Cardiac output; IABP: Intra-aortic balloon counterpulsation).

MAINTENANCE OF END-ORGAN PERFUSION

The landmark SHOCK (Should We Emergently Re-vascularize Occluded Coronaries for Cardiogenic Shock) trial demonstrated a mid to long-term survival advantage for early revascularization vs medical stabilization for managing acute myocardial infarction (AMI) complicated by CS.[1,3,4] *Post hoc* analysis of the SHOCK trial registry also confirmed the benefit of IABP for lowering in-hospital mortality.[5,6] The SHOCK investigators introduced the concept of cardiac power output [in W = mean arterial pressure (MAP) ×

CO/451] and cardiac power index (in W/m² = cardiac power output/body surface area) as novel hemodynamic parameters for the assessment and subsequent management of CS core function, therefore the mechanical support should be used to augment MAP and CO to maintain end-organ perfusion, thereby avoiding (or rationalizing) the use of supplementary vasopressor or inotrope therapy.

OPTIMIZATION OF MYOCARDIAL PERFUSION

During acute MI (AMI), the microvascular resistance is high as a result of vasoconstriction, plugging related to micro-emboli, and ischemia-reperfusion injury. In CS, this is compounded by a decrease in driving pressure and an increase in right atrial pressure.[7] Mechanical support devices should ideally facilitate myocardial perfusion by increasing the MAP and reducing right atrial pressure to overcome the higher resistance encountered in the infarct-related territory.

INTRA-AORTIC BALLOON COUNTER PULSATION (IABP)

Intra-aortic balloon counter pulsation allows increased myocardial perfusion by increasing the coronary pressure gradient from the aorta to the epicardial coronary circulation at a time when the aortic valve is closed.[8] Active deflation immediately before the onset of systole and precisely at the beginning of ISO-volumetric contraction creates a dead space in the thoracic aorta, which reduces afterload and promotes forward flow from the left venticle (LV). This causes a reduction in LV end-diastolic pressure, volume, wall tension, and work (which lowers myocardial oxygen demand) that results in increase in stroke volume, ejection fraction and CO.[8]

The blood volume displaced toward the aortic root has been calculated at 6.4% (during 1:1 inflation) and 10.0% (with 1:2 support) of the nominal balloon volume.[9] The remainder is stored in the compliant aortic wall during balloon inflation or distributed among the branches along the arch. Although this percentage appears small, it represents a significant fraction of baseline coronary flow.[9]

The benefit of IABP on high-risk patients with severe coronary disease might relate to a reduction in oxygen demand through LV systolic unloading over and above that stimulated by diastolic augmentation of coronary blood flow (CBF).[10]

EVIDENCE-BASED OBSERVATIONAL AND REGISTRY DATA

A recent US Cath PCI Registry analysis revealed that IABP use was limited to just 10.5% of all high-risk PCI procedures.[11] This could partly reflect a lack of interoperator and interhospital consensus on what is deemed high-risk. Euro Heart Survey PCI Registry of those patients revascularized for CS as a complication of AMI revealed that the IABP was only used in 24.8% of cases.[12] Again IABP use did not confer an overall survival advantage which led not to use the device routinely.

Current data from registries and retrospective analyses cannot be used to confidently support the IABP in high-risk PCI.

Some studies have shown a significant benefit of IABP in terms of in-hospital mortality[13] and freedom from periprocedural events[14,15] whereas others have shown no benefit[16] or a trend towards harm.[17]

EVIDENCE BASED RANDOMIZED TRIAL DATA

Early ST-segment elevation myocardial infarction (STEMI) trials have shown benefit when IABP was implanted postprocedure for 36 to 48 h.[18,19] But these patients were treated primarily by balloon angioplasty whereas in modern day PCI drug eluting stents are being used. There is evidence that IABP reduces mortality when combined with thrombolysis for AMI.[17]

Balloon Pump-Assisted Coronary Intervention Study-1 (BCIS-1 TRIAL). It was the first prospective, open, multicenter RCT designed to determine whether elective IABP insertion before high-risk single-vessel or multi-vessel PCI was able to reduce major adverse cardiac and cerebrovascular events at 28 days.[20] The study did not support the use of prophylactic IABP insertion before high-risk PCI. Five-year all-cause mortality data from this study is available.[21] which has shown significant survival advantage in favor of elective IABP (hazard ratio: 0.66, 95% confidence interval: 0.44 to 0.98, p = 0.039).

Counter-pulsation to Reduce Infarct Size Pre-PCI AMI (CRISP AMI) trial is a prospective, open, multicenter RCT undertaken to determine whether prophylactic IABP insertion within 6 h of pain onset and planned primary PCI (PPCI) for anterior STEMI (without CS) could reduce the mean infarct size, as measured by cardiac magnetic resonance imaging between 3 and 5 days post-intervention.[22] IABP insertion in the PPCI alone group was at the operator's discretion for indications such as persistent hypotension, overt CS, malignant arrhythmias, and AMI complications. Of note, 15 patients (8.5%) initially receiving standard care crossed over to IABP.

This shows that high-risk patients are prone to hemodynamic collapse, which supports the argument for standby MCS. With early reperfusion from PPCI having dominant effect on myocardial salvage and hence mortality, it could be argued that any further adjunctive measures would add very little to the net clinical benefit. Therefore strategy of routine prophylactic IABP implantation in PPCI of STEMI without CS cannot be advocated.

IABP-SHOCK II (INTRA-AORTIC BALLOON PUMP IN CS II) TRIAL

The trial enrolled 600 patients with CS complicating AMI proceeding to early revascularization (almost double that of the landmark SHOCK trial), who were then randomized in an open-label manner to IABP or no IABP. At 1 year, mortality remained similar in both arms (IABP group 52% vs control group 51%; p = 0.91). IABP insertion did no excess harm, with no significant differences between either group in terms of stroke, bleeding, sepsis, or peripheral ischemic complications requiring intervention.[23]

As a result, the use of IABP in CS complicating AMI has been downgraded from a previous class I indication to a class IIa and IIb recommendation in the most recent U.S. and European STEMI guidelines, respectively (Table 2).[24,25]

Impella Device

The Impella (Abiomed Inc) is placed across the aortic valve under radiographic or echocardiographic guidance. It aspirates blood from the left ventricle into the ascending aorta. Impella-mediated LV unloading reduces end-diastolic wall stress, improves diastolic compliance, increases aortic and intracoronary pressure and coronary flow velocity reserve, and stimulates a decrease in coronary microvascular resistance.[26,27] This may allow for recovery of hibernating or stunned myocardium.

The Impella 2.5 received U.S. Food and Drug Administration approval in June 2008 and can provide ante-grade flow up to 2.5 l/min (Fig. 1). The newly introduced Impella CP (known as cVAD in Europe) received U.S. Food and Drug Administration approval in September 2012 and is based on the same 2.5 platform but can provide flow up to 4.0 l/min.

The use of the Impella in high-risk PCI including CS is feasible according to registries and small single-center studies, with demonstrable improvements in CI and myocardial performance.

However, the increase in vascular access complications and the hemolysis due to the high rotational speed of the axial flow pump do not appear to be outweighed by significant gains in survival. The EUROSHOCK registry reported a 30-day mortality of 64.2% in patients presenting with CS complicating AMI, with access site complications in 24.2%.[28] The excess mortality could have been secondary to a selection bias isolating the very sickest patients with a poor hemodynamic profile and imminent risk of death. Moreover, Impella support was only instituted once CS had become refractory to high-dose inotropes and IABP. The ISAR-SHOCK (Efficacy Study of LV Assist Device to Treat Patients With Cardiogenic Shock) study randomized 25 patients with AMI complicated by CS to IABP (n = 13) or the Impella LP 2.5 (n = 12) implanted post-revascularization.[29] The Impella achieved significantly greater augmentation of CI, but this did not result in improved 30-day survival.

The **PROTECT II** (Prospective Randomized Clinical Trial of Hemodynamic Support with Impella 2.5 vs Intra-aortic Balloon Pump in Patients Undergoing High-Risk PCI) study is the largest randomized comparison of the Impella and IABP to support high-risk PCI to date.[30] The primary composite endpoint of major adverse events at hospital discharge or 30 days (whichever came sooner) in the intention-to-treat population (n = 448) was similar in both arms (Impella 35.1% vs IABP 40.1%; p = 0.277). At 90 days, there was a nonsignificant trend toward a lower major adverse event rate for the Impella (p = 0.066). At 90 days in the per-protocol population (n = 427), that trend became significant (p = 0.023), suggesting that the Impella may hold promise over the longer term.

TANDEM HEART

The Tandem Heart (Cardiac Assist, Inc., Pittsburgh, Pennsylvania) is inserted via the femoral vein and right atrium into the left atrium via a trans-septal puncture. The outflow cannula is inserted in either femoral artery and positioned at the level of the aortic bifurcation, providing left heart bypass at a flow rate of 4 l/min into the lower abdominal aorta or iliac arteries (Fig. 1). Studies of the Tandem Heart in severe refractory CS have shown the device to improve CI, MAP, and reduce pulmonary capillary wedge pressure, pulmonary artery pressure, and central venous pressure, leading to decreased filling pressures in both ventricles.[31,32] The Tandem Heart is a high-profile system so critical limb ischemia, bleeding, and vascular complications are a major concern.

EXTRACORPOREAL MEMBRANE OXYGENATION

Veno-arterial extracorporeal membrane oxygenation (ECMO) is effectively a modified cardiopulmonary bypass circuit that provides a continuous, non- pulsatile CO that can be applied percutaneously via cannulation of the femoral artery and vein (Fig. 2).[33,34] ECMO removes carbon dioxide from and adds oxygen to venous blood via an artificial membrane, thereby bypassing the pulmonary circulation. As such, it is the only PCAD that also oxygenates the blood. ECMO can provide significant hemodynamic support but has a propensity to increase LV afterload and wall stress, which in turn can increase myocardial oxygen demand and therefore limit any cardioprotective benefit (Table 3).

The system is composed of a venous reservoir, external centrifugal blood pump, membrane oxygenator, and a rewarming heparin-coated circuit. The technology has become smaller and more portable. Systemic anticoagulation with heparin is required to achieve an activated clotting time of 150 to 180s.[35] Contraindications to ECMO include significant aortic valve incompetence, severe peripheral arterial disease, bleeding diathesis, recent stroke or head trauma, and uncontrolled sepsis. A retrospective analysis of prophylactic vs standby cardiopulmonary support revealed significantly greater procedural morbidity (e.g., femoral access site complications) in the former (41% vs 9.4%, p < 0.01) but higher procedural mortality in the latter (4.8% vs 18.8%, p < 0.05).[36] The investigators suggested that standby cardiopulmonary support (CPS) was preferable in the majority although patients with LVEF <20% may benefit from a prophylactic strategy.

Early institution of ECMO for STEMI complicated by CS has been shown to significantly reduce 30-day mortality when compared with an historical cohort of patients not receiving cardiopulmonary support.[37] Observational studies and case reports constitute the evidence base on ECMO-assisted high-risk PCI.[34] All confirm the feasibility and efficacy of ECMO, but vascular complications remains problem. A reduction in platelet count, hemolysis, and a consumptive coagulopathy along with systemic heparinization can further increase the hemorrhagic risk. Since no RCT or meta-analysis data are available for ECMO, current guidelines can only be based on expert consensus (*see* Table 2).

CONCLUSION

Despite good physiological understanding, the per cutaneous cardiac assist device (PCADs) to support high-risk PCI.[11,12] reflect the equivocal results and mixed opinions coming from the current available evidence. From a clinical point, the PCADs like IABP, Impella, Tandem Heart, and ECMO should have optimal place in high-risk PCI, although they cannot be used as standard of care for every high-risk procedure. PCAD uses should be based on case-to-case selection, which patient may benefit from a particular device and subsequently to ensure MCS availability in the catheterization laboratory. This comes only from shared expertise, familiarity with and confidence in using all 4 adjunctive devices, supported by an experienced heart team.

There must be common consensus to establish and accept standardized criteria for high-risk PCI. So far, only the American College of Cardiology Foundation/American Heart Association/Society for Cardiovascular Angiography and Interventions guideline writing committee has documented these features and addressed evidence based recommendations (Table 4).

In general it is believed that the IABP, Impella, Tandem Heart, and ECMO fulfill each criterion to some degree. One should not be much eager to determine that which device is superior among these. Based on patient, anatomic, hemodynamic, and procedural characteristics that warrant adjunctive MCS may be necessary in particular case, to prepare the subject and catheterization laboratory accordingly, and then to perform the PCI.

Table 4: Current guidelines for the use of percutaneous circulatory assist devices during high-risk PCI.

American College of Cardiology/American Heart Association/Society for Cardiovascular Angiography and Interventions Recommendations

STEMI, 2013[24]	IABP can be useful for patients in cardiogenic shock after STE-MI who do not quickly stabilize with pharmacological therapy. Class IIa, Level of evidence: B	Alternative left ventricular assist. devices for circulatory support may be considered in refractory CS Class IIb, Level of evidence: C
UA/NSTEMI, 2013	IABP is reasonable in UA/NSTEMI patients for continuing or frequently recurring severe ischemia despite intensive medical therapy, hemodynamic instability pre- or post-angiography, and for mechanical complications of MI Class IIa, Level of evidence: C	No individual device recommendations

European Society of Cardiology Recommendations

PCI, 2014[38]	Short-term mechanical circulatory support in ACS patients with cardiogenic shock may be considered. Class IIb, Level of evidence: C IABP insertion should be considered in patients with hemodynamic instability/cardiogenic shock due to mechanical complications (Class IIa, Level of evidence: C) Routine use of IABP in patients with cardiogenic shock is not recommended. (Class III, Level of evidence: A)

(PCI: Percutaneous coronary interventions; STEMI: ST-segment elevation myocardial infarction; IABP: Intra-aortic balloon counterpulsation; CS: Cardiogenic shock; UA: Unstable angina; NSTEMI: Non-ST elevation MI; MI: Myocardial infarction; ACS: Acute coronary syndrome).

REFERENCES

1. Hochman J, Sleeper L, Webb J, et al. Early revascularization in acute myocardial infarction complicated by cardiogenic shock. N Engl J Med. 1999;341:625-34.
2. Van't Hof AW, Liem AL, de Boer MJ, Hoorntje JC, Suryapranata H, Zijlstra F. A randomized comparison of intra-aortic balloon pumping after primary coronary angioplasty in high risk patients with acute myocardial infarction. Eur Heart J. 1999;20:659-65.
3. Hochman J, Sleeper LA, White HD, et al. One-year survival following early revascularization for cardiogenic shock. JAMA. 2001;285:190-2.
4. Hochman J, Sleeper LA, Webb J, et al. Early revascularization and long-term survival in cardiogenic shock complicating acute myocardial infarction. JAMA. 2006;295:2511-5.

5. Sanborn TA, Sleeper LA, Bates ER, et al. Impact of thrombolysis, intra-aortic balloon pump counter pulsation, and their combination in cardiogenic shock complicating acute myocardial infarction: a report from the SHOCK trial registry. J Am Coll Cardiol. 2000;36:1123-9.
6. Hochman JS, Buller CE, Sleeper LA, et al. Cardiogenic shock complicating acute myocardial infarction-etiologies, management and outcome: a report from the SHOCK trial registry. J Am Coll Cardiol. 2000;36:1063-70.
7. Reynolds HR, Hochman JS. Cardiogenic shock: current concepts and improving outcomes. Circulation 2008;117:686-97.
8. Myat A, Mcconkey H, Chick L, Baker J, Redwood SR. The intra-aortic balloon pump in high-risk percutaneous coronary intervention: is counterpulsation counterproductive? Interv Cardiol. 2012;4:211-34.
9. Kolyva C, Pantalos GM, Pepper JR, Khir AW. How much of the intraaortic balloon volume is displaced toward the coronary circulation? J Thorac Cardiovasc Surg. 2010;140:110-6.
10. Yoshitani H, Akasaka T, Kaji S, et al. Effects of intra-aortic balloon counterpulsation on coronary pressure in patients with stenotic coronary arteries. Am Heart J. 2007;154:725-31.
11. Curtis JP, Rathore SS, Wang Y, Chen J, Nallamothu BK, Krumholz HM. Use and effectiveness of intra-aortic balloon pumps among patients undergoing high risk percutaneous coronary intervention: insights from the National Cardiovascular Data Registry. Circ Cardiovasc Qual Outcomes. 2012;5:21-30.
12. Zeymer U, Bauer T, Hamm C, et al. Use and impact of intra-aortic balloon pump on mortality in patients with acute myocardial infarction complicated by cardiogenic shock: results of the Euro Heart Survey on PCI. EuroIntervention 2011; 7:437-41.
13. Mishra S, Chu WW, Torguson R, et al. Role of prophylactic intra-aortic balloon pump in high-risk patients undergoing percutaneous coronary intervention. Am J Cardiol. 006;98:608-12.
14. Brodie BR, Stuckey TD, Hansen C, Muncy D. Intra-aortic balloon counterpulsation before primary percutaneous transluminal coronary angioplasty reduces catherterization laboratory events in high-risk patients with acute myocardial infarction. Am J Cardiol. 1999;84:18-23.
15. Briguori C, Sarais C, Pagnotta P, et al. Elective versus provisional intra-aortic balloon pumping in high-risk percutaneous transluminal coronary angioplasty. Am Heart J. 2003;145:700-7.
16. Ishihara M, Sato H, Tateishi H, Uchida T, Dote K. Intraaortic balloon pumping as the postangioplasty strategy in acute myocardial infarction. Am Heart J. 1991;122:385-9.
17. Barron HV, Every NR, Parsons LS, et al. The use of intra-aortic balloon counterpulsation in patients with cardiogenic shock complicating acute myocardial infarction: data from the National Registry of Myocardial Infarction 2. Am Heart J. 2001;141:933-9.
18. Stone G, Marsalese D, Brodie BR, et al. A prospective, randomized evaluation of prophylactic intraaortic balloon counterpulsation in high risk patients with acute myocardial infarction treated with primary angioplasty. J Am Coll Cardiol. 1997;29:1459-67.
19. Ohman EM, George BS, White CJ, et al. The Randomized IABP Study Group. Use of aortic counterpulsation to improve sustained coronary artery patency

during acute myocardial infarction. Results of a randomized trial. Circulation 1994;90792-9.
20. Perera D, Stables R, Thomas M, et al. Elective intra-aortic balloon counterpulsation during high-risk percutaneous coronary intervention: a randomized controlled trial. JAMA. 2010;304:867-74.
21. Perera D, Stables R, Clayton T, et al. Longterm mortality data from the balloon pump assisted coronary intervention study (BCIS-1): a randomized, controlled trial of elective balloon counterpulsation during high-risk percutaneous coronary intervention. Circulation. 2013;127:207-12.
22. Patel MR, Smalling RW, Thiele H, et al. Intraaortic balloon counterpulsation and infarct size in patients with acute anterior myocardial infarction without shock: the CRISP AMI randomized trial. JAMA. 2011;306:1329-37.
23. Thiele H, Zeymer U, Neumann F-J, et al. Intraaortic balloon support for myocardial infarction with cardiogenic shock. N Engl J Med. 2012;367:1287-96.
24. O'Gara PT, Kushner FG, Ascheim DD, et al. ACCF/AHA guideline for the management of ST-elevation myocardial infarction: a report of the American College of Cardiology Foundation/ American Heart Association Task Force on Practice Guidelines. J Am Coll Cardiol. 2013;61:e78-140.
25. Steg PG, James SK, Atar D, et al. ESC guidelines for the management of acute myocardial infarction in patients presenting with ST-segment elevation. Eur Heart J. 2012;33:2569-619.
26. Remmelink M, Sjauw KD, Henriques JPS, et al. Effects of mechanical left ventricular unloading by Impella on left ventricular dynamics in high-risk and primary percutaneous coronary intervention patients. Catheter Cardiovasc Interv. 2010;75:187-94.
27. Remmelink M, Sjauw KD, Henriques J, et al. Effects of left ventricular unloading by Impella recover LP2.5 on coronary hemodynamics. Catheter Cardiovasc Interv. 2007;70:532-7.
28. Lauten A, Engström AE, Jung C, et al. Percutaneous left-ventricular support with the Impella-2.5-assist device in acute cardiogenic shock: results of the Impella-EUROSHOCK-registry. Circ Heart Fail 2013;6:23-30.
29. Seyfarth M, Sibbing D, Bauer I, et al. A randomized clinical trial to evaluate the safety and efficacy of a percutaneous left ventricular assist device versus intraaortic balloon pumping for treatment of cardiogenic shock caused by myocardial infarction. J Am Coll Cardiol 2008;52:1584-8.
30. O'Neill WW, Kleiman NS, Moses J, et al. A prospective, randomized clinical trial of hemodynamic support with Impella 2.5 versus intraaortic balloon pump in patients undergoing high-risk percutaneous coronary intervention: the PROTECT II study. Circulation. 2012;126:1717-27.
31. Thiele H, Lauer B, Hambrecht R, Boudriot E, Cohen HA, Schuler G. Reversal of cardiogenic shock by percutaneous left atrial-to-femoral arterial bypass assistance. Circulation. 2001;104:2917-22.
32. Burkhoff D, Cohen H, Brunckhorst C, O'Neill WW. A randomized multicenter clinical study to evaluate the safety and efficacy of the Tandem Heart percutaneous ventricular assist device versus conventional therapy with intraaortic balloon pumping for treatment of cardiogenic shock. Am Heart J. 2006;152:469.e1-8.
33. Dardas P, Mezilis N, Ninios V, et al. ECMO as a bridge to high-risk rotablation of heavily calcified coronary arteries. Herz. 2012;37:225-30.
34. Koutouzis M, Kolsrud O, Albertsson P, Matejka G, Grip L, Kjellman U. Percutaneous coronary intervention facilitated by extracorporeal membrane oxygenation support in a patient with cardiogenic shock. Hellenic J Cardiol. 2010;51: 271-4.

35. Westaby S, Anastasiadis K, Wieselthaler GM. Ardiogenic shock in ACS. Part 2: role of mechanical circulatory support. Nat Rev Cardiol 2012;9:195-208.
36. Teirstein PS, Vogel RA, Dorros G, et al. Prophylactic versus standby cardiopulmonary support for high risk percutaneous transluminal coronary angioplasty. J Am Coll Cardiol. 1993;21:590-6.
37. Sheu J-J, Tsai T-H, Lee F-Y, et al. Early extracorporeal membrane oxygenator-assisted primary percutaneous coronary intervention improved 30-day clinical outcomes in patients with ST-segment elevation myocardial infarction complicated with profound cardiogenic shock. Crit Care Med. 2010;38:1810-7.
38. Windecker S, Kolh P, Alfonso F, et al. ESC/EACTS guidelines on myocardial revascularization: the Task Force on Myocardial Revasculasization of the European Society of Cardiology (ESC) and the European Association for Cardio-Thoracic Surgery (EACTS) developed with the special contribution of the European Association of Percutaneous Cardiovascular Interventions (EAPCI). Eur Heart J. 2014;35:2541-619.

12
Complications during Percutaneous Coronary Interventions

Vijay Trehan, Prattay Guhasarkar

Improvements in devices, increasing operator experience, the use of stents and aggressive antiplatelet therapy have significantly reduced the incidence of complications related to percutaneous coronary interventions (PCI) over the past 15–20 years. Information drawn from almost 30 years of experience allows us to estimate the risk of complications according to patient and lesion characteristics. Every physician needs to consider, if the risk to benefit ratio of the planned procedure is appropriate on the basis of these data, before performing any intervention. It is critical to be vigilant and to recognize potential complications at an early stage to try to reverse the adverse outcome, as the most common cause of all post-PCI deaths is from a procedural complication rather than from a pre-existing cardiac condition.

Complications that occur during PCI can be divided into three main groups (Table 1):
a. Cardiac related complications
b. Vascular access-site related complications
c. Other complications (For example, contrast-induced nephropathy, cerebrovascular accidents, etc.).

CORONARY ARTERY COMPLICATIONS

Complications include slow/no reflow, coronary and stent thrombosis, coronary perforation, coronary dissection and abrupt closure.

Slow/No Reflow

No-reflow is usually defined as an acute reduction in antegrade flow (TIMI 0 or 1) not attributable to abrupt closure, high-grade stenosis, or spasm of the original target lesion. No-reflow occurs as a consequence of distal embolization clogging the microcirculation, microvascular vasoconstriction and microvascular damage resulting from extensive myocardial necrosis. Two subsets of no-reflow are defined:[1] myocardial no-reflow (due to microvascular dysfunction)[2] and angiographic no-reflow (due to a non-patent epicardial coronary artery).[3,4]

Table 1: Complications of PCI.

Cardiac Related Complications

Coronary	Arrhythmias
Slow/no reflow	Ventricular tachycardia
Coronary and stent thrombosis	Complete heart block
Coronary perforation	
Coronary dissection and abrupt closure	

Vascular Access Site Related Complications

Access site bleeding and hematoma
Retroperitoneal bleeding
AV fistula
Pseudo aneurysm

Other Complications

Contrast-induced nephropathy
Cerebrovascular events
Radiation toxicity
Retained PCI equipment components
Non-access site related bleeding
Cholesterol emboli
Allergic reactions

Regardless of the mechanism, slow-flow or no-reflow after PCI is generally associated with an adverse clinical outcome, especially in the setting of ACS. The occurrence of the no-reflow varies according to the type of the interventional procedure and device utilized and varies between 0.3 % (simple balloon angioplasty)[5] (Abbo et al. 1995) and 15% (PCI during ACS)[5] (Yip et al. 2002). No-reflow phenomenon occurred in 7.7% of patients having rotational atherectomy, 4.5% after extraction atherectomy, and in 1.7% after directional atherectomy.[7] Perhaps the highest incidence of no-reflow occurs in degenerated and thrombotic vein grafts, with an incidence of 15% to 40% quoted in various studies.[5]

Various mechanical devices and pharmacological approaches have been proposed in order to prevent (Table 2) and treat the no-reflow phenomenon, although no treatment is considered universally efficacious. In Table 3, we have summarized the most utilized pharmacological strategies.

We have earlier described super-selective injections distally into the vessel or into thrombus using shaved monorail/over the wire balloons (Fig. 1). Adenosine (Fischell et al. 1998), nitroprusside (Hillegass et al. 2001), and verapamil (Piana et al. 1994) are all considered in our experience as first-line

Table 2: Prevention of slow or no flow.

Method	Remarks
Distal protection devices	Indicated in degenerated SVG grafts. Role in routine or primary PCI not established
Medications: Gp IIb-IIIa inhibitors, nicorandil, adenosine	No established role in prevention of slow or no flow
Direct stenting	Helpful with high thrombus load, prevents distal embolization of debris and microvascular dysfunction
M-guard stent	Traps the thromboembolic debris underneath a fiber net and isolates the prothrombotic intima components from the blood stream
Thrombosuction	RCT data is conflicting. The need for thrombosuction should be individualized according to the clinical setting and thrombus load

Table 3: Intracoronary drug administration regimens for treatment no-reflow.

Adenosine	:	Boluses of 18–24 mg (divided up to four doses)
Sodium nitroprusside	:	Boluses of 80–200 ug (up to 1.5 mg)
Nitroglycerin	:	Boluses of 100–200 mg (up to four doses)
Verapamil	:	Boluses of 100–250 ug (up to 1.000 mg)
Epinephrine	:	Boluses of 50–200 mg (especially in case of hypotension)
Nicorandil	:	Boluses of 2–3 mg over 30–60 s

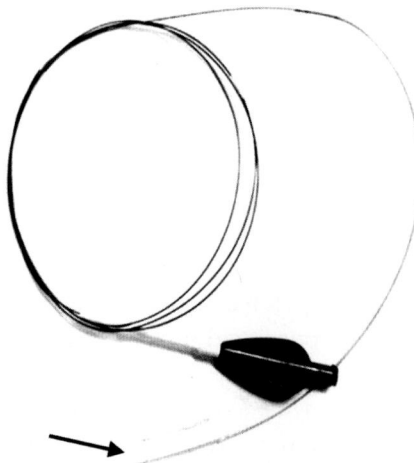

Fig. 1: Shaved PTCA balloon for super-selective injections.

agents and can be delivered distally directly as described.[8] The above technique is a very useful as double lumen catheters are not easily available and PTCA balloons can be used for this.

In order to prevent distal embolization, some recommendations should be taken into consideration:

1. Thrombus aspiration and/or direct stenting is suggested in patients with acute myocardial infarction especially in case of a high thrombus burden in culprit vessel of large calibre.
2. Embolic protection device as PercuSurge GuardWire, AngioGuard, Filter-Wire EX and others are now recommended as standard care in vein graft-PCI.[10]
3. In case of rotational atherectomy, a maximum burr to artery ratio 0.70, lower rotational speeds (140,000–160,000 rpm), and preventive use of cocktail with verapamil, nitroglycerin, heparin, and normal saline infused through the Teflon sheath of the rotational system have been advocated to reduce vasospasm and no-reflow.

Coronary and Stent Thrombosis

During PCI operators must always remain alert because longer procedures and the intentional creation of dissection planes increase the risk of spontaneous intracoronary thrombus formation. *We recommend that when using heparin, an ACT should be checked at least every hour and the value kept above 250 s during the procedure. If visible thrombus is observed, this should be removed with an aspiration device, such as a microcatheter.* Acute or subacute stent thrombosis is a relatively uncommon complication (<1 %) nowadays, since patients are now pre-treated with double antiplatelet therapy including more potent agents. Thrombosis may be related to inadequate stent expansion (in coronary bifurcation, long lesions, and chronic total occlusion) or improper anticoagulation (peri-procedural low ACT) and suboptimal angiographic result (TIMI flow 0-2), especially in some subsets of patients like the ones with acute coronary syndromes, chronic renal failure, diabetes, systemic inflammatory state, and cancer.

Optimal Anticoagulation

Anticoagulation with unfractionated heparin is most commonly utilized but attention to dosing and ACT levels is required. This is particularly the case when concomitant glycoprotein IIb-IIIa antagonists have been used. *Guidelines recommend a heparin dose 70-100 U/kg sufficient to reach an ACT of 250-300 (when using the HemoTec analyzer) or 300-350 seconds (when using the HemoChron analyzer), in glycoprotein IIb-IIIa naïve patients. In the presence of glycoprotein IIb-IIIa, heparin at 50-70 U/kg and an ACT > 200 seconds is regarded as sufficient.*[8] The association of ACT levels and PCI outcomes whilst concordant in the balloon angioplasty era (where an ACT > 250 seconds was associated with the least risk of abrupt vessel closure), have yielded conflicting data in contemporary practice.[8] Analysis of six large randomized trials suggests that an ACT of 350-375 seconds may be the optimal target. Ethnic differences may exist with Asian patients requiring 10 untis/kg less than standard doses to achieve the same ACT.[6] Heparin administration is best given centrally to assure delivery of the correct dose. ACT levels must also be checked regularly. Empirically this should be within an hour of administration and at 30 minutes intervals thereafter.

UFH does not have much role in present era of primary PCI, if bivalirudin is available. Abciximab is inferior to bivalirudin with increased risk of bleeding complications.[8] In patients undergoing elective PCI, UFH is generally adequate and bivalirudin and abciximab is not indicated.

Coronary Perforation

Perforation or frank rupture of coronary arteries, resulting from the guidewires or balloons, occurs in 0.2 to 0.6% of patients undergoing PTCA.[9] Overall mortality with coronary perforation is about 5 to 10 percent, with the main risk factors being older age, tamponade, requirement for emergency surgery and the severity of the perforation (Table 4). The adjunctive use of the platelet glycoprotein IIb/IIIa receptor antagonists during intervention does not increase the risk of adverse events in patients with a coronary perforation. However, the use of newer hydrophilic guidewires in conjunction with aggressive antiplatelet therapy is anecdotally linked to an increased risk of distal wire perforation.[6]

The Ellis classification (Table 5) is the most widely adopted method to describe coronary perforations angiographically (Ellis et al. 1994). This classification also has prognostic importance: low rates of death occur in Type 1 perforations which can be managed conservatively, whereas there is a high risk of death in Type 3 coronary perforation if it is not promptly treated.

Class I and II perforations are usually managed conservatively without any specific treatment. Class III perforations are associated with rapid

Table 4: Risk factors for coronary perforations.
High-pressure inflation of an oversized balloon (B/A ratio >1.2) or of a semi-compliant balloon inside or outside a stent
Usage of hydrophilic wires
Stenting a very calcified or fibrotic lesion without prior calcium ablation (Rotablator) or fissuring (cutting balloon)
Usage of Rotablator or directional atherectomy in very tortuous segments or following reopening of total occlusions
Combining cutting balloon and prior GPIIb/IIIa inhibitors and/or bivalirudin

Table 5: Ellis classification: Classification of coronary perforations.[6]
Type 1: A crater extending outside of the lumen only and in the absence of linear staining angiographically suggestive of a dissection
Type 2: Pericardial or myocardial blush without a 1 mm exit hole
Type 3: Frank streaming of contrast through a >1 mm exit hole
Type 4: Perforation with cavity spilling

development of tamponade (63%), the need for urgent bypass surgery (63%), and a high mortality rate (19%). *To minimize the chance of wire perforation, hydrophilic tipped or stiff wires that are used to get through difficult lesions should be exchanged for workhorse wires with softer hydrophobic tips.*

When coronary perforation occurs, the most important step is not to lose control of the situation, in particular not to lose access of the artery. In any risky situation, it remains imperative to leave the balloon at the lesion site following balloon deflation and check with a contrast injection, to confirm the presence of a perforation. In case of a perforation, immediate balloon inflation at low pressure (with the same balloon that caused the rupture) is a very important step to prevent further extravasation (Flowchart 1). When possible, prolonged balloon inflation should be attempted. Unfortunately, perfusion balloons are no longer available for those patients who develop ischemia during balloon inflation. *In the author's opinion, anticoagulation should not be immediately reversed with the wire and balloon in the vessel during the attempted perforation occlusion. Immediate reversal could lead to thrombosis throughout the whole vessel, an event that leads to a higher degree of mortality than the perforation itself.* Reversal of anticoagulation should be performed after the equipment is removed from the coronary vessel.

A turning point in the treatment of coronary perforations occurred with the introduction of covered stents (stent grafts) which allow for the percutaneous sealing of the rupture.[6]

The Following are Balloon-Expandable Covered Stents

1. *JOSTENT GraftMaster*: Stainless steel stent covered with polytetrafluoroethylene (PTFE); characterized by a wall thickness of 0.3 mm; available in sizes 3.0, 3.5, and 4.0 (6 Fr guiding catheter) and 4.5 and 5.0 (7 Fr guiding catheter). It is bulkier than the other covered stents.
2. *In Situ Direct-Stent Stent-Graft*: Stainless steel PTFE covered stent; wall thickness 0.15 mm; it is the thinnest covered stents available (starting at 1.2 mm crossing profile; available in sizes from 2.5 mm diameter to 6.0 mm; minimum guiding catheter size 6–7 Fr).

Flowchart 1: Proposed algorithm for management of coronary perforation.

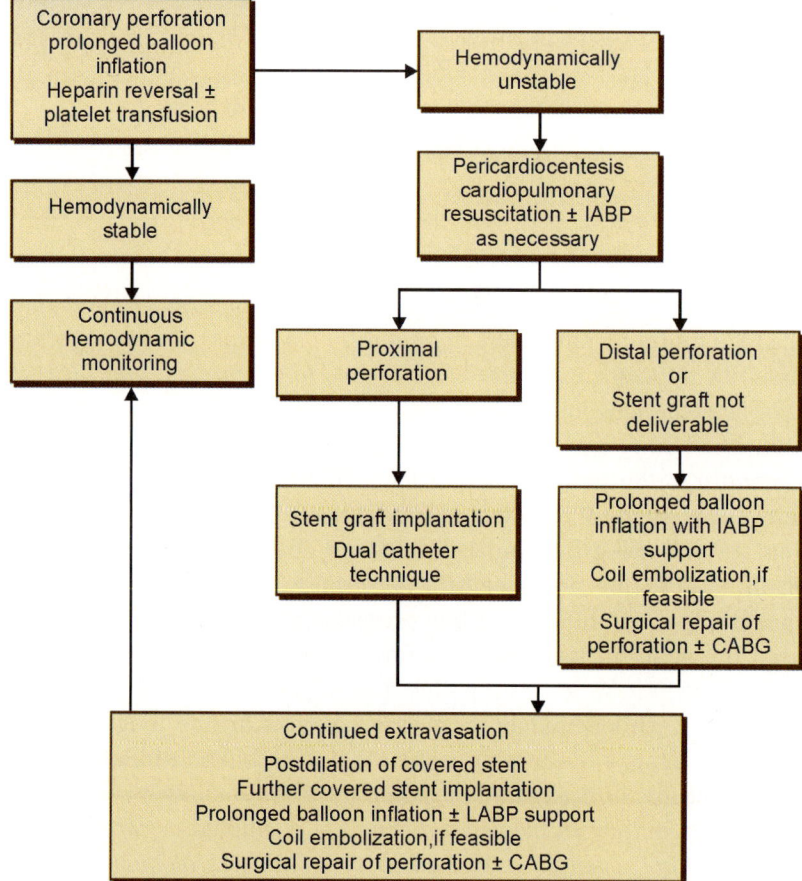

3. *Over and Under-Pericardium Covered Stent*: Stainless steel stent covered with equine pericardium (105 um thickness); highly flexible stent available in sizes 2.5, 3.0, 3.5 (6 Fr guiding catheter); 4.0 mm (7 Fr guiding catheter). Theoretically, the equine pericardium may be more biocompatible reducing the risk of stent thrombosis.
4. *PK Papyrus Covered Coronary Stent System*: Cobalt chromium stent covered with polyurethane (90 um thickness); highly flexible stent with a unique low crossing profile. It is available in sizes 2.5, 3.0, 3.5, 4.0 mm, compatible with a 5 Fr guiding catheter; and 4.5 and 5.0 mm compatible with 6 Fr guiding catheter. Theoretically, the low crossing profile reduces the stiffness of crimped stent graft by up to 58%.

All these covered stents suffer from similar limitations: they are bulkier than normal stents and show reduced flexibility and trackability, as well as an increased risk of stent thrombosis and restenosis. *In the author's opinion, it is advisable to remain skeptical of the lowest French size compatibility of the stent graft as provided by the product manufacturer and at least go for one French size higher guide catheter, to minimize the chances of a failed deliverability of the stent graft.* This is because the compatibility of stent grafts, as mentioned by the product manufacturer, is based on data with in-vitro straight tubes. In actual life, guiding catheters are not straight, negotiation of tortuous bends reduces the inner calibre of the guiding catheter and poses difficulties in the deliverability of the stent grafts. Alternatively to compensate for this, a 5 Fr mother in child catheter system can be used. It is essential to ensure the sealing of the perforation and to reduce the risk of stent thrombosis; therefore, covered stents are deployed at a reasonably high pressure (14–16 atm) with prolonged balloon inflation to allow optimal stent expansion.

The dual guiding catheter technique: A major drawback in treating a perforated vessel with a coronary stent graft is the amount of time that passes between the deflation of the sealing balloon and the final delivery of the covered stent into the lesion site. For this reason, the dual guiding catheter technique for implantation of the covered stent has been recommended (Ben-Gal et al. 2010). While the sealing balloon is inflated, the guide catheter is withdrawn slightly from the coronary ostia, and another seven or eight French guiding catheter from the contralateral femoral artery is used to engage the same coronary ostia. A coronary covered stent graft (or a coil in smaller and distal vessels) is advanced on a new wire through the second guide and placed just proximally to the sealing balloon. The sealing balloon is deflated and withdrawn proximally to allow passage of the wire and of the coronary stent graft which is deployed. The first sealing balloon, wire, and guide catheter are retrieved only after gaining adequate seal of the lesion with the covered stent graft.

When sealing of the perforation by conservative measures cannot be achieved, urgent surgery should be considered.

Coronary Dissection and Abrupt Closure

Coronary arterial dissection and consequent acute (abrupt) closure are frequent PCI complications. Usually, coronary dissections result from "controlled injury" induced by balloon dilatation. They can also result from overly vigorous attempts to advance guidewires. These problems are now much less common since stent placement is performed in most percutaneous coronary procedures. Dissections are observable in up to 50% of patients immediately after balloon angioplasty (Grossman and Baim 2006). The occurrence of dissection cannot be predicted by preintervention analysis of lesion morphology or plaque composition by intracoronary ultrasound (IVUS). Mild dissections often heal completely, although occasional late localized aneurysm formation has been described. In contrast, larger dissections are associated with an increased risk of progression to total occlusion (abrupt closure) of the treated arterial segment. The increased risk of abrupt closure and myocardial infarction associated with a large dissection has led to the routine use of stenting for any dissection. Most cases of acute closure occur within minutes of the final balloon inflation, but subacute closure can occur hours later in 0.5–1.0% of cases, typically as the heparin anticoagulation wears off. Stents can reverse abrupt closure in more than 90% of cases.

Arrhythmias

Coronary occlusion (spontaneous or iatrogenic) causes inhomogeneous myocardial cell refractory periods, prolongation of the QT interval and slow conduction particularly at the border between ischemic and nonischemic territories. Catecholamine surges, associated with intervention and also acute ischemia, produce after-depolarizations. This combination of circumstances provides the substrate for both tachy and bradyarrhythmias, both during occlusion itself and reperfusion, as action potentials and conduction normalize in a haphazard heterogeneous manner. Ventricular tachycardia (VT) and Complete heart block (CHB) are two commonly encountered arrhythmias. A few practical points are as follows:
- VT is common during interventions on the Right coronary artery (RCA). It is generally a complication of wedged coronary injections into the RCA or the conus branch. It may be caused during PCI by inadvertent administration of saline flush through the wedged coronary catheter into the RCA. VT can also be a manifestation of a reperfusion arrhythmia seen more commonly in RCA than LAD or LCX.
- CHB is more common during interventions on the RCA. Rotablation carries a higher risk compared to routine PCI. *A practical method is to cross a temporary pacing lead through the IVC, visit the RA and then park the lead in IVC. This rules out IVC interruption and can hasten RV pacing, if required.* Prophylactic RV lead placement is avoided as it can irritate the myocardium and cause arrhythmias and rarely cause RV perforation.

VASCULAR ACCESS SITE RELATED COMPLICATIONS

The common femoral artery was the most frequent access site until about 2005, at which time many interventional cardiologists started preferring the radial artery for reasons presented below.

Vascular complications at the femoral artery access site, which occur in up to 6% of cases, make up a significant portion of the morbidity associated with PCI. Minor or major hematomas and pseudo aneurysms are most common, followed by arterial laceration, retroperitoneal hematoma, arteriovenous fistula, arterial occlusion, and local infection with or without sepsis.[11] Risk factors for vascular complications include periprocedural use of high doses of heparin or fibrinolytic therapy; repeat procedure; peripheral artery disease; advanced age; obesity; duration of time that the sheath remains in place, particularly, if >15 h; use of intra-aortic balloon pump; and, in some but not all series, larger arterial sheath size and cannulation of the superficial femoral artery (Popma et al. 1993).

Access Site Bleeding and Hematoma

Access site bleeding is in part related to anticoagulation and is more frequent when antiplatelet drugs are used. Women are at higher risk for bleeding and vascular complications compared with men. This difference is not fully explained by smaller vessel or body size.

The risk of bleeding requiring transfusion is also increased in elderly patients undergoing PCI, with a rate of 9% noted in one series.[11] This risk does not appear to be influenced by whether or not a glycoprotein (GP) IIb/IIIa inhibitor was given.

Prevention of access site bleeding may be possible by reducing the intensity of anticoagulation, especially in patients receiving concomitant GP IIb/IIa inhibitors. Heparin is almost always used during PCI to reduce the risk of thrombosis, but continued therapy makes it more difficult to achieve hemostasis at the arterial access site. Some experts advocate that the dosing of unfractionated heparin during PCI should be guided by measurement of activated clotting times. Over anticoagulation, especially with concomitant administration of GP IIb/IIIa receptor blockers is associated with higher risk of hemorrhage. The use of direct thrombin inhibitors such as bivalirudin rather than heparin and a GP IIb/IIIa receptor blocker, is associated with lower risk of hemorrhagic complications.[9]

Postprocedural heparin is no longer recommended[11] since the majority of abrupt closures occur immediately after the procedure, and the incidence of other ischemic events has decreased with the use of stents and antiplatelet agents given during or immediately after PCI.

Attaining Hemostasis

The traditional approach to catheter removal from the femoral artery at the conclusion of PCI was local hand applied pressure for 15 to 30 minutes. Two alternative approaches are available: mechanical clamp compression and, more important, arterial puncture closing devices, which may increase the risk of complications.

Retroperitoneal Bleeding

Retroperitoneal bleeding represents a particularly serious type of preventable vascular complication.[12] Retroperitoneal bleeding is frequently related to artery puncture that is above the inguinal ligament and can be prevented in most cases by careful attention to anatomic landmarks and fluoroscopy of the femoral head prior to needle puncture. Even with appropriate access position, back wall punctures that exit above the inguinal ligament may result in retroperitoneal bleeding and may not be sealed by manual compression or closure devices. Injudicious advancement of the guidewire or sheath by an inexperienced operator can also traumatize the iliac artery or the lateral circumflex artery and result in bleeding in to the retroperitoneal space.[12]

The event is usually recognized by hemodynamic compromise. It can sometimes be mistaken for the more common and benign "vagal" reaction, since it may also present with profound bradycardia and associated hypotension. It is distinguished by only a transient response to initial volume loading and atropine.

Successful management depends on early recognition and volume resuscitation with crystalloid and blood. The diagnosis is usually confirmed by computed tomography imaging. The vascular surgical team should be alerted, although surgical management is not commonly needed or helpful. *We have used percutaneous methods including balloon inflation or placement of a covered stent to tamponade or seal the bleeding segment.*

Prevention of Complications

To reduce these complications attention to puncture technique is fundamental. *The use of the groin skin crease as an anatomical landmark should be avoided.* In cases where surface anatomical landmarks are difficult to ascertain fluoroscopic assisted bony landmarks or portable ultrasound can be used. *The aim should be to puncture the common femoral artery within a target zone 5 mm to 14 mm inferior to the center of the femoral head, as this gives the best chance of avoiding both the femoral bifurcation and the inferior sweep of the inferior epigastric artery.*[12]

The safety of vascular closure devices deployment can also be assessed by femoral angiography. Their use should probably be avoided if the diameter of the CFA is <5 mm, the presence of a puncture site below the common femoral bifurcation or in the presence of significant atherosclerosis. Femoral angiography can be performed before starting or at the end of the coronary procedure. If femoral angiography is performed before instrumentation of the coronaries in elective patients then this gives the opportunity for postponement, if the risk of vascular complications is deemed high.

How to Reduce Transfemoral Access Complications?

- Access using fluoroscopy (or ultrasound)
- Puncture site at or below centreline of the femoral head. Safe zone 5-14 mm below center of femoral head
- Femoral angiogram (RAO 30 and LAO 60 degrees) prior to closure
- PCI and anticoagulation only, if in the 'safe zone' (elective patients).

Radial Artery Access

For patients with acute coronary syndromes treated with PCI, many operators prefer access using the radial, rather than the femoral artery. For stable patients, either access site is acceptable. Use of the radial artery should be performed by properly trained operators who perform at least 75 interventions using the radial artery per year, as there is evidence to suggest better outcomes with higher procedural volume.

Catheterization using the radial, as opposed to the common femoral artery has the potential to reduce the risk of major access site bleeding due to the fact that the former is smaller and readily compressible. Any intervention that reduces the risk of bleeding could potentially improve outcomes given the observations of increased mortality and ischemic events in patients who bleed at the time of PCI. This is particularly true for patients undergoing catheterization for an acute coronary syndrome. However, chances of wire injury to radial artery causing occlusion and neck hematoma due to subclavian or brachiocephalic injury should be watched out for.[13]

Prevention of Complications

Although access site complications with the radial approach are dramatically reduced they are not entirely eliminated (vasospasm preventing the completion of the procedure, compartment syndrome, arterial dissection, radial avulsion, perforation or occlusion), and the technique requires a significant period of learning. Hand ischemia has not been reported after PCI, and ischemia relating to compartment syndrome or radial arterial cannula is rare. Radial artery occlusion rates of 3-5% can be reduced by procedural heparin, decreasing sheath size and the technique of perfused patent hemostasis following the end of the procedure.[13] *In the authors opinion, overall the benefit identified in studies carried out in large volume centers needs to be weighed up against the experience of the operator; a high volume femoral operator may have fewer complications than a low volume radial operator.*

Radial and other contiguous forearm arteries are particularly prone to vasospasm due to the presence of a high density of vasoconstrictor alpha receptors (predominantly alpha-1 with some alpha-2). The prevention of this complication with a pharmacological "cocktail", gentle handling of equipment and avoiding numerous exchanges is much more effective than attempts to

How to Reduce Transradial Access Complications?

- Hydration and anxiolytics
- Vessel "cocktail" (usually calcium channel antagonist and nitrate)
- Heparin (at least 3-5000 units)
- Avoid puncture through the flexor retinaculum
- Perfused patent hemostasis.

OTHER COMPLICATIONS

Contrast-Induced Nephropathy

Contrast-induced acute kidney injury (CI-AKI) represents an important cause of hospital-acquired AKI and will occur in 2–25% of patients undergoing coronary intervention (Mehran et al. 2004).[14] The incidence of CI-AKI after PCI was higher in patients with CKD associated with diabetes. Lower levels of basal hemoglobin appeared to be related to a higher risk of CI-AKI. Contrast media volume, especially if exceeding the dose adjusted for renal function, is a strong modifiable risk factor for CI-AKI (Morabito et al. 2012). There are three major causes of CI-AKI: contrast-induced acute renal failure, renal atheroemboli and hemodynamic instability with renal hypoperfusion. The most common definition of CI-AKI is a rise of serum creatinine of 0.5 mg/dL or a 25% relative rise in creatinine at 48 h after contrast exposure. Decreasing the concentration of contrast media within the tubule lumen and its contact time may diminish the direct toxicity of the contrast media. Thus, strategies to increase urine output (with high-flow hydration and Renalguard system) before, during, and after contrast media exposure are used in high-risk patients. Unfortunately, multiple clinical trials have documented the variability in the efficacy of antioxidants, N-acetylcysteine and ascorbic acid. In the MYTHOS (Induced Diuresis With Matched Hydration Compared to Standard Hydration for Contrast Induced Nephropathy Prevention) study, furosemide-induced high urine output with matched hydration significantly reduces the risk of contrast-induced nephropathy and may be associated with improved in-hospital outcome (Marenzi et al. 2012). *In the author's opinion, high-flow hydration is the best possible treatment available to prevent CI-AKI. Therefore, in our clinical practice, we give 0.9% saline at 3 mL/kg for at least 1 h prior to their procedure and for 3 h after the procedure in case of preserved left ventricular ejection fraction (LVEF). The dose is reduced at 1.5 mL/kg/h for patients with LVEF < 35%; in these patients furosemide (25–50 mg) is always given during the* *procedure.* Measuring left ventricular diastolic pressure at the beginning of the procedure is a valuable tool to guide aggressive hydration.

Cerebrovascular Events

Stroke is a rare but serious complication which can occur in 0.05–0.1% of diagnostic cardiac catheterizations and in 0.18–0.44% of patients treated with PCI.[15] Despite all the improvements in pharmacological and technical issues, the rate of stroke after cardiac catheterization has remained almost constant over the last 20 years. This is probably due to the immutability of the majority of risk factors before cardiac procedures. Advanced age, arterial hypertension, diabetes mellitus, coronary angiography performed under emergency conditions, history of stroke, renal failure, the use of an intra-aortic balloon pump, congestive heart failure and interventions at bypass grafts have been identified as risk factors for periprocedural stroke in large registries. In the PCI Registry of the Euro Heart Survey Programme (46,888 patients, 176 centers in 33 European countries), stroke was observed in 0.4% of the procedures (0.3% in elective patients and 0.6% in ACS patients). The overall in-hospital mortality was 19% for patients who developed stroke (23.2% in ACS patients) compared with 1.3% for those without stroke. In multivariate analyses hemodynamic instability, age above 75 years, history of stroke, and congestive heart failure were found to be independent predictors for periprocedural stroke in ACS, whereas only PCI of a bypass graft and renal failure could be identified as independent predictors for stroke in elective patients (Werner et al. 2013).[15]

Some concerns have been raised regarding the fact that transradial access may increase the risk of neurologic events compared with transfemoral access. However, initial reports regarding this topic suggest that radial access is not associated with an increased risk of clinically detected neurologic events, even during a period when there was a rapid evolution in the preferred access site for PCI (Ratib et al. 2012). Due to exceedingly high rates of mortality and disability, stroke after coronary angiography still has an enormous impact on the patient's prognosis and on quality of life. If patients survive this devastating complication, most of them suffer from persistent neurological deficits such as motor or speech disorders. For its low incidence and consecutively missing data from randomized clinical trials, an evidence-based treatment could not yet be established, and treatment options are generally based on case series and small studies only. Nevertheless, intra-arterial thrombolysis and mechanical embolectomy seem to be promising and relatively safe approaches in the treatment of periprocedural ischemic stroke.

Radiation Toxicity

PCI procedures can result in radiation exposure high enough to cause skin injuries in patients. In one center, the frequency of skin injuries was estimated to be 0.03%.[16] Although the number of radiation injuries due to cardiac procedures remains small, these injuries have a major impact on the patients who are affected. Early transient erythema, permanent epilation, and delayed dermal necrosis can occur at 2, 7, and 12 Gy, respectively. Of the procedures, PCI for chronic total occlusion (CTO) is a major challenge, because examination time tends to be long, and the rate of repeat PCI is relatively high. Moreover, high body mass index, history of coronary artery bypass graft surgery, and number of treated lesions were also associated with the highest patient radiation exposure.

In order to optimize patient radiation dose and minimize skin damage, the following can be done:
- Limit fluoroscopy time and the number of cine frames to the least number possible for successful completion of the procedure.
- Monitor patient radiation dose during the procedure.
- Use fluoroscopy equipment with pulsed fluoroscopy.
- Use the lowest fluoroscopic and cine dose rates necessary for each stage of the procedure.
- Rotate the gantry slightly so that the entrance beam is periodically directed at a different entrance skin site.
- Keep the image receptor (image intensifier or flat panel detector) as close as possible to the patient.
- Keep the X-ray tube as far away as possible from the entrance skin site.

When the patient's radiation dose from the procedure exceeds the institution's trigger level, clinical follow-up should be performed for early detection and management of skin injuries. Suggested values for the trigger level are a skin dose of 3 Gy, a kerma-area product of 500 Gy/cm^2 or an air kerma at the patient entrance reference point of 5 Gy (NCRP 2010). Patients who have received a substantial radiation dose should have follow-up 2–4 weeks after the procedure for detection of potential radiation injuries.

Retained PCI Equipment Components

A device inserted into the coronary tree which is not supposed to stay there permanently and cannot be removed is one of the most dramatic complications occurring in interventional cardiology. The most common trapped device is usually a burr utilized to perform rotational atherectomy (Rotablator). The Rotablator burr may be trapped because its advancement was too forceful without adequate debulking or lesion modifications or because advancement occurred at the site of a steep curve with change in angulation from way in to way out (Kokeshi phenomenon). In some cases, the trapped burr can be retrieved using simple traction, but this is potentially hazardous with possible trauma and perforation of the vessel. If a relative forceful maneuver fails to retrieve the device, possible options are advancement of the guide catheter near the trapped burr and removal of the proximal end of the Rotablator system (cut off the drive shaft and sheath of the Rotablator) to allow advancement of a second smaller guide catheter (5 Fr guiding catheter, "child-in-a-mother catheter") to come close to the trapped burr. In some situations there is the need to gain a second arterial access and to advance a balloon at the trapped burr and then inflate it in order to free the device. If during these attempts the patient develops significant ischemia, the operator may consider inserting an intra-aortic balloon pump.

Balloon fracture: Mono-rail balloons have a tendency to fracture at mono-rail to shaft junction. A clue towards the possibility of a balloon fracture is when the balloon fails to move fluoroscopically after the shaft is pulled out. *We have previously described a simple technique of retrieval of a fractured balloon by trapping the shaft of the fractured balloon with any balloon equal to or greater than the internal diameter of the guide catheter, inflated at 8 to 10 atm, followed by en-masse removal of the assembly.*[17] *Such a technique in a timely fashion is life saving and can avoid unnecessary surgery.*

Cholesterol Emboli

Cholesterol crystal embolism (CCE) is a serious complication associated with invasive vascular procedures. CCE has been estimated to occur after vascular procedures in 0.15–1.4% of cases in clinical studies.[18] It is a systemic disorder caused by the occlusion of small- to medium-sized arteries by athermanous material (150–200 mm in diameter) derived from ulcerated atherosclerotic plaques in the aorta or large feeder arteries. CCE affected predominantly elderly males, with a hypertension, history of cardiovascular disease, and aortic aneurysm. Because the abdominal aorta is the most common source of cholesterol crystals, the kidneys, intestines, and lower extremities are at prominent risk of embolization. Its course is usually subacute, occurring gradually over 4–6 weeks. In a few cases it may present with fever, thus mimicking infective endocarditis. The most common signs of CCE include livedo reticularis, gangrene and cutaneous ulcers. Acute renal failure with necrotizing glomerulonephritis is one of the most common manifestations. Generally dialysis is required in 40–60% of patients with acute or subacute renal CCE. Several drugs and therapeutic options have been used to treat CCE, including statins, corticosteroids, cilostazol and intravenous heparin. Treatment with hyperbaric oxygen therapy was also reported. Prevention of another episode involves modification of traditional risk factors such as serum cholesterol, diabetes, hypertension, and smoking. Additional percutaneous and vascular surgery procedures should be avoided, as they can induce new episodes.[18]

REFERENCES

1. Mehta RH, Harjai KJ, Cox D, et al. Clinical and angiographic correlates and outcomes of suboptimal coronary flow in patients with acute myocardial infarction undergoing primary percutaneous coronary intervention. J Am Coll Cardiol 2003;42:1739-46.
2. Ambrosio G, Weisman HF, Mannisi JA, et al. Progressive impairment of regional myocardial perfusion after initial restoration of postischemic blood flow. Circulation 1989;80:1846-61.
3. Gregorini L, Marco J, Kozakova M, et al. Alpha-adrenergic blockade improves recovery of myocardial perfusion and function after coronary stenting in patients with acute myocardial infarction. Circulation 1999;99:482-90.
4. Michaels AD, Gibson CM, Barron HV. Microvascular dysfunction in acute myocardial infarction: focus on the roles of platelet and inflammatory mediators in the no-reflow phenomenon. Am J Cardiol 2000;85:50b-60b.
5. Abbo KM, Dooris M, Glazier S. Features and outcome of no-reflow after percutaneous coronary intervention. Am J Cardiol 1995;75:778-82.
6. Dippel EJ, Kereiakes DJ, Tramuta DA, et al. Coronary perforation during percutaneous coronary intervention in the era of abciximab platelet glycoprotein IIb/IIIa blockade: an algorithm for percutaneous management. Cathet Cardiovasc Intervent 2001;52:279-86.
7. Leopold JA, Berger CJ, Cupples LA, et al. No-reflow during coronary intervention: observations and implications. Circulation 2000;102:II-604.
8. Trehan V, Girish MN, Gupta MD. Use of monorail PTCA balloon catheter for local drug delivery. J invasive cardiol 2007;19:141-3.
9. Steg PG, van't Hof A, Hamm CW, et al. EUROMAX Investigators. Bivalirudin started during emergency transport for primary PCI. N Engl J Med 2013;369:2207-17.
10. Baim DS, Wahr D, George B, et al. Randomized trial of a distal embolic protection device during percutaneous intervention of saphenous vein aortocoronary bypass graft. Circulation 2002;105:1285.
11. Johnson LW, Esente P, Giambartolomei A, et al. Peripheral vascular complications of coronary angioplasty by the femoral and brachial techniques. Cathet Cardiovasc Diagn 1994;31:165-72.
12. Mak GY, Daly B, Chan W, et al. Percutaneous treatment of postcatheterization massive retroperitoneal hemorrhage. Cathet Cardiovasc Diagn 1993;29:40-3.
13. Agostoni P, Biondi-Zoccai GG, de Benedictis ML, et al. Radial versus femoral approach for percutaneous coronary diagnostic and interventional procedures; Systematic overview and meta-analysis of randomized trials. J Am Coll Cardiol 2004;44(2):349-56.
14. Mehran R, Aymong ED, Nikolsky E, et al. A simple risk score for prediction of contrast-induced nephropathy after percutaneous coronary intervention: development and initial validation. J Am Coll Cardiol 2004;44:1393-9.
15. Werner N, Bauer T, Hochadel M, et al. Incidence and clinical impact of stroke complicating percutaneous coronary intervention results of the euro heart survey percutaneous coronary interventions registry. Circ Cardiovasc Interv. 2013; 6:362-9.
16. Wagner LK, Eifel PJ, Geise RA. Potential biological effects following high X-ray dose interventional procedures. J Vasc Interv Radiol 1994;5:71-84.
17. Trehan V, Mukhopadhyay S, Yusuf J, et al. Intracoronary Fracture and Embolization of a Coronary Angioplasty Balloon Catheter: Retrieval by a Simple Technique. Cath Cardiovas Interv. 2003;59:473-7.
18. Daimon S, Motita R, Ohtsuki N, et al. Ldl apheresis followed by corticosteroid therapy as a possible treatment of cholesterol crystal embolism. Clin Exp Nephrol 2004;4:352-5.

13 Intracoronary Assessment: Role of IVUS and OCT

G Sengottuvelu, G Raghul

INTRODUCTION

Atherosclerosis is a disease of the vessel wall and luminal narrowing is a late secondary process of atherosclerosis, hence diagnosing and treating it from the lumen profile as achieved by angiogram is bound to have limitations.

LIMITATIONS OF CORONARY ANGIOGRAM

- Inter and intra-observer variation
- Adequate knowledge of lesion morphology cannot be assessed
- Pre and post PCI guidance for stent placement is very poor
- Mechanism of Stent failure cannot be assessed with precision.

Presently intravascular ultrasound (IVUS) using sound waves and optical coherent tomography using light waves are the two technologies that achieve such a tomographic image of the blood vessels without significantly interrupting coronary blood flow. Table 1 shows characteristic features of OCT and IVUS.

IVUS

IVUS is performed during cardiac catheterization using miniature ultrasound probes mounted on the tip of a coronary catheter. The IVUS probe emits high ultrasound frequencies, typically centered at 20–50 MHz. The ultrasound signal reflected from arterial wall structures is used to generate a grey scale image which enables visualisation of the full circumference of the vessel wall.

Basic Interpretation of IVUS

- Normal coronary artery—lumen is uniform and 3 layers visible in vessel wall (Fig. 1).
- Atherosclerotic plaques—soft, low echogenicity (Fig. 2).
- Fibrous plaque—high echogenicity (Fig. 3).

Table 1: Features of OCT and IVUS.

Parameter	OCT	IVUS
Axial resolution	12-15 mm	100-200 mm
Frame rate	100 frames/s	30 frames/s
Pullback speed	20 mm/s	0.5-1 mm/s
Tissue penetration	1.0-2.0 mm	10 mm
Blood clearing	Required	Not required
Technology	Infrared light waves (1,250-1350 nm)	Ultrasound 30–40 MHz
Catheter equipment	Single rotating lens	Single rotating and multi array transducers
Physics applied	Interferometer used— high light speed	Direct measurement of back-scattered waves
Image interpretation	Grey scale and golden scale	Grey scale display
Renal dysfunction	Adds up contrast load	No issues
Complete visualization of Large vessel	Not possible	Possible
Assessment thin cap Fibroatheroma, thrombus, dissection	Superior	Can be imaged
BVS assessment	Superior	Inferior
Aorto ostial visualization	Not possible	Possible
Luminal visualization	Excellent	Limited by resolution
Positive remodeling	Usually missed	Easily picked-up
Distal vessel visualization	Not possible	Not possible
Coregistration	Available	In pipeline
3D Stent enhancement and SB crossing	Available	NA
Acquisition of image	Based on contrast injection	Easy
Interpretation	Easy	Difficult
Data	Up coming	Extensive

- Calcified plaque—high echogenicity with acoustic shadowing/reverberations (Fig. 4).

Uses

Pre-PCI Assessment

- **Assessment of plaque composition**—to decide the need for lesion preparation and appropriate devices to facilitate stent deployment. Tight lesions and chronic total occlusions require predilation before assessment.

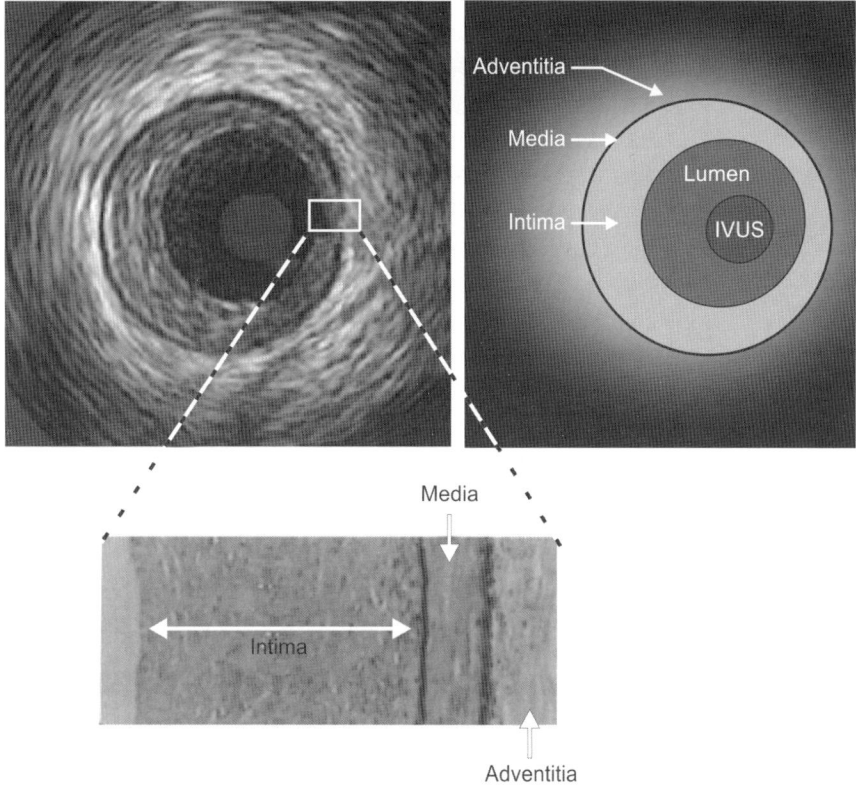

Fig. 1: Normal IVUS.

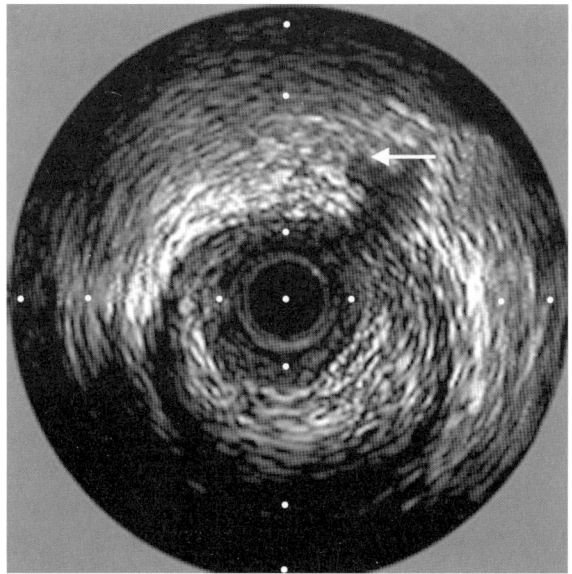

Fig. 2: Atherosclerotic plaque.

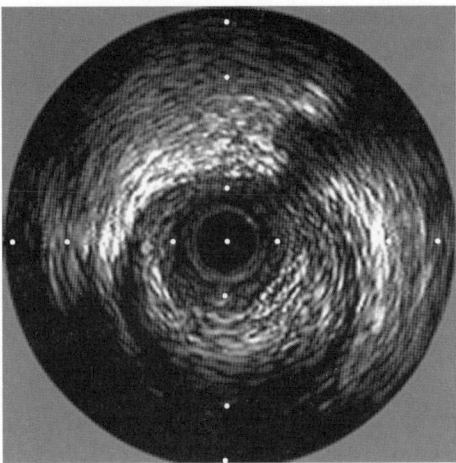

Fig. 3: Fibrous plaque.

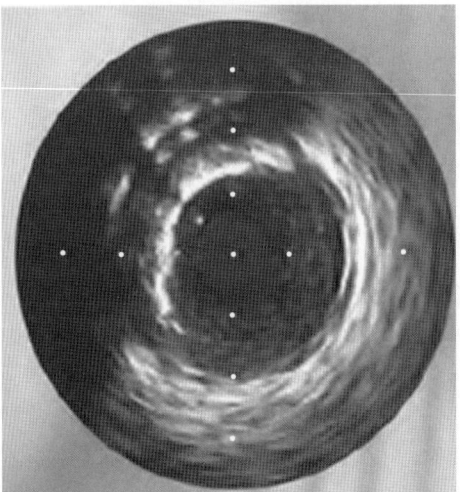

Fig. 4: Calcified plaque.

- Superficial calcium defined as subintimal or that is more nearer to intima than adventitia can be clearly shown by IVUS, but the deeper extent of the calcium cannot be measured from IVUS because of the acoustic shadowing. Nevertheless the accurate length and the circumferential extent of calcium is enough for decision making. A predominantly echolucent plaque usually yields to semi compliant balloons, whereas fibrocalcific or a calcific plaque will require cutting balloon or rotablation. Superficial calcific arcs 360° are considered for rotablation. It is ideal to do a preprocedural IVUS in restenosis and in lesions where calcium is suspected but mild on angiography.

- The lipid-laden lesions appear hypoechoic and fibromuscular lesions generate low-intensity or 'soft' echoes. Lipid-laden or fibromuscular lesions may exhibit a prominent echogenic fibrous cap which helps in identifying vulnerable plaque, but most fibrous caps are too thin to be imaged by IVUS.
- **Assess landing zones and the exact vessel diameter lesion significance.**
- IVUS criteria for optimal landing zone is a segment with a <50% stenosis. Generally accepted IVUS criteria for lesion significance is when the MLA is <4 mm² for a non-left main proximal vessel and <6 mm² for a left main.[1] There are data available now from Park et.al to show an MLA 4.8 mm² for left main and 2.75 mm² for non LM proximal coronaries can be safely left for medical management.[1] It is important to know that IVUS overestimates vessel diameter when compared to quantitative coronary angiogram (QCA) and optical coherence tomography. In spite of IVUS providing the exact diameter and length of the stent to be selected, it's positioning and deployment has to be done under angiographic guidance from the landmarks available from IVUS like the side-branch.
- **IVUS assessment of bifurcation lesions** helps in predicting side branch closure after main vessel PCI. High plaque burden in the proximal main branch segment and the degree of initial side branch stenosis are the two important factors predicting branch occlusion after main vessel stenting.

Post-PCI Assessment

- IVUS is used for both assessing the end point of PCI and to asses any suboptimal angiographic results.
- A stent strut appears as a short bright linear structure with shadows behind, whereas a strut of a bioresorbable scaffold appears as two bright lines very close to each other without shadowing.
- Quantitative parameters for optimal PCI results are a minimal stent area >90% of the mean reference lumen area without any malapposition or under expansion or edge dissections.
- Angiographic haziness within the stented area may be because of thrombus, tissue prolapse or dissection flaps and all of them can be studied accurately by IVUS. Thrombus prolapse through the stent struts in acute coronary syndrome settings are better left untouched as aggressive post dilation may lead to distal embolization and slow flow.
- IVUS is more sensitive than angiogram in detecting edge dissections but less sensitive than OCT. But in practice IVUS detected dissections have more implications with regard to further interventions than those seen by OCT. Edge dissection is identified when a flap is identified within 5 mm from the stent edge and IVUS is more sensitive to pick up angiographically silent edge dissections. IVUS criteria for a significant edge

dissections are a final lumen area <4 mm² or when the dissection angle is >60°. Flap length >0.6 mm are also considered significant.
- IVUS can identify geographical miss and ostial miss accurately that are associated with higher TLR rate and guide regarding the need for further interventions.
- Malapposition is identified when a stent strut lacks contact with the underlying wall that is not in relation to a side branch. Figure 5 showing malapposed stent
- Malapposition or incomplete stent apposition (ISA) can be acquired late after the index procedure for the following reasons:
  - Resolution of jailed thrombus after PCI during ACS
  - Positive remodelling of the vessel wall
  - Regression of underlying plaque or
  - Chronic stent recoil.
- Under expansion is considered when the minimal stent area is less than 70% of the balloon predicated maximal area, when dilated with a balloon that matched the vessel diameter at the site of under expansion (Fig. 6). Showing an under expanded stent
- Stent expansion index is the ratio between the MSA to the mean proximal and distal reference area and when this is less than 80%, then also it qualifies for stent under expansion. Both under expansion and malapposition are treated by high pressure post dilation with a noncompliant balloon, but in studies under expansion has been shown to have more events (restenosis and stent thrombosis) compared to malapposition. Calcified lesions are the most important cause for stent under expansion or malapposition. IVUS is the modality of choice in evaluating the late acquired ISA, owing to its larger field of view and deeper penetration.

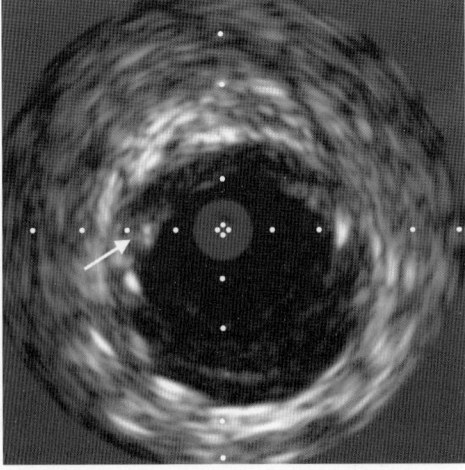

Fig. 5: Arrow showing malapposed stent.

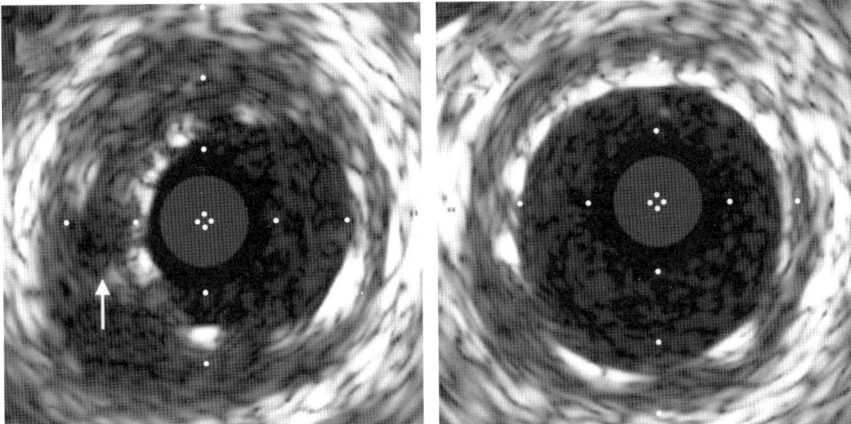

Fig. 6: Arrow showing under expanded stent right and well expanded stent after post-dilation left.

IVUS for Specific Lesion Subsets

Left Main

Assessment of left main coronary disease by angiography is difficult because of the aortic cusp opacification or "streaming" contrast obscuring the ostium, short length of the vessel may leave no normal segment for comparison, and the distal left main artery may be concealed by bifurcation or trifurcation. Ultrasound can help overcome these confounding factors. Propensity based analysis of the patient's the Main Compare trial showed that use of IVUS during LM PCI significantly reduced the 3 year mortality by preventing late stent thrombosis. IVUS-TRONCO-ICP registry also showed that an IVUS guided strategy for left main PCI significantly improved event free survival.

Bifurcation Stenting

There is minimal correlation between angiographic medina classification of bifurcation lesions and IVUS distribution of plaque. In case of LM bifurcation lesions a continuous distribution of the plaque into ostial LAD (more commonly) or the ostial LCX (less commonly) is the rule and the carina is usually spared. Pre PCI proximal main branch plaque volume is an important predictor of plaque shift causing SB stenosis and it usually requires a stent. IVUS helps in lesion assessment to plan the optimal bifurcation strategy, decide the balloon size for final kissing balloon dilation and to evaluate the final result if angiographically sub optimal. Side branch pinching secondary to carinal shift can be managed with balloon dilation alone. Though IVUS gives valuable anatomical information over angiography in bifurcation stenting FFR is best to assess the functional significance of a SB pinching. An IVUS MLA < 2.25 mm^2 or a plaque burden > 50% corresponds to FFR value of < 0.8 but its sensitivity, specificity and reproducibility are poor. The benefits of IVUS guided PCI in improving the long term outcomes after bifurcation PCI has been shown in multiple studies.

ACS

Optimal selection of stent size and landing zone is challenging during primary PCI because of the presence of thrombus and vessel spasm, and may be facilitated by using intracoronary imaging. In registry based studies it has been shown that use of IVUS during ACS increases number of additional interventions including post dilation and extra stents but the mortality and stent thrombosis were not significantly different on long term follow-up. Whether IVUS is the ideal imaging technology for the assessment of thrombotic lesions remains unclear presently.

Ostial Lesions

IVUS can be used for assessment of both aorto-ostial and non aorto-ostial lesions whereas OCT cannot be used for aorto-ostial lesions. In ostial locations exact measurement of lesion length and vessel diameter are even more important. Post stent IVUS run to helps select post dilation balloon size and to confirm ostial coverage which significantly improves the outcome. Routine use of IVUS for ostial lesions results in higher MLA and better long term outcome.

Identifying Vulnerable Plaque

According to The PROSPECT trial a minimal luminal area of <4 mm^2; a plaque burden of >70%; or lesion classified as TCFA were predictors of vulnerable plaque by IVUS.

Recommendations for IVUS

The 2011 ACC/AHA guideline for PCI has recommended[2] IVUS to be reasonable for the assessment of angiographically intermediate left main CAD, to determine the mechanism of stent restenosis and for post cardiac transplant allograft vasculopathy (Class IIa). A class IIb recommendation was for the assessment of non-left main coronary arteries with angiographically intermediate coronary stenosis (50% to 70% diameter stenosis), for guidance of coronary stent implantation, particularly in cases of left main coronary artery stenting (Level of evidence: B) and may be reasonable to determine the mechanism of stent thrombosis. IVUS for routine lesion assessment is not recommended when revascularization not being contemplated.

The expert consensus statement of the SCAI in 2013 recommended[3] that IVUS is definitely beneficial for optimisation of PCI, probably beneficial for assessing the significance of LMCA stenosis (MLA = 6 sq.mm), possibly beneficial for the assessment of plaque morphology but has no proven value for determination of non-LMCA lesion severity.

Recent Advances in IVUS by using Reconstruction with Specific Algorithms

- Virtual histology—reconstructed data about plaque morphology with colour coding
- I map—gives a reconstructed data which provides lesion morphology plaque composition in a quantitative term
- Palpography—Local strain is calculated from the gated radiofrequency traces using cross-correlation analyses, displayed in a color-coded manner. Helps in identifying vulnerable plaque
- Echogenicity uses the gray-scale IVUS data to further evaluate the distribution of the gray values within a specific coronary segment and helps to identify plaque morphology.

Limitations of IVUS:
- Interpretation must rely on visual inspection of acoustic reflections to determine plaque composition. The echogenicity and texture of different tissue components may appear quite similar
- A sonolucent luminal mass of tissue may represent intracoronary thrombus, while a nearly identical appearance may result from an atheroma with high lipid content
- Thus, IVUS is accurate in determining the thickness and echogenicity of vessel wall structures, but it is not consistently able to provide actual histology. The physical size of ultrasound catheters (currently ≈ 1.0 mm) constitutes an important limitation in imaging severe stenosis
- The resolution is lesser than that of OCT and it has a relatively longer learning curve for accurate interpretation of images when compared to OCT. Nevertheless the vast majority of literature available on intra vascular imaging is from IVUS and the present OCT criteria's are actually extrapolated from IVUS to OCT.

OCT

Optical Coherence Tomography (OCT) is an optical imaging modality that uses near-infrared light to create high-resolution images of tissue microstructure. Optical coherence tomography (OCT) guidance for coronary interventions is increasingly being used and several randomised trials are underway to show its benefits over angiography.

The advent of coregistration along with rapid acquisition, easy interpretation, instantaneous 3D reconstruction and the user friendly interface makes it an attractive tool for assisting PCI at all stages (pre-procedural lesion assessment, procedural guidance, post PCI optimization and late follow-up assessment).

Basic OCT Image Interpretation

Normal coronary artery:
- Uniform silhouette, 3 layers visible in vessel wall (Fig. 7).

Fibrous plaque:
- Homogeneous with high backscatter—signal rich and brighter pixel, finely textured, low attenuation—deeper tissue can be visualized (Fig. 8).

Calcified plaque:
- Sharp edges, heterogeneous, low backscatter—signal poor, low attenuation-deeper tissue can be visualized (Fig. 9).

Lipid plaque:
- High attenuation—low tissue penetration, diffuse shadowy edges, high backscatter on surface, Low backscatter deeper tissue cannot be visualized (Fig. 10).

Uses of OCT

Pre-PCI Assessment

1. Plaque characterization

OCT helps in assessing plaque morphology and helps in differentiating between calcific, lipid, fibro fatty and fibrous plaque, due to its high resolution helps in detailed interrogation of the superficial plaque structures such as the thin, fibrous cap and necrotic core. The in vivo visualisation of a thin fibrous cap is neither possible by angiography nor by IVUS given its limited resolution. OCT has been shown to be superior to IVUS in identifying vulnerable plaques. OCT-derived TCFA was defined as a lipid-rich plaque (lipid arc within a plaque in ≥ 2 quadrants) with a thin fibrous cap (thickness at the thinnest segment < 65 µm).[4] OCT may be able to assess inflammatory cell infiltration, primarily active macrophages, another characteristic of unstable plaque. Hence OCT has advantage of assessing high risk plaque morphology and lesion preparation by differentiating different plaques with high precision.

2. Thrombus assessment

Thrombus is well-visualized by OCT with the technique able to distinguish between different thrombus phenotypes. The sensitivity of OCT to detect thrombus higher than that of IVUS.[5,6]

OCT images for white thrombi (composed of platelets and leucocytes) produce a signal-rich mass whereas red thrombi (Fig. 11)

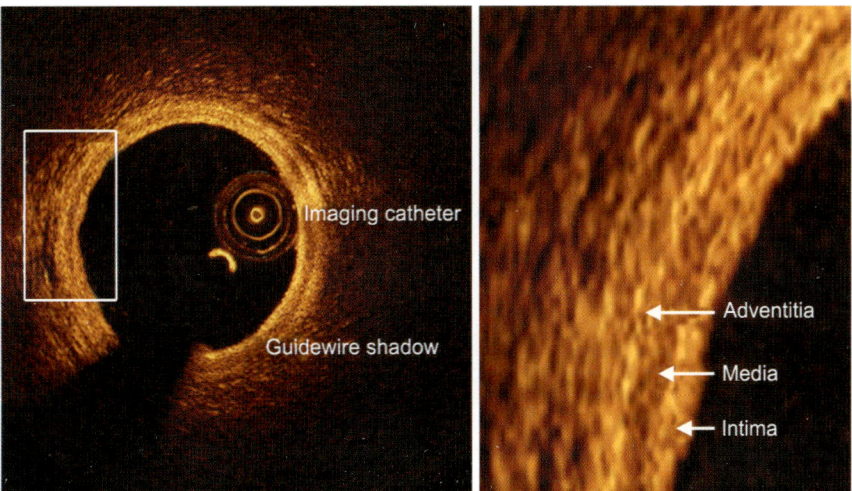

Fig. 7: Normal OCT.

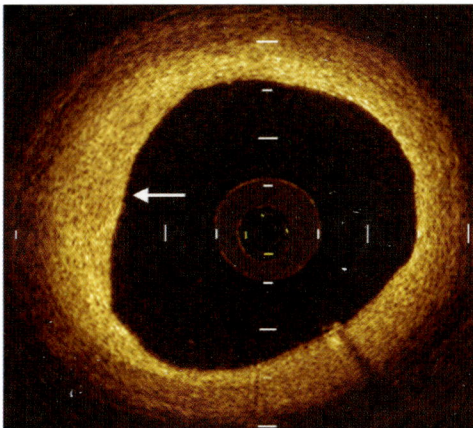

Fig. 8: OCT arrow showing fibrous plaque.

(containing mainly erythrocytes) produce high backscattering protrusions with strong signal attenuation. This gives data about plaque thrombus burden and need for further device utilization or intracoronary drug delivery to facilitate stenting.

3. **Assessment of culprit lesion in acute coronary syndromes**
   Evaluation for plaque rupture and/or thrombus in patients without angiographically evident culprit lesion.

   Evaluation of lesions with angiographic haziness: differential diagnosis between thrombus, dissection, heavy calcification.

   Determination about presence or absence of plaque (e.g. in coronary spasm).

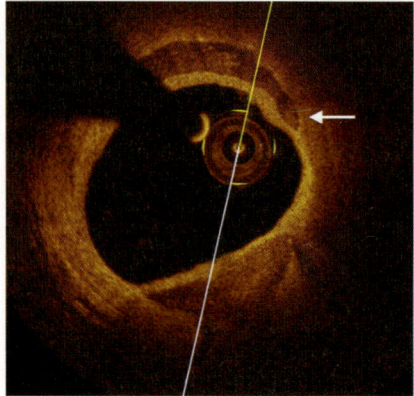

Fig. 9: Arrow showing calcific plaque.

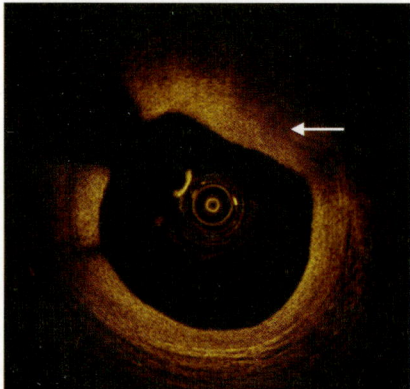

Fig. 10: Arrow showing lipid plaque.

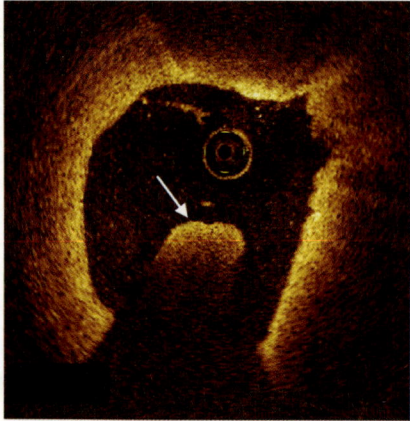

Fig. 11: Arrrow showing red thrombus.

4. **Vessel sizing and stent sizing**

OCT can provide clear delineation of the coronary lumen with an accurate measurement of reference lumen diameters, especially the proximal reference, and the minimal lumen area (MLA) at the level of the plaque which is particularly useful for the assessment of intermediate angiographic stenosis. But due to it's shallow penetration there may be a limit in the detail of the whole vessel structure visualised as compared with IVUS imaging.[7]

Assessment of plaque morphology in order to guide therapeutic strategy and device selection (rotablation, cutting balloon, etc.) Evaluation of the optimal location in the vessel for implantation of a coronary stent. Ideal landing zone according to OCT is imaged vessel should have normal 3 layered vessel atleast at an 180-degree arc. Use in bifurcation intervention (assessment of carina, ostia of side branches, stent cell geometry, tracking guide wire).

Post-PCI

Determine Stent Expansion and Apposition

OCT can provide important information, in particular, luminal diameters and area of the stented coronary segment, which correlates with the risk of restenosis.

OCT allows detailed evaluation of strut apposition to the vessel wall and stent expansion after stent deployment. As the infrared light cannot penetrate into the metal struts of the stent, the luminal surface shows a strong reflection with shadowing behind the struts and consequently improves the visibility of individual stent struts. Figure 12 showing malaposed stent. OCT is very sensitive to detect subclinical dissections and microdissections, as well as other forms of vascular injury, that may remain unnoticed by angiography or IVUS (stent edge dissection), tissue protrusion that may not be detected by either IVUS or angiography alone. Figure 13 showing edge dissection.

Rule Out Geographical Miss

Due its high resolution it precisely gives details about the geographical miss post procedure. It can reveal an incomplete coverage of the atherosclerotic lesion and therefore, the need for a second stent, or assessment of an overlapping area if multiple stents are implanted.[8]

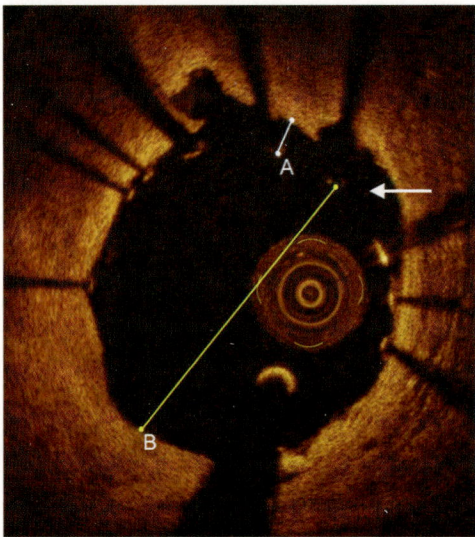

Fig. 12: Arrow showing malapposed stent.

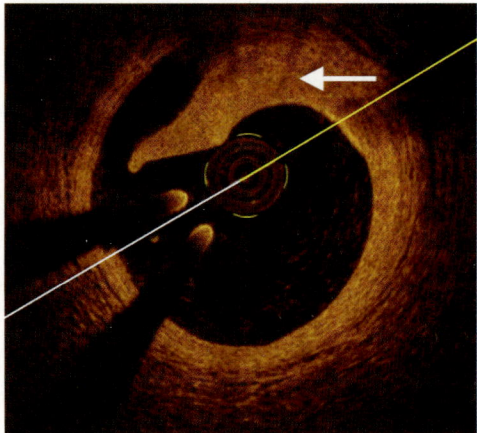

Fig. 13: OCT arrow showing edge dissection.

Follow-up Assessment of Stent Strut Coverage and ISA (Incomplete Stent Apposition)

Mid-term and long-term assessment of stent safety and efficacy: evaluation of stent restenosis (quantitative and qualitative), stent thrombosis, and stent coverage as a surrogate for vessel healing. Monitoring of the bioresorption and the healing response after implantation of bioresorbable scaffolds

Strut coverage is an important surrogate risk factor of stent thrombosis. Neo intima covering stent struts are usually < 100 μm in thickness, which is beyond the resolution of IVUS.[9]

Thus, OCT is most useful for examining patients at follow-up after DES implantation, and is capable of detecting a thin neointima due to its high resolution. Delayed arterial healing as well as incomplete endothelialization following stent implantation[10] pose high risk for very late stent thrombosis during follow up were as excessive neointimal hyperplasia poses high risk for instent restenosis and marking drug failure used in the stent. OCT provides new insights into the characteristics of the tissue covering the stent struts. The restenotic tissue of DESs, even in an early phase, also demonstrates polymorphic patterns in structure, backscatter, and composition[11,12] (Fig. 14) showing a typical restenosis.

Assessment of Biovascular Scaffolds

OCT has been extensively used to assess bioresorbable scaffolds immediately after implantation and also to follow the bioabsorption process. OCT can distinguish the rectangular polymer BVS struts that are optically transparent from the highly scattering vascular wall. Changes in the strut optical appearance at follow-up were categorized as: 'preserved box' when an intact strut footprint was present, 'open box' that marks the first OCT change in the strut footprint, dissolved 'bright box', and dissolved 'black box' that designate struts with a degraded footprint that merges into the artery wall.[13]

Limitations of OCT

1. OCT imaging needs blood-free zone to avoid attenuation by blood flow.

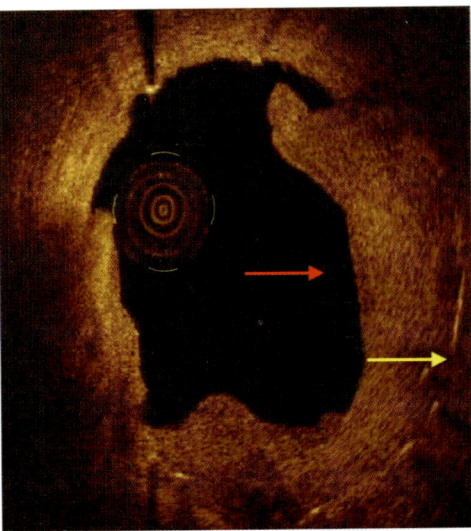

Fig. 14: Red arrow showing neointimal proliferation with restenosis and yellow arrow showing the stent implanted.

2. OCT devices has some technical limitation in some lesions including ostial disease or very tortuous lesion.
3. Penetration through the arterial wall is in the range of 2–3 mm. Sometimes, the entire plaque cannot be obtained.
4. OCT could not detect lipid pools or calcium behind thick fibrous caps, and by an inability to distinguish calcium deposits from lipid pools or the opposite.

Guidelines

The new SCAI recommendations take a step forward, indicating the technology is "probably beneficial" for determining optimal stent placement and "possibly beneficial" for assessing plaque morphology.[3]

More recent guidelines published in February 2014 by The National Institute for Health and Care Excellence (NICE)[14] suggest that the evidence on the safety of OCT to guide PCI showed good safety profile for OCT in PCI.

FURTHER READING

1. Sengottuvelu G, Rajendran R, Majumdar D. Capping spontaneous coronary artery dissection with overlapping bioabsorbable scaffolds. Heart Lung Circ. 2015 Feb;24(2):e39-40.
2. Sengottuvelu G, Erosion/malapposition of a sirolimus eluting stent - Optical coherence tomography image - A case report. Indian Heart Journal, 2012; 64(6), 610-13.
3. Sengottuvelu G, Ligthart JM, Rajendran R, 3-D optical coherence tomographic image of bifurcation lesion treated with two Absorb scaffolds. Indian Heart J. 2015 Jan-Feb;67(1):62.
4. Sengottuvelu G, Rajendran R Multimodality imaging in the evaluation of recurrent very late stent thrombosis. Asia Intervention 2015;1:124 DOI: 10.4244/AsiaInterv_V1I2A23.
5. Sengottuvelu G, Rajendran R Plaque rupture in a non-culprit artery detected by optical coherence tomography and treated with plaque capping..Indian Heart J. 2014 Nov-Dec;66(6):733-4.
6. Sengottuvelu G, Rajendran R, Dattagupta A Optical coherence tomographic image of dynamic left main coronary artery compression caused by intramural haematoma due to spontaneous coronary artery dissection - degloved artery managed with bioresorbable vascular scaffold.. EuroIntervention. 2015 Oct;11(6):659.
7. Sengottuvelu G, Rajendran R OCT during left main bifurcation PCI. Indian Heart J. 2014 Sep-Oct;66(5):557-8.
8. Sengottuvelu G, Rajendran R.Full polymer jacketing for long-segment spontaneous coronary artery dissection using bioresorbable vascular scaffolds. JACC Cardiovasc Interv. 2014 Jul;7(7):820-1.
9. Sengottuvelu G, Rajendran R. Reply: organized thrombus mimicking spontaneous coronary artery dissection. JACC Cardiovasc Interv. 2014 Dec;7(12):1458-9.

10. Sengottuvelu G, Rajendran R, Majumdar D. Optical coherence tomogram of spontaneous coronary artery dissection managed with drug eluting stent. Indian Heart J. 2014 Mar-Apr;66(2):247-8.
11. Sengottuvelu G, Rajendran R, Ravi S. Optical coherence tomographic image of an angiographically borderline lesion with a significant fractional flow reserve. J Am Coll Cardiol. 2014 May 13;63(18):1926.
12. Multimodality imaging in the evaluation of recurrent very late stent thrombosis. Asia Intervention 2015;1:124.
13. Sengottuvelu G, Robert Van-Geuns, Rajendran R. Optical coherence tomographic visualization of ten years old radial to right coronary artery anastomotic site during PCI to occluded radial graft. Heart, Lung and Circulation 2016.
14. Sengottuvelu G, Rajendran R. Optical coherence tomographic findings of myeloproliferative disorder presenting as acute myocardial infarction. Eur Heart J. 2016 Mar 16.
15. Vijayakumar subban, Gunasekaran Sengottuvelu Prevalence of parameters of suboptimal scaffold deployment following angiographic guided bioresorbable vascular scaffold implantation in real world practice—an optical coherence tomography analysis, May 2016.

REFERENCES

1. Park SJ1, Ahn JM2, Kang SJ2, Yoon SH2, Koo BK3, Lee JY2, Kim WJ2, Park DW2, Lee SW2, Kim YH2, Lee CW2, Park SW2. Intravascular ultrasound-derived minimal lumen area criteria for functionally significant left main coronary artery stenosis.ACC Cardiovasc Interv. 2014 Aug;7(8):868-74. doi: 10.1016/j.jcin.2014.02.015.
2. Glenn N. Levine, Eric R. Bates, James C. Blankenship, Steven R. Bailey, John A. Bittl, Bojan Cercek, Charles E. Chambers, Stephen G. Ellis, Robert A. Guyton, Steven M. Hollenberg, Umesh N. Khot, Richard A. Lange, Laura Mauri, Roxana Mehran, Issam D. Moussa, Debabrata Mukherjee, Brahmajee K. Nallamothu and Henry H. Ting 2011 ACCF/AHA/SCAI Guideline for Percutaneous Coronary Intervention.A Report of the American College of Cardiology Foundation/American Heart Association Task Force on Practice Guidelines and the Society for Cardiovascular Angiography and Interventions.
3. Lotfi A1, Jeremias A, Fearon WF, Feldman MD, Mehran R, Messenger JC, Grines CL, Dean LS, Kern MJ, Klein LW; Society of Cardiovascular Angiography and Interventions. Catheter Cardiovasc Interv. 2014 Mar 1;83(4):509-18. doi: 10.1002/ccd.25222. Epub 2013 Nov 13.Expert consensus statement on the use of fractional flow reserve, intravascular ultrasound, and optical coherence tomography: a consensus statement of the Society of Cardiovascular Angiography and Interventions.
4. Jang IK, Tearney GJ, MacNeill B, et al. In vivo characterization of coronary atherosclerotic plaque by use of optical coherence tomography. Circulation 2005;111:1551-1555.
5. Jang IK, Tearney GJ, MacNeill B, et al., In vivo characterization of coronary atherosclerotic plaque by use of optical coherence tomography, *Circulation*, 2005; 111:1551–5.
6. Tanaka A, Imanishi T, Kitabata H, et al., Lipid-rich plaque and myocardial perfusion after successful stenting in patients with non-ST-segment elevation acute coronary syndrome: an optical coherence tomography study, *Eur Heart J*, 2009;30:1348–55.

7. Yamaguchi T, Terashima M, Akasaka T, et al., Safety and feasibility of an intravascular optical coherence tomography image wire system in the clinical setting, *Am J Cardiol,* 2008;101:562–7.
8. Tanabe K, Serruys PW, Degertekin et al. TAXUS II Study Group. Incomplete stent apposition after implantation of paclitaxel eluting stents or bare metal stents: insights from the randomized TAXUS II trial.Circulation, 2005;111:900-5.
9. Matsumoto D, Shite J, Shinke T, et al. Neointimal coverage of sirolimus-eluting stents at 6-month follow-up: evaluated by optical coherence tomography. Eur Heart J 2007;28:961-967.
10. Finn AV, Nakazawa G, Joner M, et al., Vascular responses to drug eluting stents: importance of delayed healing, *Arterioscler Thromb Vasc Biol,* 2007;27:1500–10.
11. Gonzalo N, Serruys PW, Okamura T, et al. Optical coherence tomography patterns of stent restenosis. Am Heart J 2009;158:284-293.
12. Nagai H, Ishibashi-Ueda H, Fujii K. Histology of highly echolucent regions in optical coherence tomography images from two patients with sirolimus-eluting stent restenosis. Catheter Cardiovasc Interv 2010;75:961-963.
13. Serruys PW, Ormiston JA, Onuma Y, et al. A bioabsorbable everolimus-eluting-coronary stent system (ABSORB): 2-year outcomes and results from multiple imaging methods. Lancet 2009;373:897–910.
14. Optical coherence tomography to guide percutaneous coronary intervention. NICE interventional procedures guidance [IPG481], 2014. Available at: www.nice.org.uk/ Guidance/IPG481 (Accessed 1 July 2014).

14 Role of FFR in Evaluation of Coronary Artery Disease

CG Bahuleyan, Shifas Babu

INTRODUCTION

Fractional flow reserve (FFR) is the gold standard for invasive assessment of functional significance of coronary artery lesions. FFR guided percutaneous coronary intervention (PCI) has been shown to be superior to angiography guided PCI in terms of outcomes like death, myocardial infarction (MI) and repeat revascularization. Recently, European Society of Cardiology (ESC) has upgraded FFR to Class-I A indication in multi-vessel PCI. Presence and extent of myocardial ischemia is the major determinant of clinical outcomes from coronary artery disease (CAD).[1,2] Although coronary angiography has been widely used for detection of ischemia, there are several limitations recognized. FFR estimation is a reliable method which will give prompt and accurate lesion specific information on the ischemic potential of both left main (LM) as well as non-LM stenoses.

TECHNIQUE OF FFR ESTIMATION

- Patient should be fasting, avoid caffeine containing drinks, theophylline containing drugs at least 12 hours before the procedure.
- Can be measured using 5 Fr or 6 Fr guiding catheter.
- Therapeutic anticoagulation as per PCI protocol.
- A 0.014" pressure wire system (Certus, Aeris) provided by St Jude medical, Minneapolis, Minnesota or (Prime wire) Volcano Therapeutics, Rancho Cordova, California could be used.
- Remove the pressure wire with its plastic hoop from the packet, place it on the Cath table on an even surface, fill with saline and keep it filled for approximately 1 minute.
- The pressure wire is removed from the plastic hoop, connected to the pressure analyzer, calibrated and zeroed to atmospheric pressure.
- Ensure that the guiding catheter is flushed and no contrast is retained.
- Intra coronary (IC) nitroglycerin 200 mcg. should be given to minimize vascular tone.

- Make the required small curve at the tip of the pressure wire gently and introduce into Y connector using a thin needle. The wire is advanced to the proximal coronary artery.
- Remove the introducer needle, close the Y connector tightly and electronically equalize the wire by keeping the sensor just outside the tip of the guiding catheter. It is advisable to wait 5 to 10 seconds in this position to ensure absence of drift.
- The lesion is crossed and the wire sensor is kept at least 30 mm distal to the lesion. The wire tip should not be parked in a small branch.
- Ensure the guiding catheter is co-axial and preferably disengaged from the coronary ostium to avoid pressure damping.
- Hyperemia is induced with IV adenosine 140 mcg/kg/min or IC bolus 200 mcg for left coronary artery (LCA); 100 mcg for right coronary artery (RCA). IV administration can be done through a central vein or a proximal arm vein. Commonly used hyperemic agents are shown in Table 1. The ratio of mean distal pressure Pd to mean proximal pressure Pa (Pd/Pa) during maximal steady state of hyperemia indicates FFR (Fig. 1). It is usually measured 2 minutes after adenosine IV infusion or 10–15 seconds after IC administration.
- If the response to standard IV dose (140 mcg/kg/min) is inadequate, the dose could be increased to 180 mcg/kg/min.
- If the FFR value is close to 0.80, a repeat FFR could be done during the same diagnostic procedure.
- After completion of the PCI, FFR can be repeated. Pijls et al. have shown that a post PCI FFR > 0.95 is associated with a lower rate of adverse outcome.[3]
- Finally the FFR wire is pulled back to the guiding catheter to verify that Pa and Pd are equal and absence of drift is ensured.
  - FFR measurement is done only when a steady state of maximum hyperemia is achieved.
  - Proper technique is to be observed to keep up the accuracy of FFR measurement.

Table 1: Commonly used hyperemic agents.

Epicardial Vasodilatation	
Isosorbide dinitrate	200 mcg intracoronary bolus
Microvascular vasodilatation	
Adenosine	LCA -200 mcg , RCA 100 mcg intracoronary bolus 140 mcg/kg/min intravenous infusion
Papaverine	8 mg in the RCA,12 mg in the LCA intracoronary bolus
Nitroprusside	0.6 mcg /kg intracoronary bolus
Regadenoson	400 mcg intravenous slow bolus in 10 seconds

Chapter 14: Role of FFR in Evaluation of Coronary Artery Disease

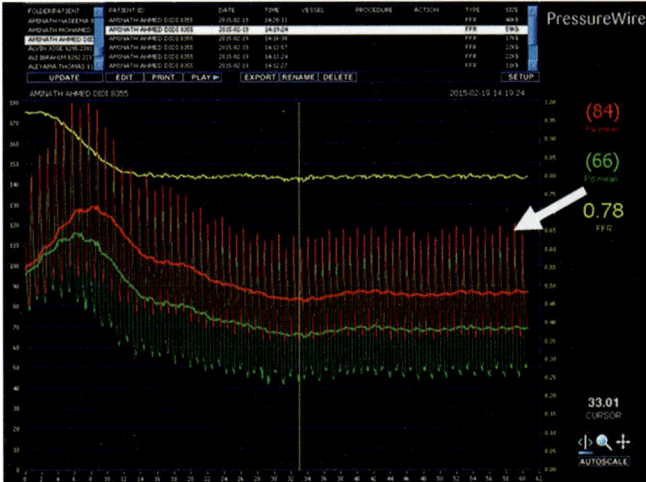

Fig. 1: Maximal steady state of hyperemia and FFR measurement. Horizontal Pd/Pa line (arrow) indicates steady state of maximum hyperemia. FFR is measured during this time.

- Trained catheterization laboratory (cath lab) staff dedicated to FFR measurement is mandatory.

COMMON PITFALLS DURING FFR ESTIMATION

- Submaximal Hyperemia is suspected when there is no characteristic response to adenosine like symptoms of chest tightness, palpitation, fall in systolic and diastolic pressure by at least 20% of the resting value and rise in heart rate more than 10% from baseline. Careful attention to the concentration of adenosine infused and avoidance of possible loss of adenosine through improper IV line connection will help to correct the inadequate hyperemia. However, in some individuals, adenosine insensitivity still remains to be a cause. In such patients, alternate vasodilator has to be considered.
- Guiding catheter induced alteration in the aortic pressure can occur when there is ostial stenosis of the coronary artery, when deep catheter engagement happens during hyperemia or when a large guiding catheter is used (Figs. 2A and B). Guiding catheter with side holes may be avoided because it influences proximal coronary pressure and also interferes with IC administration of the vasodilator.
- Pressure drift can occur during long procedures. It can be suspected when Pa and Pd have exactly the same morphology with preservation of aortic notch in the distal pressure (Figs. 3A and B). Once the drift is suspected re-equalization of the pressures by pulling back the pressure wire and keeping the sensor just outside the guiding catheter is recommended.

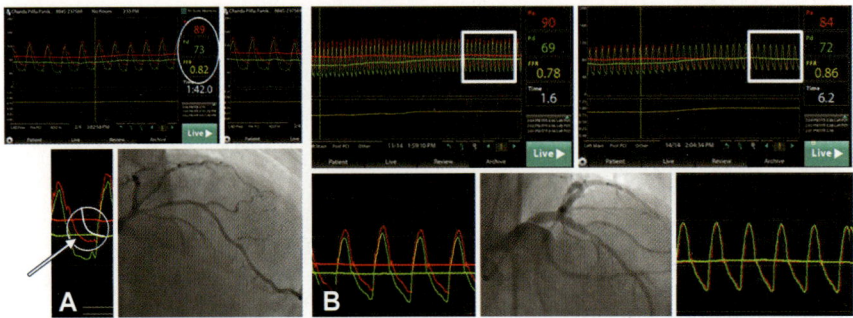

Figs. 2A and B: Effect of guiding catheter induced alteration in the aortic pressure. FFR in Proximal LAD Lesion. (A) Aortic pressure waveform alteration (arrow) with guide catheter engagement showed an FFR = 0.82. (B) FFR after catheter disengagement and correction of pressure waveform (arrow) showed significant FFR of 0.78.

FFR IN INTERMEDIATE LESION

One of the common indications of FFR estimation is to decide the functional significance of angiographic intermediate stenosis (50–70% diameter stenosis). FFR has been shown to be more accurate than exercise electrocardiography, myocardial perfusion imaging (MPI) and stress echocardiography for the detection of hemodynamically significant angiographic intermediate lesions.[4] It is considered superior to imaging techniques like intravascular ultrasound (IVUS) or optical coherence tomography (OCT) to decide whether a lesion is to be treated or not.

Fractional flow reserve (FFR) cut-off value of ≤ 0.75 was derived by comparing FFR against a series of noninvasive tests. DEFER study was designed to find the outcome difference of treating FFR negative lesions (FFR ≥ 0.75) with either PCI (PCI performance group) or PCI deferral (Defer group).[5] Five years outcomes showed similar event-free survival for the deferred and the performance group, confirming lack of advantage of doing PCI for lesions with FFR of ≥ 0.75 (79% in the defer group and 73% in performance group (p = 0.52)).[6] Fifteen years follow-up revealed that the death was not different between the groups. The rate of MI was significantly lower in the defer group (2.2%) compared with the performance group (10.0% p = 0.03).[7]

It has been observed that ischemia still exists for lesion with FFR between 0.76 and 0.80 and these values represent a grey zone. The decision to treat such lesions should be taken with consideration of anatomical and morphological aspects of the lesion, patient characteristics like diabetes mellitus, typical versus atypical angina and results of noninvasive tests for ischemia. The FAME studies adopted FFR cut-off value of ≤ 0.80 and better outcomes were demonstrated for FFR guided PCI.[8] Currently, the cut-off value of ≤ 0.80 has been recommended in clinical practice guidelines and this is applicable for LM as well as non-LM lesions.

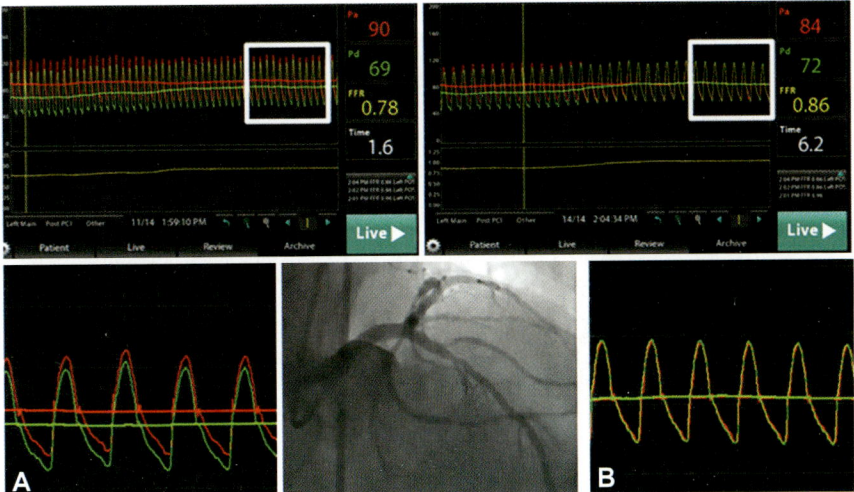

Figs. 3A and B: Pressure drift. (A) shows a pressure drift and a FFR of 0.78 in the proximal LAD lesion (note the Pd and Pa look identical). (B) Repeat FFR after re equalization of the pressure wire showed a FFR of 0.86.

- Currently utilized FFR cut off value is ≤0.80 for LM and non-LM lesions
- Decision to treat lesions with FFR values in the gray zone should take into consideration lesion characteristics, clinical features and non-invasive test results for ischemia.

FFR IN MULTIVESSEL DISEASE

The prognosis of patients with multivessel disease (MVD) could be improved by PCI with the use of current generation drug eluting stents (DES). This depends on correcting the impact of ischemia by treating lesions with ischemic potential. Noninvasive testing for detection of ischemia has limitations in the setting of MVD, due to overlap of ischemic zones, masking of areas of hypoperfusion due to balanced ischemia and lack of concordance with the coronary artery distribution. In contrast, FFR offers a readily available accurate and lesion specific information of ischemia in cath lab.[9,10]

FAME trial randomized patients with MVD to a strategy of angiography guided versus FFR guided PCI (FFR cut-off value used was ≤0.80). At 1 year; significantly lower rate of composite end point of death, non-fatal MI, and repeat revascularization was seen in the FFR guided PCI group.[8] After 2 years, a significant 34% reduction in the composite endpoint of death and MI and 37% reduction of MI alone was observed.[11] FFR driven group had been implanted fewer stents than the angio guided group. When anatomical and functional syntax score was calculated in 45% of patients with MVD in the FAME trial, 32% of patients with higher-risk were reclassified

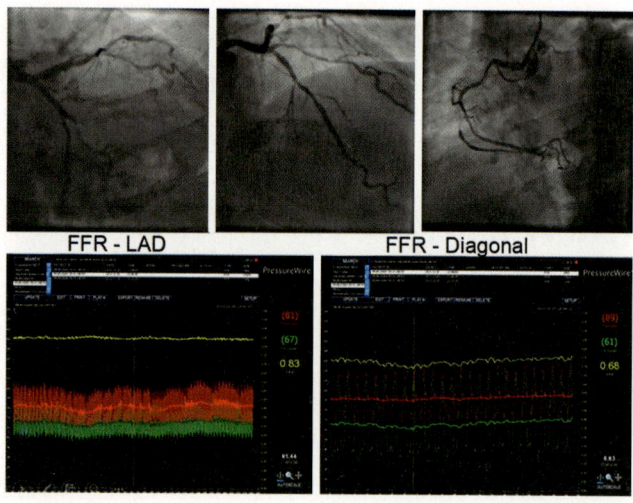

Fig. 4: Multivessel disease. Multivessel disease. FFR of LAD lesion is 0.82. Hence PCI to Diagonal, OM and RCA can be considered in this case.

as lower-risk group and this approach better identified the risk for adverse events following PCI.[12] Example of MVD with FFR assessment is shown in Figure 4.
- PCI could be considered a feasible option in many patients with MVD if FFR based strategy is adopted.
- During diagnostic angiography, FFR estimation could be done. All lesions with angiographic stenosis of 40 to 90% in MVD may be considered for FFR estimation.

FFR IN LEFT MAIN DISEASE

Angiography has several limitations in determining severity of LM stenosis. In situations when noninvasive test results are inconclusive and angiography reveals intermediate stenosis of LM, FFR estimation is useful in taking the decision of revascularization. A cut-off value of ≤ 0.80 is accepted for FFR evaluation of LM stenoses. Hamilos et al. tested this concept in 213 patients with angiographically equivocal LM stenosis. When FFR was > 0.80, patients were treated medically (n = 138), and when FFR was ≤ 0.80 coronary artery bypass graft (CABG) surgery was performed (n = 75). Five years follow-up did not reveal statistically significant difference in survival and event-free survival between medically treated group and those who have undergone CABG (90 vs 85% p = 0.48; 74 vs. 82% p = 0.50).[13] An important observation from this study was that 23% of lesions judged less than 50% at angiographic analysis turned out to be significant after FFR evaluation. An example of FFR evaluation in a moderate LM stenosis is shown in Figure 5.

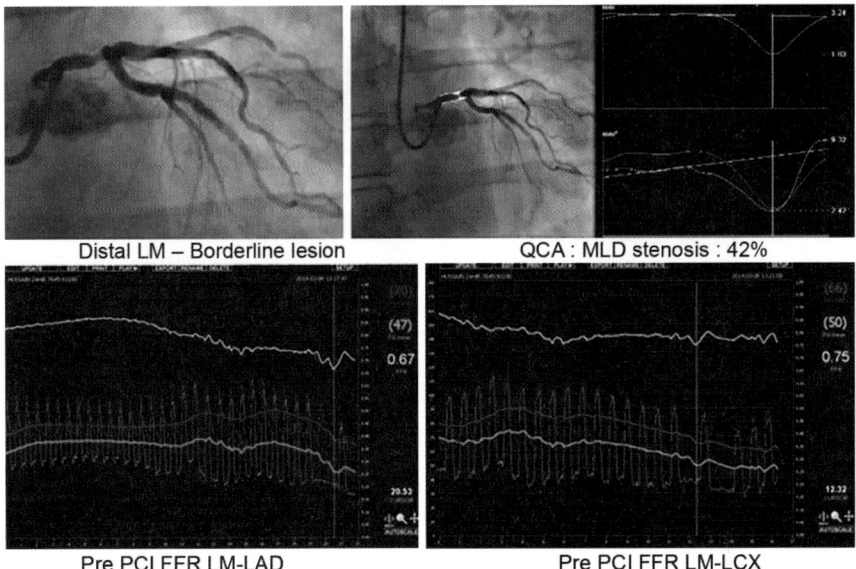

Fig. 5: LM-FFR. QCA of distal LM lesion 42%. FFR done both to LAD (0.67) and LCX (0.75).

Fractional flow reserve is utilized in the evaluation of ostial, shaft and distal LM lesions. In the case of ostial lesions equalization of pressures is done by disengaging the catheter and keeping the wire sensor in the aorta. FFR evaluation of distal LM lesion should be done from both left anterior descending (LAD) artery and left circumflex (LCX) artery separately. The catheter pressure wave form should be carefully monitored during hyperemia. It is mandatory to use IV adenosine for FFR assessment of LM. This allows complete disengagement of the guiding catheter from the ostium, as well as performing pull back recording in case of associated lesions in either LAD or LCX. In case of additional downstream significant lesion in proximal LAD, measuring FFR of LM lesion by keeping pressure wire in the LCX is inaccurate.[14] A pressure wire kept deep down in the LAD will give the sum of FFR across LM and LAD lesions (summed epicardial FFR). A pull back recording determines the pressure drop across the lesions, and the lesion with greatest pressure drop is treated first and FFR is repeated afterwards[15] (Fig. 6). Treating LAD stenosis first and then assessing LM stenosiles severity may not be the choice in many cases. It is desirable to know the severity of LM stenosis before deciding the treatment strategy. In such cases IVUS may be performed to assess LM stenosis by the criteria of minimal luminal area (MLA) so as to make appropriate decisions.

In the scenario of chronic total occlusion (CTO) of right coronary artery (RCA) and borderline LM lesion with plenty of collaterals from left coronary artery (LCA) to RCA, the FFR of LM may appear to be significant (<0.80).

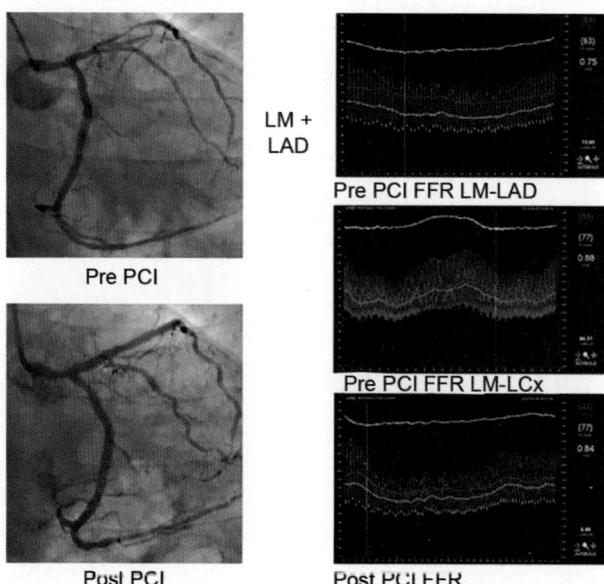

Fig. 6: LM and LAD disease. Intermediate lesion of distal left main associated with proximal severe LAD stenosis. Pre PCI FFR done both to LAD and LCX. After stenting the LAD FFR is 0.84, indicates that LM stenosis is not significant.

Successful PCI of RCA- CTO reverses the impact of collaterals and repeat FFR will reveal that LM stenosis is not significant (>0.80).

FFR is useful determining the functional significance of angiographically borderline LM stenosis and the cutoff value is ≤0.80.

In distal LM stenosis, FFR should be obtained from LAD and LCX separately.

In case of coexistent significant proximal LAD or LCX stenosis, pressure wire pull back information will be useful.

FFR IN SERIAL LESION AND DIFFUSE DISEASE

When an epicardial artery is having two or more moderately severe lesions separated by 10–20 mm of irregular or nearly normal segment, FFR can be utilized to decide which lesion is to be treated. During maximum hyperemia the first stenosis limits the maximum flow across the distal lesion and vice versa. Pijls and De Bruyne have demonstrated this phenomenon in experimental animal model.[15,16] As the severity of the distal stenosis increases, it reduces the flow across the proximal lesion and FFR becomes higher (>0.80). Hence FFR of individual lesions cannot be accepted to decide the treatment in serial lesions.[16]

In case of serial lesions, FFR wire is placed in the vessel with the sensor distal to the distal lesion and if the FFR is ≤0.80, the pressure wire pull back

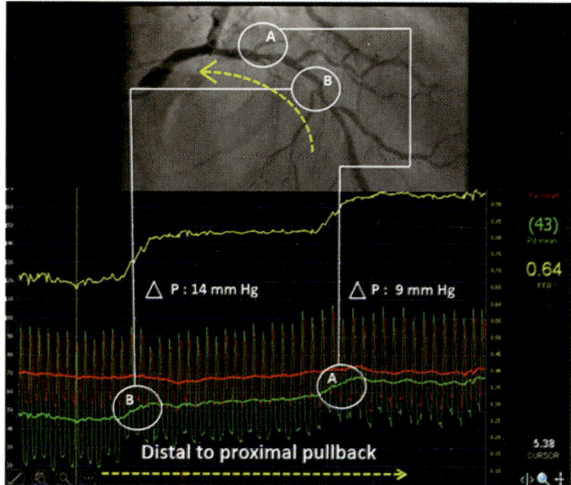

Fig. 7: Serial lesion assessment. LAD shows 2 serial lesions (A and B). Summed FFR is 0.64. Pull back tracing showed maximum ΔP at lesion B (14 mm Hg). Lesion B is to be stented first and then repeat FFR to find out the significance of lesion A.

is done slowly while maximum hyperemia is maintained. The lesion with maximum pressure gradient is stented first. After treating the first lesion, if the FFR remains abnormal, do the pull back again and stent the next lesion with the largest pressure gradient. Kim has shown the safety and efficacy of pull back technique in decision making in the treatment of serial lesions.[17] An example of serial lesion assessment (Fig. 7).

In diffuse coronary disease, continuous pressure wire pull back from distal to proximal with maximum hyperemia helps to decide the treatment options. If the FFR is ≤0.80 and the pull back reveals a continuous and gradual pressure recovery the patient can be better treated medically. If focal pressure drop is found in diffuse disease, spot stenting may be done to cover that segment. Example of a diffuse disease treated with focal stenting (Fig. 8).

Serial lesions: FFR of individual lesions cannot be accepted to decide which lesion is to be treated. Pressure wire pullback with maximum hyperemia is recommended and the lesion with higher pressure shift (ΔP) will be treated first.

FFR IN BIFURCATION LESIONS

The side branch (SB) narrowing is difficult to be assessed by angiography because of overlap with the main branch, stent strut across the side branch and foreshortening. Visual-functional mismatch is common in bifurcation disease especially overestimation of ostial side branch stenosis. Koo et al.

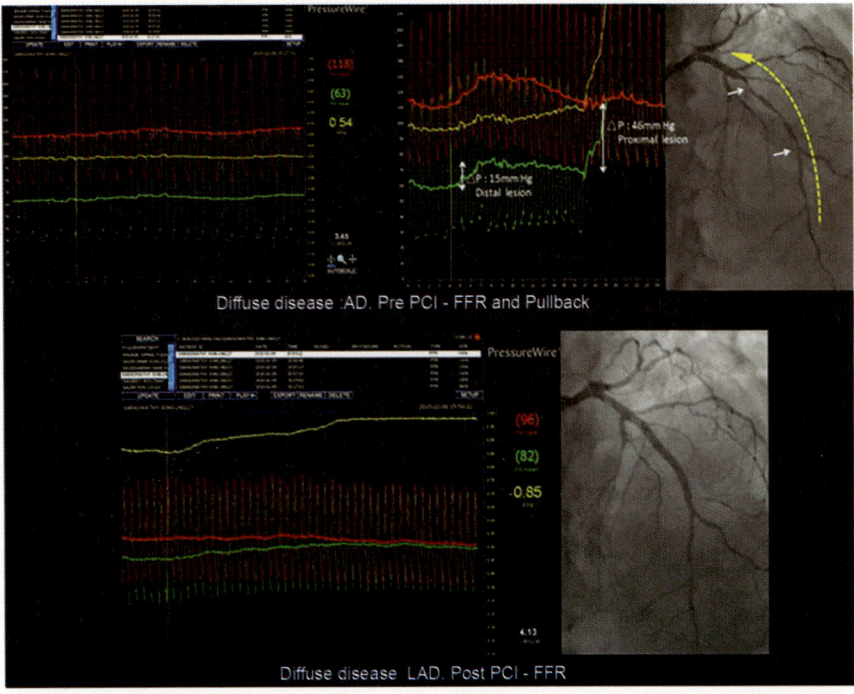

Fig. 8: Diffuse disease treated with focal stenting. Baseline FFR of diffuse LAD stenosis is 0.54. Pullback tracing showed ΔP in mid LAD (arrows). After stenting the segments with pressure shift FFR became 0.85 and pullback showed gradual recovery of pressure difference indicative of residual diffuse disease.

compared FFR to angiography in 97 jailed side branch lesions after stenting and found that no lesion with < 75% stenosis had FFR < 0.75 and only 27% of 73 lesions with stenosis > 75% were functionally significant.[18] When IVUS and FFR were compared in SB ostial lesions, a statistically significant cut-off value of MLA correlating with FFR could not be found.[19] Therefore FFR assessment of the jailed SB may be an accurate method to decide the need for SB intervention. This strategy can reduce unnecessary complex interventions and associated complications. Preintervention SB FFR cannot reliably predict the functional significance of jailed side branch due to the influence of main branch stenosis and the dynamic geometric changes during PCI. FFR interrogation of a SB after PCI can be technically challenging as the wire characteristics are different from the usual coronary wires. The measurement of FFR is not indicated in small side branches or branches in which revascularization is clinically not needed. Similarly in very tortuous, heavily calcified or diffusely diseased side branch lesions, benefit of FFR estimation is less evident; moreover procedural risk is likely to be higher. The DK CRUSH-VI trial compared FFR versus angiography guided SB intervention in 320 patients with true bifurcation lesions. FFR guided group underwent FFR of the SB after main branch stent deployment. 1-year target vessel revascularization and stent thrombosis rates were similar in both groups, with identical 1-year major adverse cardiac event (MACE) rates of 18.1% (hazard ratio [HR] 0.91, 95% confidence interval [CI], 0.48-1.88; P = 1.00).[20]

FFR IN ACUTE CORONARY SYNDROME (ACS)

Fractional flow reserve has limited application in ACS setting, especially in ST- Elevation MI (STEMI). Variable grades of microvascular dysfunction in the infarct related artery (IRA) territory leads to reduced maximum achievable flow and higher FFR across the IRA stenosis. After 3–5 days the microvascular dysfunction recovers and the FFR becomes lower. De Bruyne et al. compared FFR in 57 patients with MI >6 days old to single photon emission computed tomography (SPECT) before and after PCI. Patients with positive SPECT before PCI had a significantly lower FFR than patients with negative SPECT. The FFR cut-off in the IRA observed was 0.78.[21] Samady et al. performed FFR and SPECT in 48 patients 3-7 days after MI and the optimal FFR cut-off value of IRA stenosis observed was 0.78.[22] When patients with acute MI present 3–5 days after the event, FFR could indicate the functional significance of the IRA lesion.

Fractional flow reserve has been measured in 112 non-culprit stenoses in patients with ACS (75 STEMI, 26 NSTEMI) in the acute phase as well as at 35 ± 24 days later. Only 2 out 112 stenoses showed a change in FFR on follow-up (FFR >0.80 during ACS became 0.75 at follow-up).[23] FFR could be done in the non-culprit vessels in acute MI to decide the need for intervention. Leessar et al. showed better 1 year clinical outcome in 70 patients with NSTE-ACS with FFR guided revascularization.[24] Two years follow-up of FAME study revealed only 1 out of 513 or 0.2% deferred lesions based on FFR developed late MI.[11] In FAMOUS-NSTEMI trial 350 NSTEMI patients were randomly assigned to FFR-guided or angiography-guided management. At 12 months, revascularization remained lower in the FFR-guided group [79.0 vs. 86.8%, difference 7.8% p = 0.054] [25] FFR appears to be safe and accurate in evaluating both culprit and non-culprit vessels in NSTE-ACS.

FFR IN GRAFT DISEASE

Fractional flow reserve assessment of CABG conduit is complicated by: (1) Competing flow (and pressure) from both the native and conduit vessels, (2) Presence of collaterals from long-standing native coronary occlusion and (3) Potential for microvascular abnormalities due to ischemic fibrosis and scarring, preexisting or bypass surgery-related MI or chronic low flow ischemia. Aqel et al. studied the use of FFR to assess the functional significance of saphenous vein graft (SVG) lesions and showed that FFR <0.75 has a negative predictive value of 85% and accuracy of 70% for the detection of ischemia when compared to stress MPI.[26] Assessment of FFR for an SVG lesion is similar to that for native lesions. The pressure sensor is zeroed and subsequently positioned distal to the anastomosis of the graft into the native vessel. FFR is measured during hyperemia. The FFR reflects only the functional significance of the SVG lesion if the native vessel is occluded. Currently, the cut-off value of ≤0.80 recommended in clinical practice guidelines is applicable for Graft disease also. If both native vessel and SVG have lesions, pressure pullback during maximal hyperemia should be performed on each lesion. The stenosis with the greatest pressure gradient (ΔP, not FFR) should be treated first. FFR can be repeated in the non-treated lesion with consideration for revascularization if the FFR remains <0.80. In a study of 223 patients with stable or unstable angina and intermediate stenosis of a bypass graft, Di Serafino and colleagues showed that the major adverse cardiac and cerebrovascular events (MACCE) occurred in 28% of the FFR-guided PCI group versus 51% of the angiography-guided PCI group (HR 0.33, 95% CI, 0.11-0.96; p = 0.043).[27]

IMPACT OF COLLATERALS ON THE ASSESSMENT OF FFR

Fractional flow reserve estimation may be done reliably even in the presence of collaterals. Distal coronary pressure during maximal hyperemia is dependent both on the antegrade flow as well as the flow through the collaterals. FFR depends on the amount of myocardium supplied by the particular artery. This concept is important when assessing intermediate lesions in arteries which supply collaterals (donor artery) to the territory of an artery with CTO. FFR may give false positive results in such situations. Successful CTO-PCI may reverse an ischemic donor artery FFR to normal FFR.[28] Hence it is preferable to recanalize the CTO whenever feasible in order to avoid unnecessary stenting of intermediate donor artery stenosis.

SUMMARY

Fractional flow reserve estimation is the currently available most accurate method to assess the functional significance of coronary artery stenosis in the cath lab. It is reliable, reproducible, easily obtainable and lesion specific. Use of FFR helps to avoid unnecessary intervention and make PCI more safe and effective. Large amount of clinical trial results have supported its use in elective PCI, for various anatomic spectrum of CAD. Recently data is emerging to define its possible role in the revascularization of patients with ACS.

REFERENCES

1. Shaw LJ, Iskandrian AE. Prognostic value of gated myocardial perfusion SPECT. J Nucl Cardiol. 2004;11:171-85.
2. Metz LD, Beattie M, Hom R, et al. The prognostic value of normal exercise myocardial perfusion imaging and exercise echocardiography: a meta-analysis. J Am Coll Cardiol. 2007;49:227-37.
3. Pijls NH, Klauss V, Siebert U, et al. Coronary pressure measurement after stenting predicts adverse events a follow-up: A multicentre registry. Circulation. 2002;105(25)2950-4.
4. Pijls NH, De Bruyne B, Peelsk, et al. Measurement of fractional flow reserve to assess the functional severity of coronary artery stenosis. N Engl J Med. 1996;334:1703-98.
5. Bech GJ, De Bruyne B, Pijls NH, et al. Fractional flow reserve to determine the appropriateness of angioplasty in moderate coronary stenosis: a randomized trial. Circulation. 2001;103:2928-34.
6. Pijls NHJ, van Schaardenburgh P, Manoharan G, et al. Percutaneous coronary intervention of functionally non-significant stenosis: 5-year follow-up of the DEFER study. J Am Coll Cardiol. 2007;49:2105-11.
7. Zimmermann FM, Ferrara A, Johnson NP, et al. Performance of percutaneous coronary intervention of functionally non-significant coronary stenosis: 15-year follow-up of the DEFER trial. Eur Heart J. 2015;36(45):3182-8.
8. Tonino PAL, De Bruyne B, Pijls NHJ, et al. Fractional flow reserve versus angiography for guiding PCI in patients with multivessel coronary disease (FAME study). N Engl J Med. 2009;360:213-24.
9. Pijls NH, van Son JA, Kirkeeide RL, et al. Experimental basis of determining maximum coronary, myocardial, and collateral blood flow by pressure measurements for assessing functional stenosis severity before and after percutaneous transluminal coronary angioplasty. Circulation. 1993;87:1354-67.
10. De Bruyne B, Baudhuin T, Melin JA, et al. Coronary flow reserve calculated from pressure measurements in humans. Validation with positron emission tomography. Circulation. 1994;89:1013-22.
11. Pijls NH, Fearon WF, Tonino PA, et al. Fractional flow reserve versus angiography for guiding percutaneous coronary intervention in patients with multivessel coronary artery disease: 2-year follow-up of the FAME (Fractional Flow Reserve Versus Angiography for Multivessel Evaluation) study. J Am Coll Cardiol. 2010;56:177-84.
12. Nam CW, Mangiacapra F, EntjeEntjes R, et al. Functional SYNATX Score for risk Assessment in Multivessel Coronary Artery Disease. J Am Coll Cardiol. 2011;58(2):1211-18.
13. Hamilos M, Muller O, Cuisser T, et al. Long-term clinical outcome after fractional flow reserve-guided treated in patients with angiographically equivocal left main coronary artery stenosis. Circulation. 2009;120:1505-12 (PMID:19786633).
14. Kern MJ. When does a left anterior descending stenosis alter flow across a left main segment?: Interpreting left main fractional flow reserve with downstream obstruction. Circ Cardiovasc Interv. 2013;6:128-30.
15. Pijls NHJ, de Bruyne BG Bech GJ, et al. Pressure measurement to assess the hemodynamic significance of serial stenosis within one coronary artery validation in humans. Circulation. 2000;102:2371.

16. De Bruyne B, Pijls NHJ, Heyndrickx GR, et al. Pressure-derived fractional flow reserve to assess serial epicardial stenosis, theoretical basis and animal validation. Circulation. 2000;101:1840.
17. Kim HL, Koo BK, Nam CW, et al. Clinical and physiological outcomes of Fractional flow pressure guided percutaneous coronary intervention in patients with serial stenosis within one coronary artery. JACC Cardiovasc Interv. 2012;5(10):1013-18.
18. Koo BK, Park KW, Kang HJ, et al. Physiological evaluation of the provisional side-branch intervention strategy for bifurcation lesions using fractional flow reserve. Eur Heart J. 2008;29:726-32.
19. Koh JS, BK, Kim JH, et al. Relationship between fractional flow reserve and angiographic and intravascular ultrasound parameters in ostial lesions: major epicardial versus side branch ostial lesions. JACC Cardiovasc Interv. 2012;5:409-15.
20. Chen SL, Ye F, Zhang JJ, et al. Randomized comparison of FFR guided and angiography-guided provisional stenting of true coronary bifurcation lesions: the DK CRUSH-VI Trial (Double Kissing Crush Versus Provisional Stenting Technique for Treatment of Coronary Bifurcation Lesions VI). JACC Cardiovasc Interv. 2015;8:536-46.
21. De Bruyne B, Pijls NHJ, Bartunek J. et al. Fractional flow reserve in patients with prior myocardial infarction. Circulation. 2001;104:157-62.
22. Samady H, Lepper W, Powers ER, et al. Fractional flow reserve of infarct–related arteries identifies reversible defects on noninvasive myocardial perfusion imaging early after myocardial infarction. J Am Coll Cardiol. 2006;47:2187-93.
23. Ntalianis A, Sels JW, Davidavicius G, et al. Fractional flow reserve for the assessment of nonculprit coronary artery stenoses in patients with acute myocardial infarction. JACC Cardiovasc Interv. 2010;3:1274-81.
24. Leesser MA, Abdul Baki T, Akkus N, et al. Use of fractional flow reserve versus stress perfusion scintigraphy after unstable angina. Effect on duration of hospitalization, cost, procedural characteristics and clinical outcome. J Am Coll 2003;41:115-21.
25. Layland J, Oldroyd KG, Curzen N, et al. Fractional flow reserve vs. angiography in guiding management to optimize outcomes in non-ST segment elevation myocardial infarction: the British Heart Foundation FAMOUS-NSTEMI randomized trial. Eur Heart J. 2015 Jan 7;36(2):100-11.
26. Aqel R, Zoghbi GJ, Hage F, et al. Hemodynamic evaluation of coronary artery bypass graft lesions using fractional flow reserve. Catheter Cardiovasc Interv. 2008;72:479-85.
27. Di Sarafino L, De Bruyne B, Mangiacapra F, et al. Long-term clinical outcome after fractional-flow reserve-versus angio-guided percutaneous coronary intervention in patients with intermediate stenosis of coronary artery bypass grafts. Am Heart J. 2013;166:110-18.
28. Sachdeva R, Uretsky BF. The effect of CTO recanalization on FFR of the donor artery. Catheter Cardiovasc Interv. 2011;77:367-69.

15 Cardiac MRI and Cardiac CT: Indispensable Tools for the Diagnosis of Coronary Artery Disease

Bhavin Jankharia, Parang Sanghavi, Aamish Kazi

INTRODUCTION

Coronary artery disease (CAD) affects 7 to 13% of urban and 2 to 7% of the rural populations in India and produces a significant disease burden.[1] Accurate evaluation of CAD helps improves outcomes. Early diagnosis of CAD can help institute aggressive measures to control disease and prevent progression to ischemic heart disease.[2]

Cardiac Magnetic resonance imaging (MRI) and cardiac computerized tomography (CT) in the last two decades have made great technological leaps that have allowed both of them to make a difference in the evaluation of CAD. Both of them have different indications and uses that we will discuss in the next few pages.

CARDIAC CT

For many years, this was the holy grail of imaging. While electron beam CT scanners (EBCT) had the temporal resolution to allow evaluation of the calcium content of the coronary arteries,[3] it was with the advent of four slice CT scanners,[4] with a slow heart rate of around 60, that it was possible to achieve a temporal resolution that could summate the coronary arteries over a few heart-beats and allow visualization of the coronary arteries. The current 256 and 320 slice scanners allow even faster acquisition of images, though good quality studies still need a low, steady heart rate and can be achieved with 64-slice CT scanners as well.

CA SCORING

This was the first modality to evaluate CAD risk. Outcome data over more than two decades has shown that a calcium score of 0 is associated with an extremely low coronary event risk.[5] As the calcium score increases, the event risk rises. It is an independent risk factor for coronary events and event-free survival. It is a modality ideally situated for mass screening.

- Plain scan
- Low radiation
- Easy to interpret.

CORONARY ANGIOGRAPHY (CCA)

This requires intravenous contrast administration, a low heart rate as far as possible and a steady heart rate for the best images.

CCA is performed in the following situations:

To Rule Out Coronary Artery Disease

In patients with medium to high risk of coronary artery disease, who are otherwise asymptomatic or have equivocal symptoms or results of ECG or stress test, CCA is the modality of choice to evaluate the status of the coronary arteries. Outcome data is now available and shows that a normal coronary angiogram has a negligible coronary event risk with a negative predictive value approaching 100%[6] (Fig. 1).

CCA is also used in emergency rooms to triage chest pain. A "triple rule-out" study helps rule out coronary artery disease, pulmonary thromboembolism and aortic aneurysm with dissection.[7]

Stents

In-stent evaluation is still an issue. The larger the stent, the easier it is view the lumen (Fig. 2). The faster scanners with iterative reconstructions have

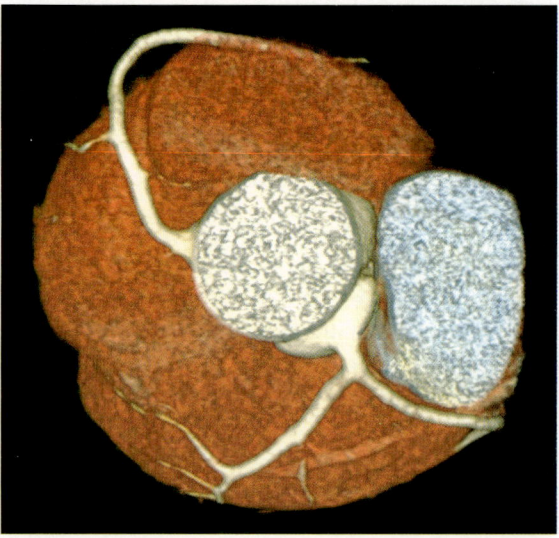

Fig. 1: Volume rendered coronary CT angiogram (CTA) shows normal coronary arteries.

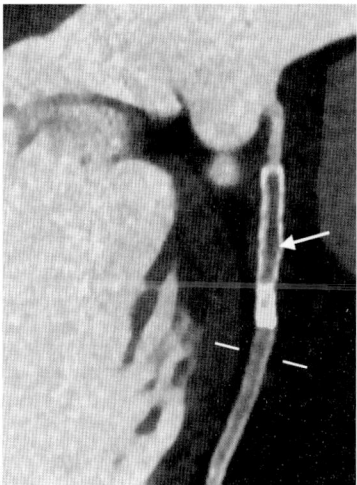

Fig. 2: Maximum intensity projection (MIP) CTA of the left anterior descending artery (LAD) using an iterative reconstruction algorithm shows in-stent occlusion (arrow).

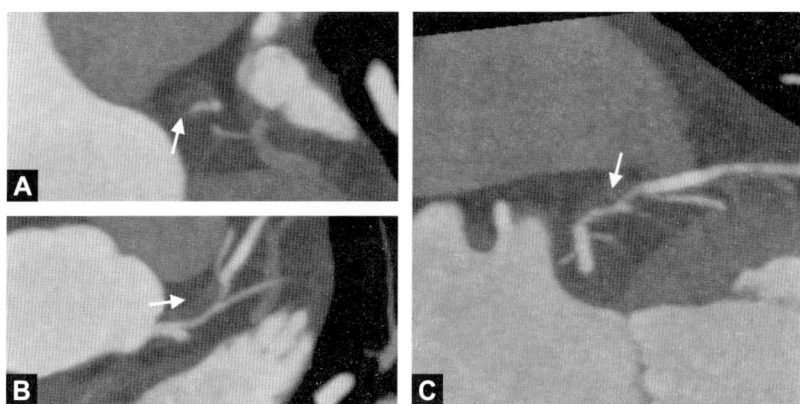

Figs. 3A to C: MIP images in cross-section (A) and in two perpendicular longitudinal planes (B and C) shows a complex plaque (arrows) with a lipid core (arrow in A) with significant stenosis.

improved the ability to see the in-stent lumen (Figs. 3A to C), though with small stents, there are still issues.[8] While CCA is used in some instances to evaluate in-stent lumen, especially in patients with equivocal symptoms, often the reason to do CCA is to evaluate the rest of the vessels, with the same clinical indication as above.

Plaque Evaluation

Cardiac CT is an excellent modality to evaluate plaque composition. The newer dual energy scanners with iterative reconstruction techniques have

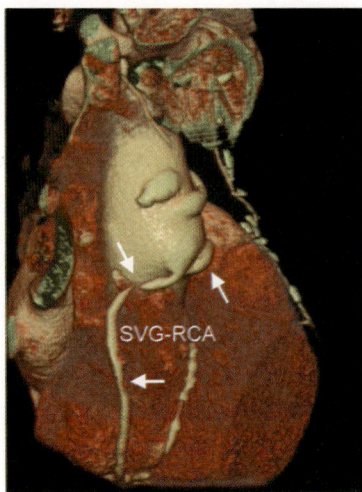

Fig. 4: VRT CT angiogram shows 2 occluded venous grafts (fat white arrows). The saphenous vein graft (SVG) to the posterior descending artery (PDA) shows focal severe stenosis (arrow) with another 50% stenosis more distally (arrow).

made plaque analysis (*see* Figs. 3A to C) more robust, though clinical utility is still suspect.[9] The analysis of plaque-at-risk using CCA is being evaluated in multiple clinical trials, but clinical utility may still be a few years away.[10]

Perfusion[11]

The newer scanners allow perfusion studies to be performed, but given the increased radiation and the availability of other equally good or better modalities with tested outcome data, it is unlikely that CT perfusion will assume an important role at least in the near future.

Following Bypass Surgery

Cardiac CT allows accurate evaluation of grafts, both venous and arterial and can serve as the first modality to evaluate graft patency, anastomotic site pathology and abnormalities of the post-graft vessel. A recent meta-analysis shows a sensitivity and specificity of 99% each for graft occlusion and 98% each for evaluation of >50% graft stenosis[12] (Fig. 4).

Cardiac MRI (CMR)

In the late 1990s, with the advent of faster gradients and balanced gradient sequences, it became easy to perform cardiac MRI studies in clinically acceptable times. This led to the use of cardiac MRI in myocardial, valvular and pericardial pathologies with an impact on management in many situations.

Coronary Arteries

While the first multi-center study on the use of CMR in the evaluation of coronary arteries showed good results, in practice, the visualization of coronary arteries by CMR is a time-consuming affair even with the use of whole heart techniques.[13]

Perfusion

Adenosine stress perfusion by CMR is a robust technique that is not inferior to nuclear medicine techniques.[14] The temporal and spatial resolution are now better and outcome data has shown results that are superior to nuclear medicine perfusion. Perfusion is usually combined with viability imaging, which improves the clinical utility of this test.

Viability Imaging

The discovery that 5-7 minutes after injection of gadolinium, it was possible to visualize infarcts (Fig. 5), paved the way for the use of CMR in the assessment of viability after a coronary event. Today CMR is the gold standard for viability imaging and accurately predicts the presence of stunned, hibernating and non-viable segments, allowing correct clinical decision-making regarding revascularization, in patients with coronary artery stenoses and severe ischemia/infarction[15] (Fig. 6).

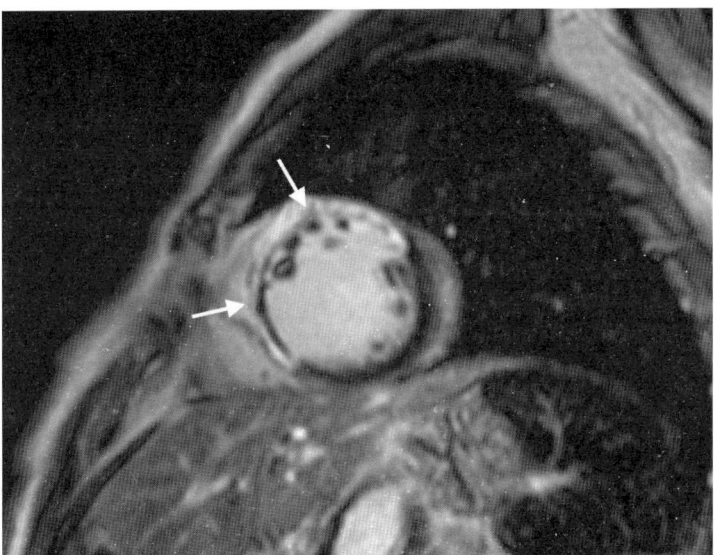

Fig. 5: Short axis (SA) mid-cavity, inversion recovery (IR) image obtained 7 minutes after intravenous (IV) gadolinium (Gd) injection shows a full-thickness LAD territory infarct involving the anterior wall and septum (arrows).

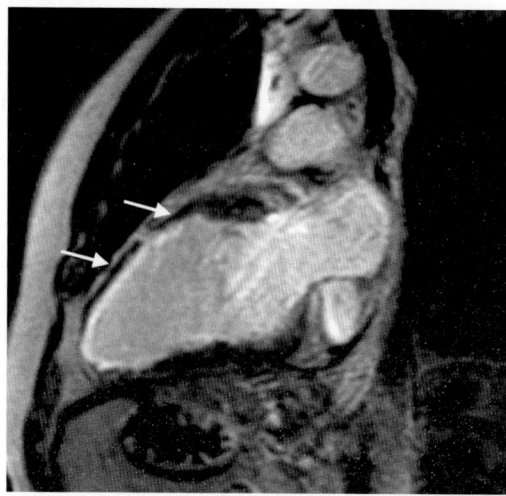

Fig. 6: 4-chamber (4C) IR image obtained 8 minutes after IV Gd injection shows an anterior wall infarct involving < 50% of the thickness of the myocardium (arrows), suggesting hibernating, potentially viable myocardium, in this patient with LAD occlusion and akinesia of the septum.

CONCLUSION

Cardiac CT is anatomic tool that can be used in early diagnosis of CAD (calcium scoring) and in diagnosing coronary artery disease (cardiac CT angiography). Cardiac MRI is a functional tool that allows assessment of perfusion defects and is the gold standard for viability imaging.

REFERENCES

1. Krishnan MN. Coronary heart disease and risk factors in India - on the brink of an epidemic? Indian Heart Jour 2012;64:364.
2. Shah N, Soon K, Wong C, et al. Screening for asymptomatic coronary heart disease in the young 'at risk' population: Who and how? IJC Heart Vascul 2015;6: 60.
3. Sechtem U. Electron beam computed tomography: on its way into mainstrem cardiology? Eur Heart Jour 2000;21:87
4. Achenbach S, Giesler T, Ropers D, et al. Detection of coronary artery stenoses by contrast-enhanced, retrospectively electrocardiographically gated, multislice spiral computed tomography. Circulation 2001;103:2535.
5. Greenland P, Bonow RO, Brundage BH, et al. ACCF/AHA 2007 clinical expert consensus document on coronary artery calcium scoring by computed tomography in global cardiovascular risk assessment and in evaluation of patients with chest pain: a report of the American College of Cardiology Foundation Clinical Expert Consensus Task Force (ACCF/AHA Writing committee to update the 2000 Expert Consensus Document on Electron Beam Computed Tomography) developed in collaboration with the Society of Atherosclerosis Imaging and Prevention and Society of Cardiovascular Computed Tomography. JACC 2007;49:378.

6. Mowatt G, Cook JA, Hillis G, et al. 64-Slice computed tomography angiography in the diagnosis and assessment of coronary artery disease: systematic review and meta-analysis. Heart 2008;94:1386.
7. Frauenfelder T, Appenzeller P, Karlo C, et al. Triple rule-out CT in the emergency department: protocols and spectrum of imaging findings. Eur Rad 2009;19:789.
8. Taylor AJ, Cerqueira M, Hodgson JM, et al. ACCF/SCCT/ACR/AHA/ASE/ASNC/NASCI/SCAI/SCMR 2010 Appropriate Use Criteria for Cardiac Computed Tomography. A Report of the American College of Cardiology Foundation Appropriate Use Criteria Task Force, the Society of Cardiovascular Computed Tomography, the American College of Radiology, the American Heart Association, the American Society of Echocardiography, the American Society of Nuclear Cardiology, the North American Society for Cardiovascular Imaging, the Society for Cardiovascular Angiography and Interventions, and the Society for Cardiovascular Magnetic Resonance. Jour Cardiovasc Computed Tomogr 2010;4:407e1-33.
9. Obaid DR, Calvert PA, Gopalan D, et al. Dual-energy computed tomography imaging to determine atherosclerotic plaque composition: a prospective study with tissue validation. Jour Cardiovasc Computed Tomogr 2014;8:230.
10. Latif MA, Cury R, Akhlaq M, et al. A systematic review and meta-analysis: prevalence of coronary plaque high-risk features (low attenuation, enlarged diameter or positive remodeling, napkin ring, and spotty calcification (lens) in acute coronary syndrome as assessed by coronary computed tomographic angiography (CTA). JACC 2016;67:1736.
11. Varga-Szemes A, Meinel FG, De Cecco CN, et al. CT myocardial perfusion imaging. Am J Roentgenol 2015 Mar;204:487.
12. Barbero U, Innaccone M, d'Ascenzo F, et al. 64 slice-coronary computed tomography sensitivity and specificity in the evaluation of coronary artery bypass graft stenosis: a meta-anaylsis. Int J Cardiol 2016;216:52.
13. Sakuma H. Coronary CT versus MR angiography: the role of MR angiography. Radiology 2011;258:340.
14. Coelho-Filho OR, Rickers C, Kwong RY, et al. MR myocardial perfusion imaging. Radiology 2013;266:701.
15. Rajiah P, Desai MY, Kwon D, et al. MR imaging of myocardial infarction. Radiographics 2013;33:1383.

16
Radionuclide Studies in Cardiology

Vikram R Lele

INTRODUCTION

Nuclear Cardiology uses radioisotopes to study the function of the heart. The radioisotopes are labeled to different compounds which study specific functions of the heart, such as perfusion, metabolism, contraction, receptors, etc. The radiolabeled compounds are injected intravenously and the passage through the heart is imaged with the help of Gamma cameras. Two technologies are available: SPECT or Single Photon Emission Computed Tomography, which uses shortlived isotopes like ^{99m}Technetium and 123-Iodine labeled with different compounds and rotating Gamma cameras which generate tomographic images of the heart. The other technology is PET-CT or Positron Emission Tomography which uses very shortlived isotopes (which decay within minutes to hours) of 11C, 13O, 15N and 18F produced in a machine called Cyclotron and which are imaged with special PET camera. Both these technologies and isotopes are available in India. Table 1 enumerates the scope of Nuclear Cardiology, and the various aspects of cardiac pathophysiology which can be studied.

In India, mainly SPECT myocardial perfusion studies are performed. Viability studies are performed with PET using 18F-FDG.

Table 1: Scope of nuclear cardiology.
• Myocardial perfusion
• Myocardial metabolism
• Myocardial contraction
• Myocardial innervation
• Myocardial infarction
• Atherosclerosis, apoptosis imaging
• Imaging gene therapy

Table 2 summarizes the radiopharmaceuticals used in nuclear cardiology and their utility.

Table 2: Isotopes and clinical utility of SPECT and PET technologies.

Radiopharmaceuticals	Study	Information obtained
SPECT 99mTc-MIBI (Methoxy Isobutyl isonitrile)	Myocardial perfusion	Detection of myocardial ischemia and infarction Quantification of extent and severity of myocardial ischemia
	Myocardial infarction	Identifying vascular territories of ischemia Risk stratification and prognosis
PET 13NH3 82 Rubidium		Absolute quantification of myocardial flow in ml/gm/min Coronary Flow Reserve (CFR) estimation
Same as above	Myocardial function	Left ventricular ejection fraction (LVEF) at rest and stress Left ventricular diastolic function Left ventricular phase analysis for dyssynchrony quantification
123I-MIBG (Meta Iodo Benzyl Guanidine)	Adrenergic innervation	Detection of adrenergic denervation. Prediction of arrhythmic events in dilated ventricles
SPECT 99mTc-MIBI (Methoxy Isobutyl Isonitrile) **PET** 13NH3 82 Rubidium 18F-FDG	Myocardial viability Combination of resting perfusion scan (SPECT or PET radiopharmaceuticals) And metabolism scan (PET with 18F-FDG)	Assessment of presence of and quantity of viable myocardium in patients with left ventricular failure for decision about revascularization (stunned and/ or hibernating myocardium)

MYOCARDIAL ISCHEMIA

The principal use of Nuclear Cardiology is in the detection and quantification of myocardial ischemia. This is done by performing a myocardial perfusion scan (**MPS**). Infect MPS is the gold standard for myocardial ischemia detection. Over the last many years, several studies have documented the diagnostic and prognostic utility of MPS for myocardial ischemia. It should be clearly understood that MPS is for detection of myocardial ischemia and NOT coronary artery disease. The presence of coronary disease (stenosis) is

inferred if ischemia is documented. Coronary stenosis may be present **without** presence of significant ischemia and ischemia may be present **without documented** epicardial coronary stenosis. Therefore, proper management of coronary artery disease requires documentation of both anatomic stenosis and presence of ischemia. Several studies including COURAGE and FAME have confirmed that management strategies based on anatomical stenosis alone are no longer appropriate and ischemia has to be considered in management.

Principle of MPS

During stress, there is coronary vasodilatation due to increased demand of myocardium for perfusion due to increased workload. A radiotracer injected during peak stress will pass through the coronary arteries and enter the myocardium perfused by these arteries. It is retained in the myocardium due to its pharmacologic properties (binding to mitochondria or cytosol elements) allowing imaging at a later time. The images obtained indicate the perfusion at the time of injection at peak exercise. In arteries which are stenosed, lesser amount of tracer will pass through and enter the myocardium as compared to normally dilated arteries. This gives rise to different amount of tracer uptake in different parts of myocardium, with high uptake in normally perfused myocardium and low uptake in myocardium supplied by stenosed arteries (perfusion defects). When injected at rest, this heterogeneity in uptake is not apparent since there is no increased demand and tracer passes equally through all arteries. Thus, perfusion defects on stress with normal perfusion at rest are hallmark of 'reversible or inducible ischemia'.

Table 3 enumerates indications for performing Myocardial Perfusion Scan (MPS).

Table 3: Who should go for MPS?

1. Patients with abnormal baseline ECG (LBBB, LVH, Digitalis, WPW syndrome) where treadmill stress test interpretation is difficult
2. Women: High rates of false positive stress test results
3. Patients unable to perform treadmill stress test (severe arthritis, neurological disorders, lack of motivation. Pharmacological stress with Adenosine/Dobutamine can be done)
4. Asymptomatic or mildly symptomatic individuals with risk factors for ischemic heart disease
5. Patients with diagnosed coronary artery disease by angiography; for risk stratification and for evaluation of physiological significance of coronary stenosis
6. Postangioplasty for evaluation of restenosis
7. Postcoronary bypass surgery for patency of grafts
8. Postmyocardial infarction for risk stratification and viability assessment

Preparation for MPS
1. Patient fasting for 4 hrs.
2. Stop beta blockers for 48 hrs. Before study and nitrates for 12 hrs.
3. No tea, coffee or caffeine containing foods for 24 hrs. before scan (chocolates, colas).

Procedure
Myocardial perfusion scans are performed using SPECT technology (201 Thallium, 99mTc-MIBI, and 99mTc-Tetrofosmin). A resting injection of the radiopharmaceutical is given. A resting perfusion scan is then performed. The patient is then taken for stress (treadmill, bicycle or pharmacological). A full stress as per Bruce protocol is performed with standard end points for termination of stress. A second injection of the radiopharmaceutical is given at peak stress. For pharmacological stress, Adenosine is the preferred stressor (140 mcg/kg/min infusion for 4-6 minutes with injection of radiopharmaceutical at 2-3 minutes of infusion). A stress image of myocardium is obtained after a while. The rest and stress images (reconstructed in standard short axis, vertical and horizontal long axis orientation) are then reviewed side by side. Stress images are inspected for presence of perfusion defects, their site, extent and severity and the rest images are viewed to see if these defects disappear (Table 4). Gating the images using ECG gating signal permits analysis of left ventricular ejection fraction (LVEF) both at stress and rest, along with analysis of diastolic function (Fig. 1).

Based on the scan findings the scans are categorized as 'low risk, intermediate risk, or high risk'. This risk stratification has been validated over several studies and is well accepted (Table 5).

The prognostic value of an MPS is well established. A low risk scan confers a cardiac event risk of <1% (myocardial infarct, death) over 2 years. Patients with a 'low risk scan' pattern can be managed medically in spite of abnormal coronary angiography.

A high risk scan, on the other hand, confers a risk of >8% for cardiac events. Patients with a high risk scan pattern should be sent for coronary angiography (if not already done) with an aim of revascularization (Fig. 2).

Table 4: Findings on the scan and their interpretation.

Stress image	No perfusion defect	Perfusion defect	Perfusion defect	Perfusion defect
Rest image	No perfusion defect	No perfusion defect	Perfusion defect of same size	Smaller perfusion defect
Interpretation	Normal	Inducible ischemia	Infarction or attenuation artifact	Mixture of ischemic and infarcted myocardium

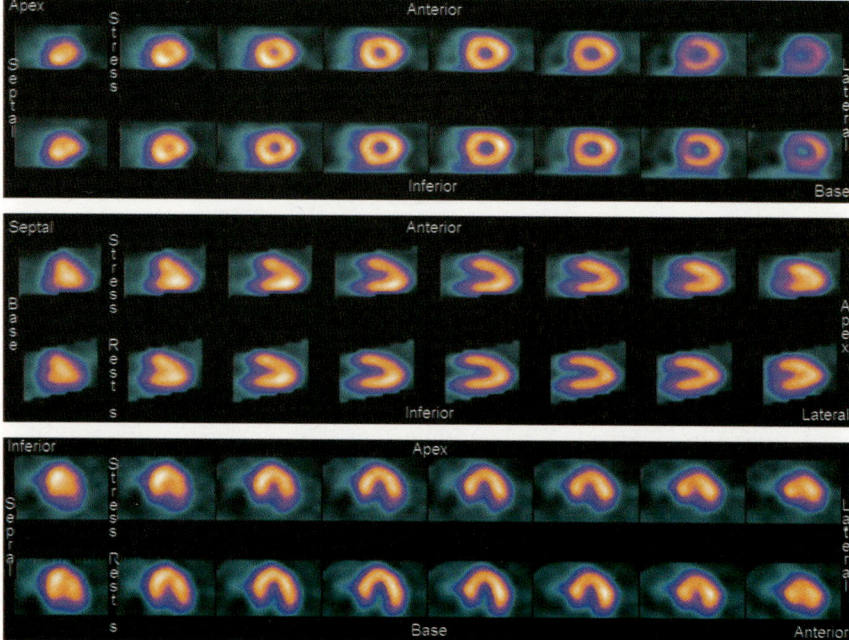

Fig. 1: A normal, low-risk myocardial perfusion scan. Top two rows show stress short axis (upper row) and rest short axis (lower row) images from apex to base showing homogenous perfusion with no perfusion defects. Middle two rows showing stress (upper row) and rest (lower row) vertical long axis images from septum to lateral wall. Bottom two rows showing stress (upper row) and rest (lower row) horizontal long axis images from inferior to superior.

Table 5: Risk stratification.
Low-risk scan
Normal scan OR
Small perfusion defect <10% of the myocardium
Intermediate-risk scan
Medium perfusion defect involving 10-20% of the myocardium OR
Small perfusion defect plus LV dilatation or lung uptake of tracer
High-risk scan
Large perfusion defect >20% of myocardium OR
Medium perfusion defect plus transient dilatation or lung uptake of tracer

The amount of ischemic myocardium has important implications for therapy. Large volume of data suggest that if >12.5% of myocardium is ischemic, then interventional revascularization strategies (CABG, PTCA) will have superior outcomes compared to medical therapy alone.

SPECT MPS suffers from certain drawbacks. If all arteries are similarly narrowed (balanced triple vessel disease), the radiotracer will pass equally through all the arteries giving rise to a normal appearing stress image with

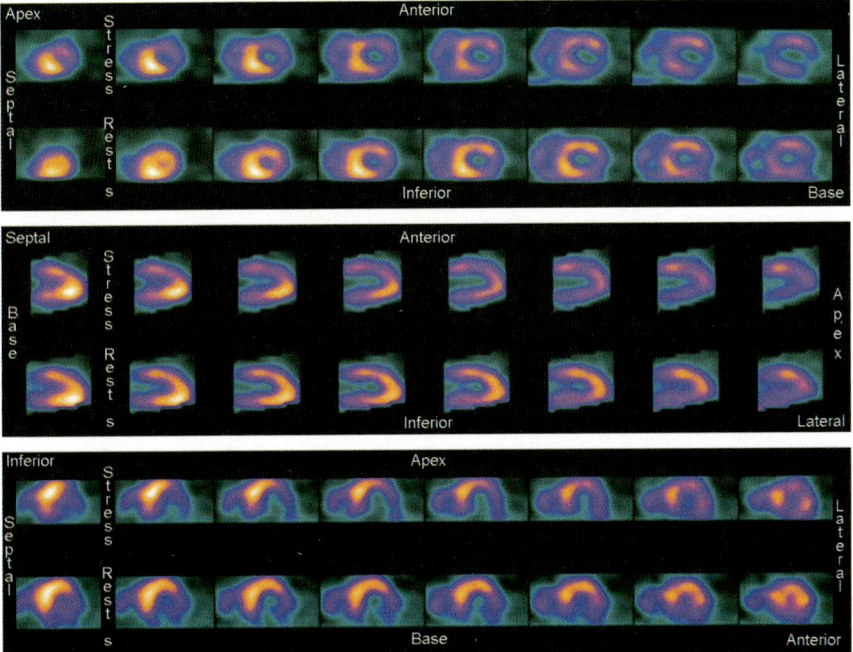

Fig. 2: Abnormal 'high risk scan' pattern with large area of inducible ischemia in all territories, TID, along with lateral wall infarct. The orientation is the same as mentioned for figure 1.

no perfusion defects. The ability to detect perfusion defects on SPECT MPI depends on different severity of stenosis in arteries causing perfusion defects of different severity and extent in vascular territories. So, one may get a relatively 'normal perfusion' in balanced triple vessel disease. To avoid this pitfall, ancillary findings on the scan such as lung uptake of tracer (indicating pulmonary congestion), transient dilatation of the left ventricle on stress (TID, Transient ischemic dilatation), fall in LVEF on stress compared to rest are searched for as surrogate markers of severe myocardial ischemia inspite of 'normal perfusion'. In obese patients, SPECT MPS is subject to attenuation artifacts causing interpretation difficulties.

SPECT MPS is also unable to quantify absolute myocardial blood flow or measure coronary flow reserve (CFR).

PET MPS using Rubidium -82 or 13N-Ammonia gives ability to measure absolute myocardial perfusion and CFR.

Most anatomic imaging modalities, like catheter coronary angiography and CT coronary angiography focus on epicardial coronary vessels, ignoring the huge subterranean microvasculature where the coronary disease begins. Endothelial dysfunction forms an important component of microvascular disease. The resolution of angiography is insufficient to image this microvasculature. Two parameters useful to interrogate this microvasculature are absolute myocardial blood flow (MBF) in ml/gm/min and the Coronary Flow Reserve (CFR). PET MPS is the current gold standard for MBF and CFR measurements.

Recently, Fractional Flow Reserve (FFR) measured by catheter angiography is being increasingly used to determine the physiological significance of the coronary stenosis. FFR is a pressure-based measurement, being the ratio of aortic root pressure to the pressure across a stenosis. An arbitrary cut-off of 0.80 is taken to decide physiological significance of stenosis, with values < 0.80 indicating physiologically significant stenosis.

CFR measured by PET is a flow-based reserve, being the ratio of flow during maximal vasodilatation (adenosine induced) to flow at rest. A value of 2.5 is considered normal and values of 1.5 and below are seen as ischemic thresholds. There is a discordance between CFR and FFR in 40% of the lesions. This is because CFR measures global disease while FFR measures only segmental disease. Presence of global disease may significantly affect the significance of segmental FFR, making CFR a more important measurement for clinical decisions than FFR.

Currently, PET MPS is available only in a few centers in India (AIIMS, Delhi, HCG, Bengaluru and PGI, Chandigarh). PET MPS with 13N-Ammonia requires onsite Cyclotron to produce the shortlived isotope, making it a very expensive technology available in only a few centers. Rubidium -82-based MBF and CFR can be done at any PET-CT center, requiring a Rubidium generator, less expensive than cyclotron-based studies.

PET MPS gives higher quality images, not prone to attenuation artifacts in obese patients and gives the MBF and CFR estimations which are so vital in management decisions. Several studies have demonstrated clinical utility of CFR measurements (Table 6).

Table 6: Clinical applications of PET, MPS and CFR estimation.

Impaired CFR in early coronary atherosclerosis
- Hypertension
- Hyperlipidemia
- Diabetes
- Smoking

Impaired CFR in coronary stenosis and advanced coronary atherosclerosis
- Evaluation of functional significance of coronary lesions (intermediate lesions)
- Detection/delineation of multivessel coronary artery disease
- Track disease progression/regression

Impaired CFR in nonatherosclerotic microvascular disease
- Syndrome X
- Cardiomyopathies (HCM, DCM)
- Hypertensive heart disease

Several studies document reduction in CFR in hypertension, hyperlipidemia, diabetes and smoking in absence of epicardial disease with return to normal values on treatment, making it a powerful tool to show effect of therapy.

PET MPS will probably be the best modality in the near future for diagnosis and management of coronary artery disease.

MYOCARDIAL VIABILITY

In patients presenting with cardiac failure with low LVEF, several studies indicate the importance of demonstrating viable (stunned or hibernating) myocardium versus scarred myocardium. Nonrandomized observational studies have demonstrated better clinical outcomes with revascularization strategies in patients with viable myocardium as opposed to medical management, with worse outcomes with revascularization in the absence of viable myocardium.

Viability can be assessed by nuclear scans, low-dose dobutamine ECHO and cardiac MRI.

Of all the available modalities, 18F-FDG (Fluorodeoxyglucose) PET scan is the most sensitive method for detecting viable myocardium.

Viable myocardium retains the ability to use glucose for metabolism while dead, scarred myocardium does not. 18F-FDG is a PET tracer analogue of Glucose, which is picked up my normal and viable myocardium. To assess viability, a combination of a resting perfusion scan (PET or SPECT MPS) and metabolism scan (18F-FDG PET) is used (Fig. 3).

A severe perfusion defect demonstrated on the MPS (infarct), which shows uptake of 18F-FDG, is indicative of infarcted but viable myocardium (perfusion-metabolism mismatch), while a sever perfusion defect, which does not pick up 18F-FDG, is non-viable, scarred myocardium (perfusion-metabolism match).

Classically, definition of hibernating myocardium is one which recovers its function on revascularization. Therefore, improvement in LVEF after revascularization has been taken as the final proof for viability. By this definition, low-dose dobutamine ECHO is the most predictive test for improvement in LVEF post revascularization, since akinetic/hypokinetic segments which demonstrate improved contraction on low-dose dobutamine are most likely to recover function after revascularization. Many of the areas demonstrating viability on 18FDG PET may not show improvement in LVEF post revascularization, leading many to label the test as too sensitive and not specific for predicting post revascularization LVEF improvement.

However, it is now realized that improvement in LVEF is dependent on several factors, like duration of hibernation, severe LV remodeling, completeness of revascularization, perioperative infarction, and graft restenosis,

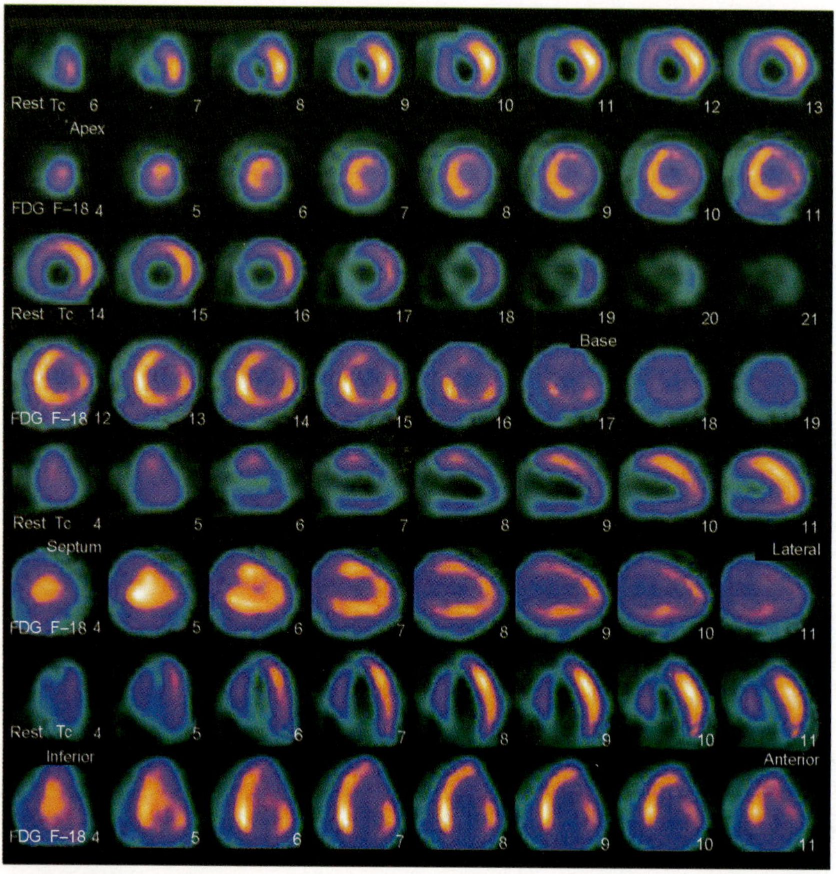

Fig. 3: Viability study using resting MPS (99m$_{Tc}$-Tetrofosmin) and FDG PET. Row 1 and 3 short axis perfusion images from apex to base. Row 2 and 4 are short axis metabolism images. Row 5 and 6 are vertical long axis images from septum to lateral wall for perfusion and metabolism respectively. Row 7 and 8 are horizontal long axis images from inferior to anterior wall for perfusion and metabolism respectively. Images show perfusion defect in septum anterior wall and inferior wall with maintained metabolism (perfusion metabolism mismatch) indicating viable myocardium.

time at which improvement in LVEF is assessed. Most studies have assessed improvement in LVEF at 3-6 months. Studies have shown that long-standing hibernation may require longer times for recovery of LVEF after successful revascularization, sometimes even 2-3 years. It is also clear that patients show improvement in symptoms, exercise capacity, reduction in arrhythmias inspite of no improvement in LVEF.

Therefore, having the most sensitive technique (FDG-PET) for demonstrating viability is of vital importance to make decisions for revascularization.

Currently, the decision about which modality to use for demonstrating viability will depend on local availability of PET scans and MRI, local expertise and confidence of the referring cardiologist on the reports.

In view of established and emerging literature, FDG PET is undoubtedly the most sensitive modality for detecting viable myocardium.

MYOCARDIAL INNERVATION

Noninvasive assessment of cardiac presynaptic sympathetic nerve activity is possible with 123I-MIBG SPECT and 11C-HED (metahydroxyephedrine) PET. These analogues of norepinephrine share the same reuptake and storage mechanisms as naturally occurring norepinephrine but do not undergo metabolism by COMT or MAO unlike native norepinephrine. 11C carazolol or 11C CGP or 18F-Flurocarazolol are useful in imaging postsynaptic beta adrenoreceptor expression and density. The combination of 11C HED and 11C CGP permits imaging of both pre- and postsynaptic sympathetic function. The cardiac sympathetic nervous system plays an important role in the pathophysiology of many cardiac diseases including congestive heart failure and arrhythmias, hypertrophic and dilated cardiomyopathy, myocardial infarction, myocarditis and in Parkinson's disease. Regional uptake and washout of the radiotracer are expressed as heart to upper mediastinum (H/M) ratio in the early and late images of 123I-MIBG SPECT. A low H/M ratio strongly predicts poor outcome. In dilated cardiomyopathy, reduced uptake and increased washout are closely related to LV dysfunction. In congestive heart failure, a decrease in H/M ratio accompanies worsening of CHF. Treatment with ACE inhibitors has shown to reduced washout.

Diabetic autonomic neuropathy can be detected by scintigraphy in the early stages of the disease. Patients with good control show decreased denervation over a three-year period compared to those with poor control of the disease. The surgical procedure of cardiac transplantation causes autonomic denervation of the donor heart as shown by absent tracer uptake on 11C HED PET imaging. Over a period of time, regional reappearance of sympathetic nerve fibers can be documented by tracer retention >7.5% indicative of presynaptic catecholamine uptake sites. Reinnervation has a beneficial on-exercise performance of the transplanted heart. In myocardial infarct patients, a larger area of sympathetic denervation compared to the perfusion defect provides the electrophysiological substrate for re-entrant arrhythmias. Regional heterogeneities in β-adrenergic receptor number and reuptake occur in subjects with sudden cardiac death, and may be predictive for future events.

Genetic variations in β-adrenergic receptors have major implications in terms of future development of CHF and early associated mortality. As newer third-generation beta blockers like carvedilol become available, it will become increasingly important to identify markers predictive of drug efficacy for individual heart failure patients, based on sympathetic nerve imaging.

CONCLUSION

Nuclear cardiology has established itself as a very important diagnostic tool in the management of heart disease. By its unique ability to study physiological processes and their alteration in health and disease, it provides important diagnostic and prognostic information vital for making appropriate management decisions. Information from anatomical modalities should be combined with physiological information from nuclear cardiology techniques for full understanding of disease pathophysiology and appropriate management.

SUGGESTED READING

Barry Zaret, George Beller. Clinical Nuclear Cardiology: State of the Art and Future Directions, 4th edition, Elsevier Mosby. 2010, 896 pages.

Diwakar Jain, Harry Lesig, Influence of 99mTc-Tetrofosmin SPECT myocardial perfusion imaging on the prediction of future adverse cardiac events. Journal of Nuclear Cardiology.16;4:August 2009.

Gould KL, Johnson NP, Bateman TM, et. al., Anatomic versus physiologic assessment of coronary artery disease. Role of coronary flow reserve, fractional flow reserve, and positron emission tomography imaging in revascularization decision-making. J Am Coll. Cardiol. 2013 Oct 29;62(18):1639-53.

Mouaz H Al-Mallah, Arkadiusz Sitek, Stephen C Moore. Assessment of Myocardial Perfusion with PET and PET-CT. Journal of Nuclear Cardiology. 2010; 17: 498-513.

William Wijns, Bernard De Bruyne, What does the clinical cardiologist need from noninvasive cardiac imaging: is it time to adjust practices to meet evolving demand?:14;3,May 2007.

17 Balloon Mitral Valvuloplasty

Manjunath CN, Nagaraja Moorthy

INTRODUCTION

Though the prevalence of rheumatic fever is declining rheumatic mitral stenosis continues to be an important health issue especially developing countries. Balloon mitral valvuloplasty is an established treatment modality in selected patients with gratifying short and long-term results. This chapter discusses all the aspects of this procedure along with technical details and tips and tricks.

Keywords

Rheumatic heart disease, Mitral stenosis, Valvuloplasty, Septal puncture, Inoue balloon, Wilkin's score.

ANATOMIC CONSIDERATIONS

The mitral valve (MV) apparatus is a complex structure consisting of annulus fibrosus, mitral leaflets, chordae tendinae, papillary muscles, and the posterior wall of LV. The normal mitral valve area (MVA) is 4.0–6.0 cm². MS occurs when stenosis of the valve occurs from leaflet thickening, commissural fusion (Figs. 1A and B), and chordal shortening/fusion ultimately resulting in increased pulmonary capillary wedge pressure, an elevated pulmonary vascular resistance, and right ventricular dysfunction. As the severity of MS increases, cardiac output becomes subnormal at rest and fails to increase during exercise. When the MVA is reduced to 1.5 cm² or less, symptoms may become severe and complications may develop.

BALLOON MITRAL VALVULOPLASTY

Historical Aspect

The treatment of MS has been revolutionized since the development of balloon mitral valvuloplasty (BMV). In 1982, Kanji Inoue, a Japanese cardiac surgeon, performed first BMV using a balloon with differential compliance.[1]

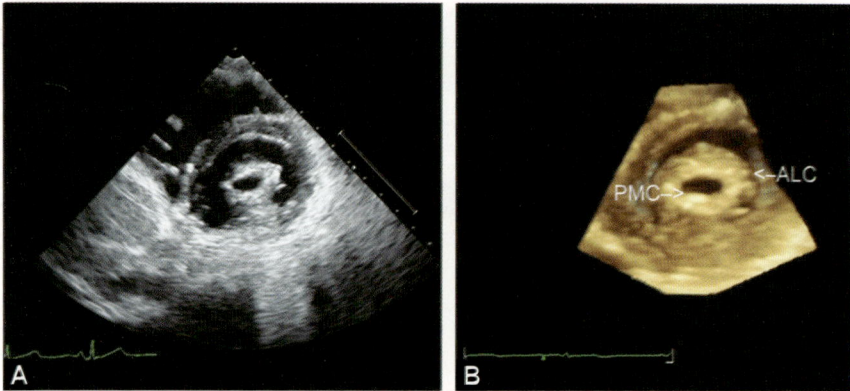

Figs.1A and B: Transthoracic 2D (A) and 3D (B) echocardiogram showing thickened mitral valve with bi-commissural fusion giving "fish-mouth" appearance.

Though various techniques were described and practiced in the past like "Double balloon technique", "Multitrack technique" and "Metallic commissurotomy" are almost abandoned due to risks and complications involved when compared to "Inoue Balloon Technique". Inoue's single-balloon technique has become the most popular method for performing BMV in most parts of the world. The mechanism of BMV is split of fused commissures.

Indications and Recommendations for Percutaneous Balloon Mitral Valvuloplasty (BMV)

Indications for BMV have been formulated by the American College of Cardiology (ACC) and the American Heart Association (AHA).[2,3]

Class I recommendations are as follows:

1. Symptomatic patients with severe MS (MVA ≤1.5 cm^2, stage D) and favorable valve morphology in the absence of left atrial thrombus or moderate-to-severe MR (Level of Evidence: A).
2. Asymptomatic patients with moderate or severe MS and valve morphology that is favorable for BMV who have pulmonary hypertension (pulmonary artery systolic pressure greater than 50 mm Hg at rest or greater than 60 mm Hg with exercise) in the absence of left atrial thrombus or moderate to severe MR (Level of Evidence: C).

Class IIa recommendations are as follows:

1. Asymptomatic patients with very severe MS (MVA ≤1.0 cm^2, stage C) and favorable valve morphology in the absence of left atrial thrombus or moderate-to-severe MR (Level of Evidence: C).

Class IIb recommendations are as follows:

1. Asymptomatic patients with severe MS (MVA ≤1.5 cm^2, stage C) and valve morphology favorable for BMV in the absence of left atrial thrombus or moderate-to-severe MR who have new onset of AF (Level of Evidence: C).

2. Symptomatic patients with MVA greater than 1.5 cm^2 if there is evidence of hemodynamically significant MS based on pulmonary artery wedge pressure greater than 25 mm Hg or mean MV gradient greater than 15 mm Hg during exercise (Level of Evidence: C).
3. Symptomatic patients (NYHA class III to IV) with severe MS (MVA ≤1.5 cm^2, stage D) who have a suboptimal valve anatomy and who are not candidates for surgery or at high risk for surgery (Level of Evidence: C).

Contraindications

The following are contraindications for BMV (i.e. class III recommendations):
1. BMV is not indicated for patients with mild MS (level of evidence: C)
2. BMV should not be performed in patients with moderate to severe MR or left atrial body thrombus, Bi-commissural calcium (level of evidence: C) However using modified over the wire technique BMV can safely be done in patients with Type Ia, Ib and IIa LA/LAA thrombus after 8–10 weeks of anticoagulations.

PERIPROCEDURAL CARE

Preprocedural Planning

Physical examination is an important initial step in assessing the pliability of the valve. Accentuation of the first heart sound (S1) occurs when the MV leaflets are pliable. Marked calcification of the valve may make S1 softer. The opening snap (OS) of the MV most readily audible at the apex; if present, may indicate that the MV has at least some mobility.

Role of Echocardiography in BMV: Valve Assessment and Case Selection

Echocardiography is the primary modality of evaluation in patients who is planned for BMV. It is essential for the pre-procedural evaluation of patients, case selection, intraprocedural monitoring, and the postprocedural assessment and follow-up. The primary aim of echocardiographic assessment is to find the suitable valve for BMV and identify high-risk echocardiographic features which may result in complications. The echocardiographic scoring system developed by Wilkins et al (*see* Table 1) is useful for estimating likely outcomes of BMV.[4]

In this system, points are given for leaflet mobility, valve thickening, subvalvular thickening, and valvular calcification. The final score is determined

Table 1: Echocardiography scoring system (Wilkins score) to predict outcome of mitral balloon valvuloplasty.

Grade	Mobility	Thickening	Calcification	Subvalvular thickening
1	Highly mobile valve with only leaflet tips restricted	Leaflets near normal in thickness (4–5 mm)	A single area of increased echo brightness	Minimal thickening just below the mitral leaflets
2	Leaflet mid and base portions have normal mobility	Midleaflets normal, considerable thickening of margins (5–8 mm)	Scattered areas of brightness confined to leaflet margins	Thickening of chordal structures extending to one-third of the chords
3	Valve continues to move forward in diastole, mainly from the base	Thickening extending through the entire leaflet (5–8 mm)	Brightness extending into the midportions of the leaflets	Thickening extended to distal third of the chords
4.	No or minimal forward movement of the leaflets in diastole	Considerable thickening of all leaflet tissue (<8–10 mm)	Extensive brightness throughout much of the leaflet tissue	Extensive thickening and shortening of all chordal structures extending down to the papillary muscles

The total score is the sum of the four items and ranges between 4 and 16.

by adding the points for each of the components (maximum, 16 points). A score of 8 or lower is usually associated with excellent immediate and long-term results for BMV, whereas scores higher than 8 are associated with less impressive results, including the risk of development of MR.

Another important factor in determining the suitability of the valve for BMV is the absence of commissural calcification. Calcification of both commissures is considered as absolute contraindication for BMV as it poses increased risk of leaflet tear. The presence of predominant subvalvular fibrosis and calcification results in suboptimal results from BMV.

Though several echocardiographic scoring systems have been proposed as a guide to the selection of patients for BMV, no single parameter is able to predict success or complications independently. These criteria should be used, therefore, only as a guide in selection of patients for BMV.

PATIENT PREPARATION

Usually, BMV is done with the patient under local anesthesia and conscious sedation. The patient remains in the supine position during the procedure.

TECHNIQUES

Approach

Currently, the antegrade approach with transseptal catheterization is more widely used. It is usually performed through the femoral vein; or, rarely, through the jugular vein approach.

Choice of Technique

Though various techniques were described and practiced in the past like "Double balloon technique", "Multitrack technique" and "Metallic commissurotomy" are almost abandoned due to risks and complications involved when compared to "Inoue Balloon Technique."

Inoue Balloon Technique

The Inoue balloon technique, first described in 1984,[1] is the most commonly employed technique today. Since then wide experience has now been acquired by a number of groups worldwide. In developing countries Inoue prototype Accura Balloon (Vascular Concepts) is routinely used with comparable success rate.

Vascular Access

A 7-French sheath is inserted in the right femoral vein for transseptal access; a 5-French sheath is placed in the right or left femoral artery for left-heart catheterization. After bolus administration of 1000 U heparin, right heart catheterization is performed. Two pressure transducers are required for simultaneous left atrial, left ventricular pressures. A pigtail catheter is placed in the aortic root (Left/Non-coronary sinus), and aortic pressures are obtained.

Transseptal Puncture

Transseptal catheterization is the vital component of BMV. The danger of the transseptal approach lies in the possibility that the needle and catheter will puncture an adjacent structure (e.g., the coronary sinus, the posterior wall of the right atrium, or the aortic root). To minimize the risk of complications, the operator must have a detailed knowledge of the regional anatomy of the atrial septum. The steps of septal puncture are listed in Table 2.

Equipments for Septal Puncture

The essential instruments include a preshaped transseptal sheath with introducer (Mullins sheath) and a preshaped transseptal puncture needle (Brockenbrough Needle).

Table 2: Steps of septal puncture.
Step-1: Mullins sheath with Brockenbrough needle positioned in SVC. Pigtail catheter positioned in aorta at the level of aortic valve.
Step-2: Mullins sheath with Brockenbrough needle withdrawn into the right atrium to lie half to one vertebra below the level of the pigtail catheter in AP projection
Step-3: Brockenbrough needle rotated to 4-5 o' clock position. Optimal position confirmed in AP, RAO and lateral/ LAO projection. (Refer above described fluoroscopic land marks)
Step-4: Left atrial entry by probing/puncture around fossa ovalis site with tip of Mullins sheath or tip of Brockenbrough needle.
Step-5: Confirm left atrial entry by withdrawal of oxygenated blood, pressure recording showing LA pressure tracing and by contrast injection into LA chamber

Landmarks for septal puncture: Transseptal puncture if usually done under fluoroscopic guidance. There are certain fluoroscopic landmarks which are used to identify the location of fossa ovalis (Figs. 2A to D). The pigtail marks the location of aortic valve. In AP view the fossa ovalis lies inferior and medial to aortic valve. To select optimal transseptal puncture site, 2 imaginary lines are drawn: (1) the vertical mid line and (2) the horizontal M line. The point of intersection of vertical "mid line" and horizontal "M line" locates the site of septal puncture. Usually the intersection point will be half to one vertebral body below the horizontal line drawn from the aortic root in the vertical midline.

In most institutions the septal puncture is done in LAO 40 degrees, or in left lateral projection as shown in Figure 2C. In these projections the ideal septal puncture site corresponds to the midpoint between the pigtail catheter placed in aortic sinus and the spine. The position should also be confirmed in RAO 30 degrees projection (Fig. 2D).

Dilatation of IAS Puncture Site

After septal puncture, a coiled-tip guide wire is placed into the left atrium. Later the septal dilator (14F polyethylene tube with a thinner tip 70 cm in length) is advanced over the coiled-tip wire to facilitate the entry of Inoue balloon catheter. Once the catheter is safely placed in the left atrium, heparin (usually 100 U/kg) is administered for anticoagulation. Anticoagulation time is monitored during the procedures to maintain appropriate levels of anticoagulation.

Selection of Balloon Catheter

The most commonly used balloon catheters during BMV are the triple lumen Inoue balloon catheter (Toray International America Inc.) and the

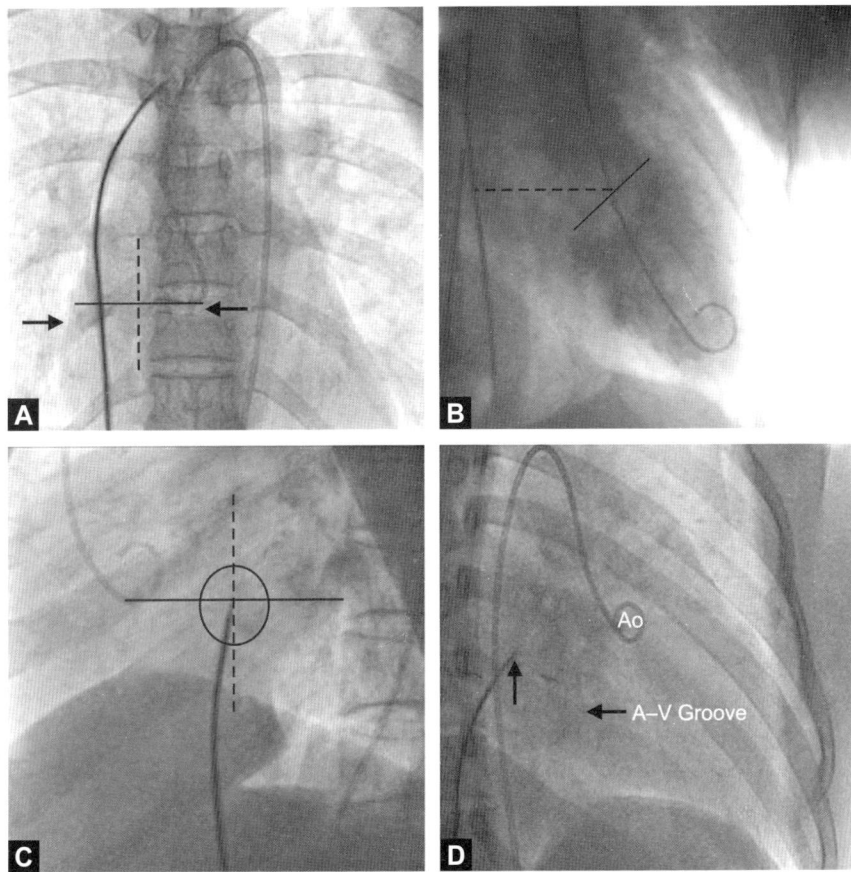

Figs. 2A to D: Fluoroscopic landmarks for septal puncture: (A) An imaginary horizontal line is drawn from point T to point L where the line intersects the lateral border of the left atrium. The dotted vertical line crossing the midpoint between T and L is the midline. (B) The M-line is obtained using the left ventriculogram with a stop frame RAO view. The target site for septal puncture is located at the intersecting point of the vertical "midline" and horizontal M-line: Fluoroscopic landmark for septal puncture in LAO projection and (C) the target site for septal puncture is located at the intersecting point of the vertical "midline" and horizontal M-line: Fluoroscopic landmark for septal puncture in LAO projection and (D) in RAO projection.

double lumen Accura balloon catheter (Vascular Concepts, Halstead, UK). Both Accura and Inoue balloon mitral valvotomy balloons are effective in providing relief from hemodynamically significant mitral stenosis in terms of gain in valve area and reduction in transmitral gradient.[5] A balloon catheter system for accomplishing BMV consists of the following devices: Inoue/Accura balloon catheter, metallic stiffening cannula (18 gauge, 80 cm in length) for stretching and stiffening the Inoue balloon catheter, guidewire for BMV (0.028 inches in diameter, 180 cm in length), dilator (14F polyethylene tube with a thinner tip 70 cm in length) for dilating the puncture site of the femoral vein and atrial septum, and a stylet (wire with J-shaped tip, 0.038 inches in diameter, 80 cm in length) for directing the Inoue balloon toward the mitral orifice.

The balloon diameter size is chosen on the basis of the patient's weight, height, body surface area. Most commonly the reference size of the balloon is calculated according to Hung's formula;[6] the patient's height (cm) is rounded to the nearest zero and divided by ten and ten added to the ratio to yield the reference size (mm), e.g., if the patient's height is 158 cm, then reference diameter will be 160/10 + 10 = 26 mm.

In case of pliable, non-calcified valves with mitral regurgitation of ≤1+, a balloon catheter with a nominal reference size calculated according to Hung's formula can be used. In contrast in patients with high-risk features of developing severe MR (valvular calcification, severe subvalvular stenosis, and nonpliable valves), a balloon catheter two size smaller than reference size is selected. However after each dilatation echocardiography should be reviewed for new appearance of significant MR or worsening of pre-existing MR before the next inflation.

At authors' institution initial inflation is done at 2 mm less than the reference diameter and size is upgraded after carefully assessing hemodynamics and MR. The balloon catheter upsizing should be "**guided, guarded and gated** " to achieve optimal results.

Crossing the Mitral Valve

In the next step, the Inoue/Accura balloon catheter is advanced over the coiled-tip wire. The stylet is inserted in the balloon catheter, and the stylet is given 2-3 anticlockwise rotations so that the balloon catheter with stylet is moved together toward the MV orifice. Once the balloon is close to the valve bobbing movement or "wood pecking sign" of the balloon may be observed. Several techniques are described for entering MV like (1) the vertical method, (2) the direct method, (3) sliding method (4) posterior loop method and (5) Modified over the wire technique.

Once the balloon catheter has been inserted into the left ventricle, the distal portion of the balloon is inflated with contrast media (Diluted 1:1) using a specially graduated syringe. The catheter is then pulled until resistance is felt when the balloon catheter aligns across the MV and inflate the balloon fully to expand the proximal part of the balloon. Figures 3A to F illustrate step by step demonstration of the BMV procedure.

After each dilatation, the operator should obtain the left atrial pressure and the mitral gradient. If the transmitral pressure gradient does not decrease, the balloon size is increased in 1-mm increments until the pressure gradient decreases or substantial worsening of mitral regurgitation occurs (Figs. 4A and B). In addition, 2-dimensional echocardiographic

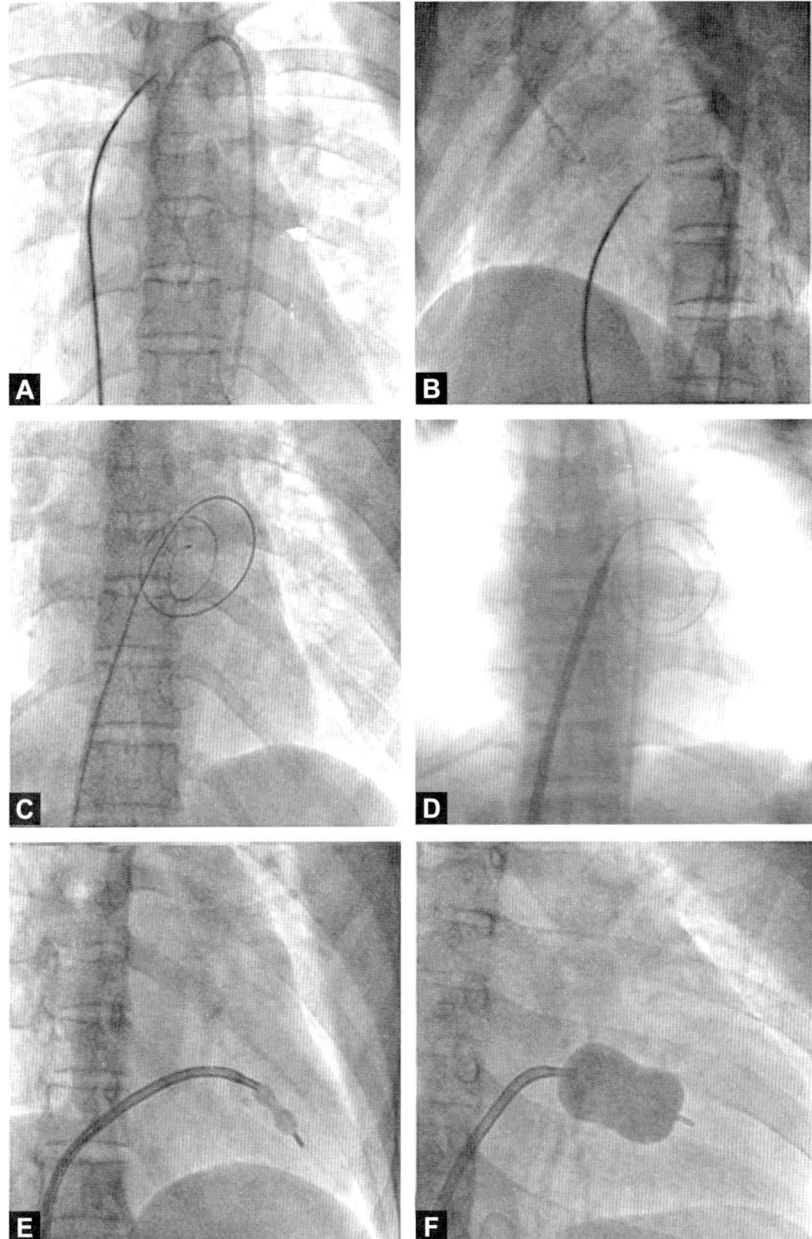

Figs. 3A to F: Salient steps of BMV: (A) Pig tail catheter in aorta, (B) Septal puncture using Brockenbrough needle, (C) Coiled wire in LA after septal puncture, (D) Septal dilatation with 14F dilator, (E) Inoue balloon LA entry assisted with stylet, (F) Fully inflated Inoue balloon across mitral valve.

observations are performed after each dilatation. To assess MV orifice area after each dilatation, planimetry of the valve orifice with 2-dimensional

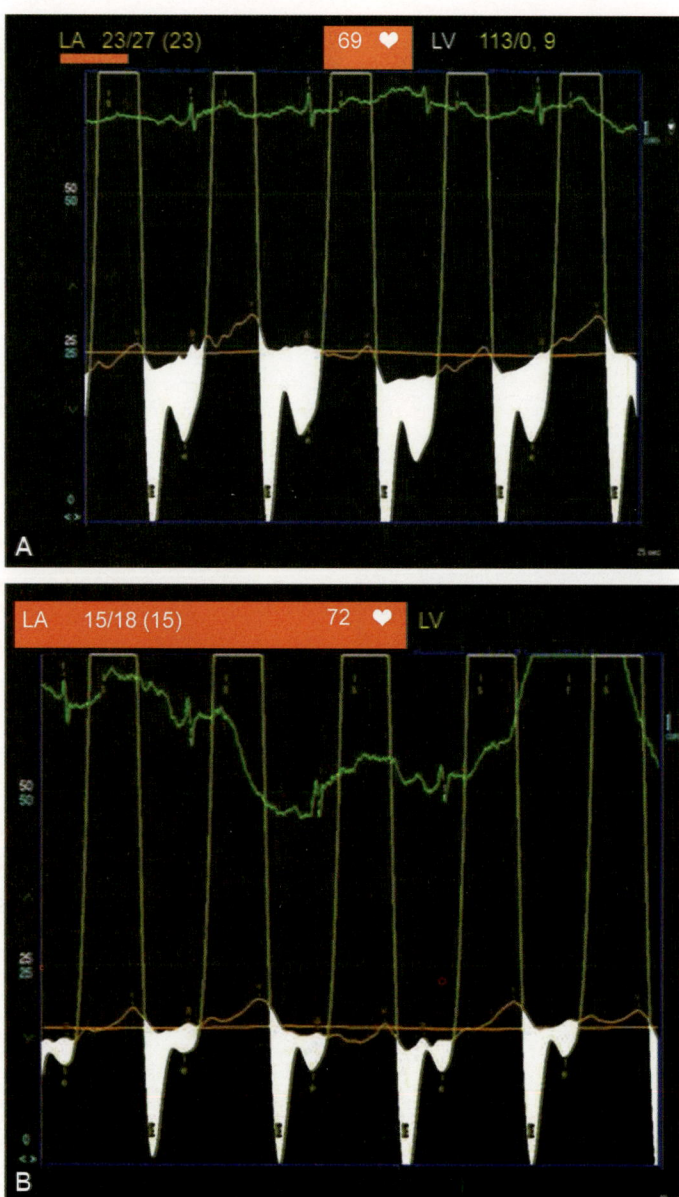

Figs. 4A and B: Simultaneous tracings of pulmonary capillary wedge pressure and left ventricular pressure in a patient with mitral stenosis before (A) and after (B) valvuloplasty. The preprocedural mean LA pressure was 23 mm Hg and post procedural mean LA pressure was 15 mm Hg.

echocardiography should be adopted rather than the pressure half-time method on continuous Doppler waveform, because pressure half-time–derived orifice area might be inaccurate in this acute setting.

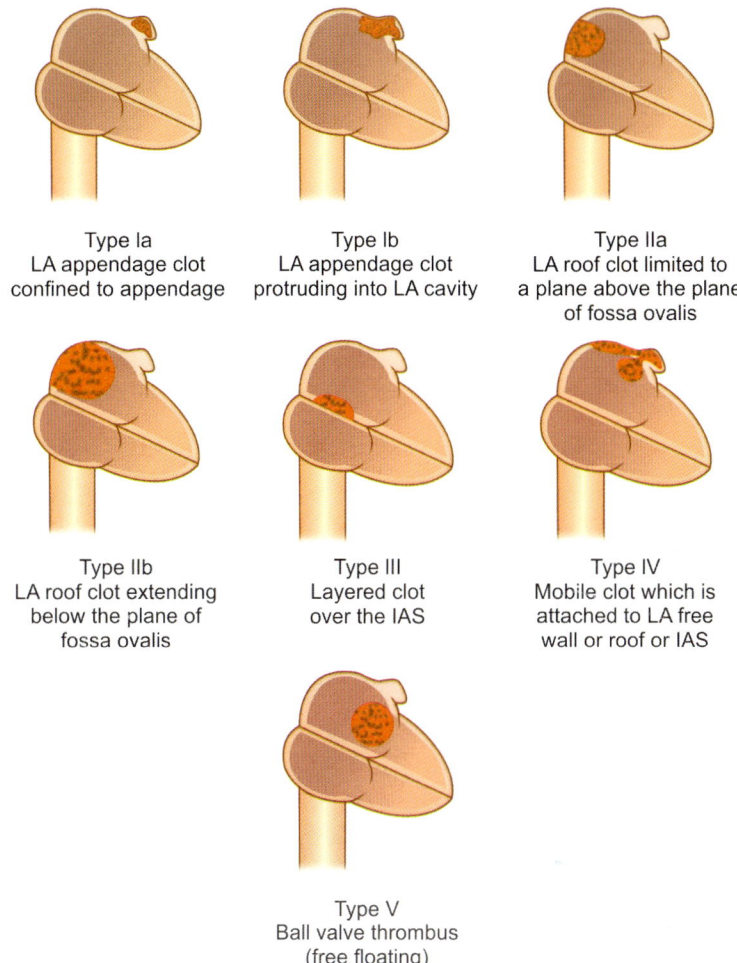

Fig. 5: Classification of left atrial clot by Manjunath et.al. (Diagrammatic representation).[7]

BMV IN DIFFICULT SCENARIOS

BMV in LA/LAA Clot

LA thrombus in patients with MS has long been regarded as a contraindication for BMV. In selected patients of mitral stenosis with LA thrombus (type Ia, Ib, and IIa) (Fig. 5),[7] BMV can be performed safely with the modified over the wire technique (Figs. 6A to F).[7]

Our modification of the over-the-wire technique is safe, effective, and does not require any additional accessories. This technique involves direct positioning of a coiled Inoue wire into the left ventricle through the Mullin sheath followed by introduction of an Inoue catheter over the wire as illustrated in Figures 6A to F.

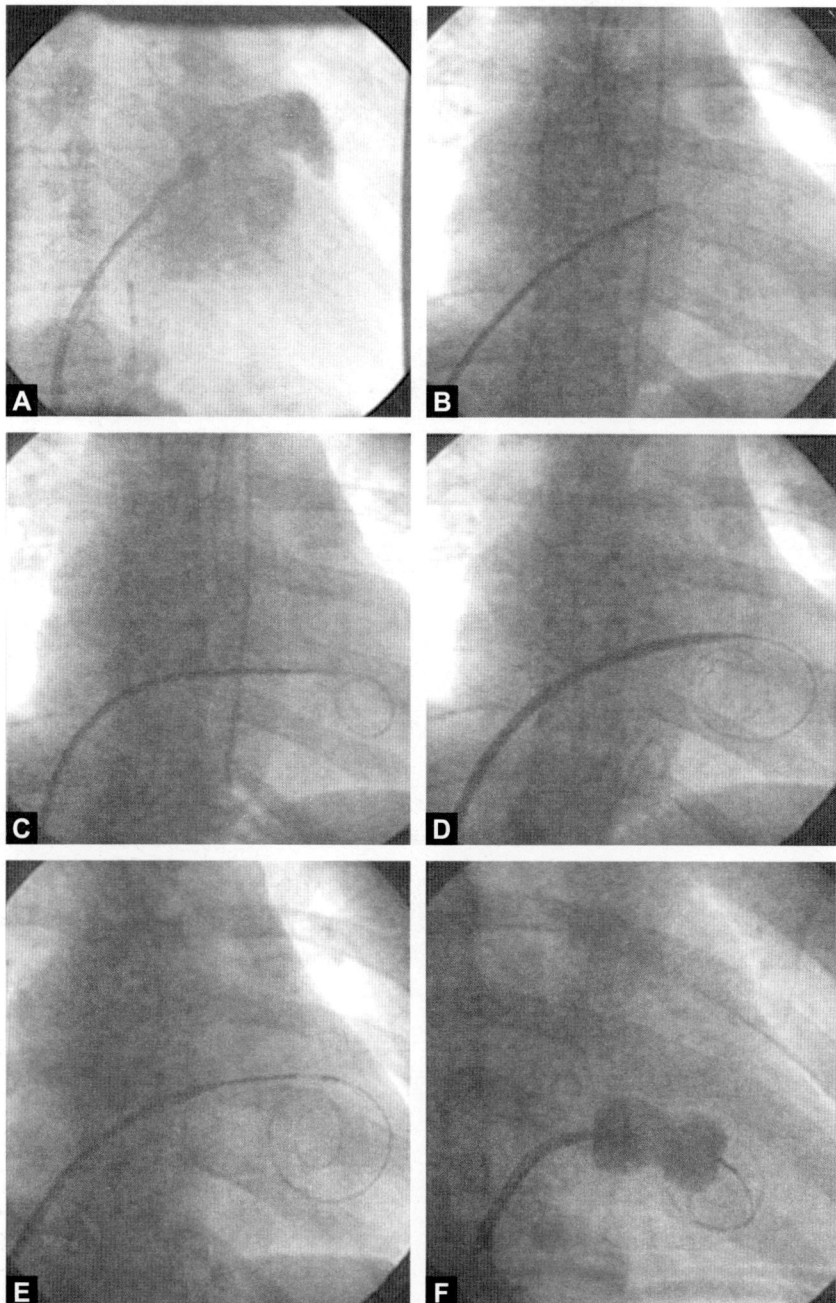

Figs. 6A to F: Over-the-wire technique described by Manjunath et. al.[22] Cine recordings showing the position of LA appendage and the steps involved in modified over the wire technique: (A) Position of the left atrial appendage. (B) Mullins sheath near the mitral valve. (C) Coiled guidewire directly introduced into left ventricle. (D) Septal dilatation over the coiled guidewire. (E) Accura balloon over the coiled guidewire crossing the mitral valve. (F) Accura balloon inflation.

BMV in Giant LA/IAS Aneurysm

In patients with giant LA and septal aneurysm; technical difficulties may be encountered in performing the transseptal puncture and crossing the MV orifice. In such situations increasing the curvature of the Brockenbrough needle or probing around the fossa ovalis may assist in safe septal puncture. When difficulty is encountered in crossing mitral valve either changing the shape of the stylet, "reverse loop entry", "modified over the wire technique"[8] (Figs. 6A to F), balloon flotation catheter assisted entry or deliberate low septal puncture methods may be opted to enter LV.

BMV in Severe Subvalvular Disease

Severe subvalvular stenosis may also cause difficulty in entering the Inoue balloon into LV. In such situations predilating and releasing submitral apparatus stenosis using peripheral angioplasty balloon (short length balloons with 6–8 mm in diameter) may facilitates subsequent entry of 12F Inoue balloon catheter. This can be achieved either through antegrade approach or retrograde approach. However utmost care should be taken not to cause chordal or papillary muscle rupture.

BMV in IVC Interruption/IVC Anomalies through IJV Approach

In certain congenital or acquired anomalies of the inferior vena cava or ilio-femoral veins may preclude transfemoral approach and transjugular approach to transseptal BMV is a useful alternative in such patients with venous anomalies. Land marks for septal puncture are derived from Inoue's angiographic method in frontal projection. Alternatively levophase injection of pulmonary arteriogram may be utilized to delineate interatrial septum. Deliberate high atrial puncture facilitates balloon crossing into the left ventricle in jugular approach. However, trans-jugular approach is technically challenging as may be considered as an alternative approach to femoral approach in when the anatomical variations warrant.

BMV in Juvenile Mitral Stenosis

In comparison with adults, children and adolescents with rheumatic mitral stenosis more often have severe pulmonary hypertension and very high transmitral gradient but less often have atrial fibrillation and left atrial dilation. Careful attention to procedural details—use of a balloon diameter smaller than the typically recommended size, stepwise increases in balloon diameter, meticulous pressure-gradient measurement, and watch for MR after each dilatation—is important in these young patients. BMV in young patients is effective, safe and provides better immediate results than in adults particularly with regard to acute complications. Although indexed MVA was larger than in adults, freedom from restenosis and from clinical events at 10 years was no different from adult populations.

BMV in Pregnancy

Majority of patients with moderate to severe MS worsen during pregnancy due to increased intravascular volume and increase in heart rate. Symptoms occur in 25% of patients, become apparent by 20th week and aggravate at the time of labor and delivery. Without intervention maternal mortality is significantly higher [6.8%] for those in NYHA classes III and IV, particularly during labor and delivery. Optimal timing of BMV is end of 2nd trimester or beginning of third trimester during which radiation risk to the fetus is negligible. BMV should be performed by experienced operators with abdominal and pelvic shielding and with minimum radiation exposure and should be avoided during the first trimester.

COMPLICATIONS OF BMV

Most of the adverse complications relevant to this procedure occur during the procedure (i.e. during the process of interatrial septum puncture, manipulation of the Inoue balloon catheter in the left atrium, and commissurotomy of the MV by Inoue balloon catheter). Major complications with regard to the Brockenbrough puncture are related to penetration of the Brockenbrough needle into the adjacent structure (i.e ascending aorta and the postatrium pericardial space). Procedural mortality ranges from 0–3% in most series. Table 4 lists complications during BMV and management options.

Pericardial Effusion/Tamponade

The most common serious complication is hemopericardium, with an incidence of 0 to 2.0%. When hemopericardium or rupture into the space surrounding the aortic root occurs, protamine sulfate should be administered to promote spontaneous hemostasis and may need emergency pericardiocentesis. In cases with massive pericardial effusion not responding to pericardiocentesis and autotransfusion may need surgery.

Acute Mitral Regurgitation

In most cases, the degree of mitral regurgitation slightly increases after PBMV without requiring surgical intervention. The mechanism of MR could be excessive tearing of the commissures(s) or the posterior/anterior leaflet, or rupture of the subvalvular apparatus.

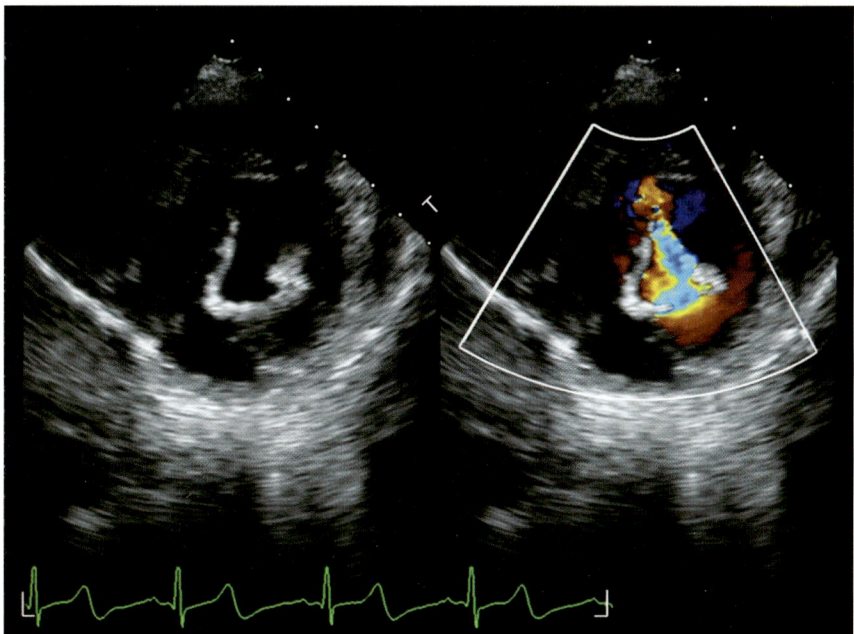

Fig. 7: Transthoracic echocardiography showing post BMV anterior mitral leaflet tear and severe mitral regurgitation.

The incidence of acute severe MR following BMV in our study[9] is 1.3%. Anterior mitral leaflet tear (Fig. 7) is the most common cause for severe MR. The severity of submitral disease appears to be one of the important risk factors predisposing to severe MR. A strategy of early MVR, preferably within 24 hours of onset of severe MR, is recommended for optimal outcome.

Stroke, Embolism

The frequency of embolic events related to mitral valvuloplasty ranges from 0.5 to 5.0%. It is critical to rule out LA/LAA thrombus prior to BMV.

Residual Atrial Septal Defect

The frequency of residual atrial septal defects after BMV ranges from 10 to 90% in different series and these are typically small and restrictive shunts. In our study[10] incidence of residual atrial septal defect within 48 hours of PTMC by TEE color flow Doppler imaging is 66.5%. Majority of the defects closes spontaneously and a residual defect is observed in 8.7% patients at 6 months.

Table 3: Definition of successful BMV.

1. ≥ 50% increase in the mitral valve area (MVA)
2. Increase in mitral valve area to ≥ 1.5 cm^2
3. Significant fall in LA pressure and Transmitral gradient (Figs. 4A and B)
4. Mitral regurgitation not more than Grade II
5. At least one of the commizures is visible split
6. No major complications

Table 4: Complications during BMV.

Complications	Incidence	Management
Pericardial effusion/ tamponade	0.5 to 12.0%	1. Pericardiocentesis 2. Reversal of heparin with protamine 3. Autotransfusion 4. BMV through 2nd puncture to reduce LA pressure 5. Surgical closure of perforation when conservative strategy fails
Acute severe MR requiring surgery	0.9–2%	Early MVR, preferably within 24 hours is recommended for optimal outcome.
Acute embolism/ stroke	0.5 to 5.0%	Conservative management ? Intra-arterial lysis
Residual atrial septal defect	At 48 hrs: 60–70% At 6 months: 8–10%	Conservative in almost all cases

Immediate Results of BMV

After PBMV, MVA approximately doubles in most successful cases. Mitral valve anatomy as assessed by 2-dimensional echocardiography is a strong predictor of the immediate results of PBMV (Table 3). The previously described Wilkins score has a discriminant cut-off point at 8 according to analyses of the immediate results of PBMV. Whatever echo scoring system is used, older age, smaller valve area, previous commissurotomy, or baseline mitral regurgitation should be considered as potential predictors for poor immediate outcome with a similar predictive strength as valve calcification.

Long-term Results

Most patients with initial procedural success report significant functional improvement. The best results of BMV are observed in young patients who have MS with favorable anatomic characteristics (i.e. pliable noncalcified valves and moderate impairment of the subvalvular apparatus). Suboptimal immediate results lead to relatively early intervention. The incidence of restenosis after a successful procedure ranges from 2 to 40% in different studies, at time intervals ranging from 3 to 10 years. Reportedly, the freedom from restenosis rates were 85% at 5 years, 70% at 10 years, and 44% at 15 years and were significantly higher (i.e. 92% at 5 years, 85% at 10 years, and 65% at 15 years) for patients with optimal morphology.[11,12] Depending on the anatomy, restenosis can be treated either with repeat PMBV or with surgical MV replacement.

CONCLUSION

Although the incidence of rheumatic fever and the prevalence of rheumatic heart disease as sequelae are decreasing in most Asian countries, a small but substantial occurrence of rheumatic MS still exists. Since its introduction, percutaneous mitral commissurotomy has demonstrated good immediate and midterm results and has replaced surgical mitral commissurotomy as the preferred treatment of rheumatic MS in appropriate candidates. The need for adequate understanding of indications, BMV procedures, complications and assessment of results cannot be overemphasized.

REFERENCES

1. Inoue K, Owaki T, Nakamura T, Kitamura F, Miyamoto N. Clinical application of transvenous mitral commissurotomy by a new balloon catheter. J Thorac Cardiovasc Surg. 1984; 87:394–402.
2. Nishimura RA, Otto CM, Bonow RO, Carabello BA, Erwin JP III, Guyton RA, et al. AHA/ACC guideline for the management of patients with valvular heart disease: executive summary: a report of the American College of Cardiology/American Heart Association Task Force on Practice Guidelines. Circulation 2014;129(23):e521-643.
3. Bonow RO, Carabello BA, Chatterjee K, de Leon AC Jr., Faxon DP, Freed MD, et al. ACC/AHA 2006 guidelines for the management of patients with valvular heart disease: a report of the American College of Cardiology/American Heart Association Task Force on Practice Guidelines (Writing Committee to Develop Guidelines for the Management of Patients With Valvular Heart Disease. J Am Coll Cardiol. 2006;48(3):e1-148.
4. Wilkins GT, Weyman AE, Abascal VM, et al. Percutaneous balloon dilatation of the mitral valve: an analysis of echocardiographic variables related to outcome and the mechanism of dilatation. Br Heart J. 1988;60:299-308.
5. Manjunath CN, Dorros G, Srinivasa KH, Patil CB, Venkatesh HV, Gowda C, et al. The Indian experience of percutaneous transvenous mitral commissurotomy: comparison of the triple lumen (Inoue) and double lumen (Accura) variable sized single balloon with regard to procedural outcome and cost savings. J Interv Cardiol 1998;11:107–12.
6. Hung JS, Lau KW. Pitfalls and tips in Inoue balloon mitral commissurotomy. Cathet Cardiovasc Diagn 1996;37:188-99.
7. Manjunath CN, Srinivasa KH, Ravindranath KS, Manohar JS, Prabhavathi B, Dattatreya PV, et al. Balloon mitral valvotomy in patients with mitral stenosis and left atrial thrombus. Catheter Cardiovasc Interv. 2009;74(4):653-61.

8. Manjunath CN, Srinivasa KH, Patil CB, Venkatesh HV, Bhoopal TS, Dhanalakshmi C. Balloon mitral valvuloplasty: our experience with a modified technique of crossing the mitral valve in difficult cases. Cathet Cardiovasc Diagn 1998;44: 23–6.
9. Nanjappa MC, Ananthakrishna R, Hemanna Setty SK, Bhat P, Shankarappa RK, Panneerselvam A, et al. Acute severe mitral regurgitation following balloon mitral valvotomy: echocardiographic features, operative findings, and outcome in 50 surgical cases. Catheter Cardiovascular Interv. 2013;81(4):603-8.
10. Manjunath CN, Panneerselvam A, Srinivasa KH, Prabhavathi B, Rangan K, Dhanalakshmi C. et al. Incidence and predictors of atrial septal defect after percutaneous transvenous mitral commissurotomy - atransesophageal echocardiographic study of 209 cases. Echocardiography 2013;30(2):127-30.
11. Fawzy ME, Shoukri M, Al Buraiki J, Hassan W, El Widaal H, Kharabsheh S, et al. Seventeen years' clinical and echocardiographic follow up of mitral balloon valvuloplasty in 520 patients, and predictors of long-term outcome. *J Heart Valve Dis.*2007;16:454–60.
12. Fawzy ME, Shoukri M, Hassan W, Nambiar V, Stefadouros M, Canver CC. The impact of mitral valve morphology on the long-term outcome of mitral balloon valvuloplasty. Catheter Cardiovasc Interv. 2007;69:40–46.

18 Pulmonary and Aortic Balloon Valvuloplasty

Bharat Dalvi, Kshitij Sheth, Shreepal Jain

PULMONARY BALLOON VALVULOPLASTY

First described by Morgagni in 1761, valvar pulmonary stenosis (PS) is one of the common congenital heart defects (CHDs) and may also be associated with other CHDs.

Incidence: Valvar PS constitutes approximately 7% of all CHDs. There is no specific sex predilection. In isolated PS, the recurrence risk is reported to be 1.7–3.7%.

Valvar PS occurs frequently in patients with Noonan syndrome, and has been described in Williams-Beuren syndrome, neurofibromatosis, 22q11 deletion syndrome, Alagille and rarely congenital Rubella syndrome.

Embryogenesis: Calcineurin/Nfatc1 signaling in secondary heart field (SHF) is essential for semilunar valve development. The absence of SHF calcineurin causes increased apoptosis of conal cushion mesenchyme, leading to failure or abnormal development of semilunar valves.

Pathology: Classical valvar PS is characterized by a normal sized valve annulus and a thin, pliant, conical or dome shaped membrane with 3 well defined but incomplete raphae extending from the central narrow opening. Obstruction is mainly secondary to incomplete opening of the leaflets (Figs. 1A and B). There is associated post stenotic dilatation of the main pulmonary artery (MPA) usually extending into the left pulmonary artery (LPA).

Dysplastic pulmonary valve, seen in up to 20% of patients, is characterized by hypoplastic annulus, 3 distinct thick immobile cusps without any commissural fusion. There is usually no post stenotic dilatation of the MPA. Majority of these valves have the leaflets tethered to the wall of the MPA and also associated supravalvular narrowing of the MPA.

Moderate and severe degree of stenosis is associated with right ventricular (RV) myocardial hypertrophy. Localized hypertrophy of the infundibular region develops in some producing an element of subvalvar obstruction.

Pathophysiology: In long standing moderate to severe PS, systolic coronary flow to RV myocardium is reduced leading to subclinical infarction and subendocardial fibrosis.

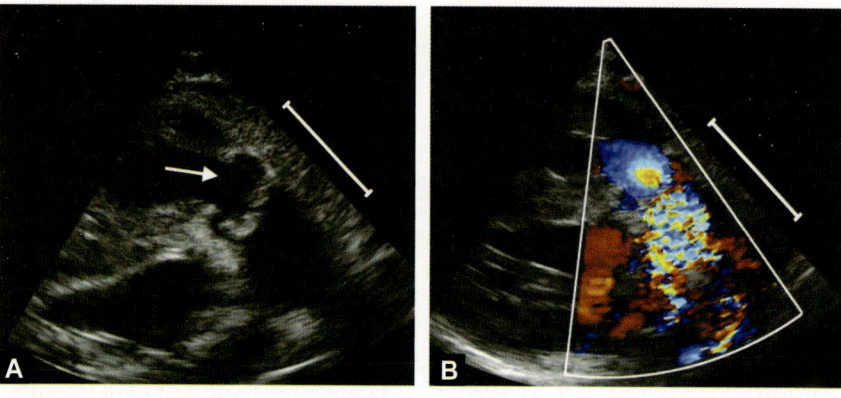

Figs.1A and B: Two-dimensional echocardiogram in parasternal long axis view with anterior sweep depicting a typical doming pulmonary valve (arrow) (A). Color Doppler echocardiogram showing flow acceleration beginning at the level of pulmonary leaflets (B).

Although a hypertrophied RV is initially able to maintain normal stroke volume, it eventually may dilate and fail. In those with a patent foramen ovale (PFO) or Atrial septal defect (ASD), cardiac output might be maintained via right to left shunt at atrial level at the cost of desaturation.

Critical PS: Neonates with critical PS are characterized by severely hypertrophied RV with hypoplastic cavity, systemic or supra-systemic RV pressures, central cyanosis secondary to right to left atrial shunt and duct dependent pulmonary blood flow.

CLINICAL FEATURES

Symptoms: Majority patients are incidentally diagnosed after a murmur is detected on routine examination. Those with long standing moderate to severe stenosis tend to present with exertional dyspnea and fatigue owing to inability of the RV to maintain adequate cardiac output during exertion.

Neonates with critical PS present with severe cyanosis at birth and worsen after closure of Patent Ductus arteriosus (PDA). In those with severe tricuspid regurgitation, there is associated heart failure.

Signs: Growth and development may be impaired in patients with Noonan's or Rubella syndrome. Typical facies may be seen in syndromes like Williams, Noonan's and Alagille. Central cyanosis may be detected for reasons described above.

Peripheral pulse although usually normal, may be reduced in severe PS with RV failure.

The 'a' wave in jugular venous pressure (JVP) tends to be progressively larger with increasing severity of PS due to stronger atrial contraction. With development of tricuspid regurgitation and RV failure, the 'v' wave becomes more prominent with a brisk 'y' descent.

Palpation in moderate and severe PS may reveal a palpable thrill in the 2nd and occasionally 3rd left intercostal space (LICS), radiating upward and toward the left.

On auscultation, a normal S1 is followed by a high-pitched, sharp pulmonary ejection click (PEC) sound, heard maximal in the 2nd LICS. The click is not heard in those with dysplastic valve. S1-PEC interval decreases with increasing severity of PS and PEC may be difficult to separate from S1 in severe PS. Intensity of PEC decreases with deep inspiration and increases on expiration.

Murmur is ejection systolic type heard maximally in 2nd LICS and radiating upward and to the left. With increasing severity, the murmur peak tends to occur later in systole and even extending beyond A2.

S2 in PS is usually split, with the degree of splitting being proportional to the severity of stenosis. Pulmonary component (P2) tends to become softer with increasing severity.

Neonates with critical stenosis tend to have softer systolic murmur as a result of reduced RT output across the pulmonary valve. P2 is usually not audible in such cases.

Electrocardiographic Findings: Right axis deviation, R:S ratio in lead V1 > 4:1 and R > 20 mm are common findings in moderate PS. With severe stenosis, further rightward axis deviation, high R wave amplitude in lead V1 and deep S waves in the left precordial leads, with an R:S ratio <1 in V6, can be seen. Presence of q wave in V1 signifies dilatation of the right atrium. Leftward QRS axis in the presence of valvar PS is a hallmark of Noonan's syndrome.

In those with critical PS or severe PS with hypoplastic RV cavity, the QRS axis tends to be relatively leftward than expected (+30 to +70 degrees) with evidence of left ventricular hypertrophy.

Radiological Findings: Cardiac size is usually normal except in cases with Tricuspid Regurgitation (TR) and RV failure or in neonates with critical PS. Most notable finding is a prominent main pulmonary artery (PA) segment secondary to post stenotic dilatation.

Echocardiographic Findings: A 2-dimensional echocardiogram (2DE) with color Doppler study is the now the investigative modality of choice for confirming the diagnosis of PS (Figs. 1 and 2). It can help in assessing the valve morphology along with its severity, exact site of stenosis, RV size and function, tricuspid valve function and presence and direction of atrial level shunting. Doppler derived peak gradient correlates well with catheterization measured gradient in PS.

Cardiac Catheterization: Catheterization is now mainly reserved for interventional purpose (Figs. 3 and 4). Important hemodynamic information that can be obtained includes RV systolic pressure, gradient across the pulmonary

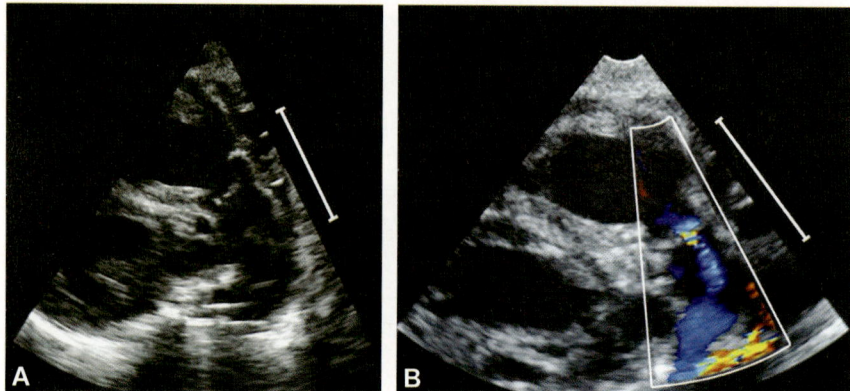

Figs. 2A and B: Two-dimensional (A) and color (B) echocardiographic images from parasternal long axis view with anterior sweep in a newborn with critical pulmonary stenosis depicting doming pulmonary valve with a narrow jet of blood flow across the valve into pulmonary artery.

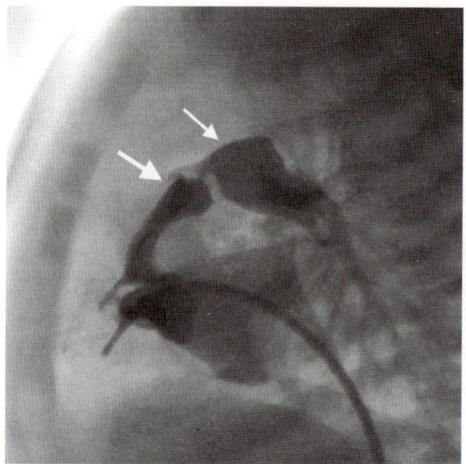

Fig. 3: Right ventricular angiogram in lateral view demonstrating a typical doming pulmonary valve with thin leaflets (arrow) and narrow jet of flow across it along with post stenotic dilatation of the main pulmonary artery (thick arrow).

valve and presence of infundibular component that can be detected with the help of an end-hole catheter. PA pressure is usually normal or may be low in severe PS. Elevated RV end diastolic pressure is suggestive of severe RV hypertrophy with diastolic dysfunction.

DIFFERENTIAL DIAGNOSIS

Moderate and severe PS need to be differentiated from small to moderate sized VSD and moderate to severe aortic stenosis. Neonatal critical PS needs

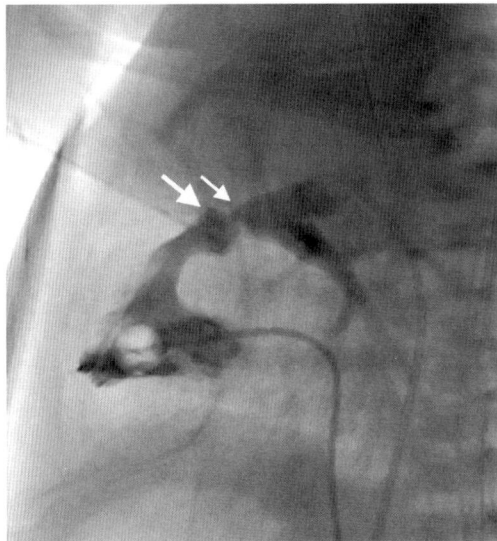

Fig. 4: Right ventricular angiogram in lateral view demonstrating a dysplastic pulmonary valve (arrow) with tethering and supravalvular narrowing (thick arrow) and absence of significant post stenotic MPA dilatation.

to be differentiated from Ebstein's anomaly with functional pulmonary atresia and pulmonary atresia with intact ventricular septum.

MANAGEMENT

1. *Balloon pulmonary valvuloplasty (BPV)*: First described by Kan and associates in 1982, is now the therapeutic modality of choice for moderate and severe PS with typical doming pulmonary valve as well as the initial therapy for dysplastic valve. Balloon diameter is chosen as 1.2-1.4 times the angiographically measured pulmonary annulus size. Mechanism of obstruction relief involves commissural splitting after balloon inflation. As a result, pulmonary regurgitation (PR) is a natural consequence of the procedure and an indirect indicator of adequate dilatation. Occasionally some residual gradient may be noted across the infundibular region due to dynamic obstruction (Figs. 5A and B).

   As per the American Heart Association scientific statement, class I indications for BPV include critical PS and valvar PS with catheter measured or echocardiographically measured peak instantaneous gradient of ≥ 40 mm Hg or clinically significant valvar PS with evidence of RV dysfunction.

   At mid-term follow-up (<2 years), restenosis is observed in 8–10% of patients. In the long-term follow-up, the freedom of reintervention is reported as 88% and 84% at 5 and 10 years, respectively. Reported

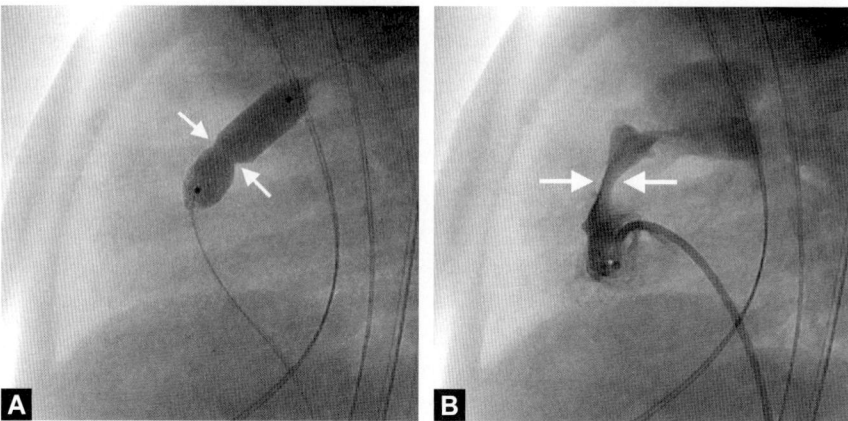

Figs. 5A and B: Balloon dilatation of the pulmonary valve being performed with the balloon positioned across the annulus suggested by the waist (arrows) (A). Infundibular spasm (thick arrows) noted after the balloon dilatation, which may be responsible for transient persistence of gradient across the right ventricle to pulmonary artery (B).

incidence of adequate obstruction relief in those with dysplastic valve ranges from 35–65%.

Critical PS in a newborn poses technical challenges during transcatheter intervention. Entering the hypoplastic RV or crossing the Tricuspid valve (TV) in the presence of TR can pose some difficulties. Using a preshaped hard end of 0.035" Teflon coated wire can help overcome this difficulty. Use of a long 4Fr sheath has a tendency to look into the RV inflow and therefore can help in entering the RV. In case these do not work, the other option is to keep the catheter in the right atrium and try and cross the TV and then the pulmonary valve with a 0.025" angled glide wire or a 0.014" soft tipped coronary wire. Sometimes, despite having an optimum wire position, the balloon refuses to track along the wire as it curves in the RV inflow and then in the RV outflow. Tyshak II Mini with its extremely low profile can help overcome this problem. All the balloon should be dry prepared in order to maintain their profile. In some newborns, even Tyshak II Mini faces resistance while going through the two curves of the RV inflow and outflow. In such an event, it is worth trying the loop the wire in the RA and then try to track the balloon over the loop similar to what one would do while approaching from the internal jugular vein. The other option is to pass the guidewire through the PDA and snare it through the aorta to form a venoarterial loop. This stabilizes the wire and helps in tracking the balloon even in the most difficult circumstances. In critical PS, immediate effective gradient reduction is achieved in more than 90% patients. However, 5–10% patients are unable to maintain adequate forward flow across the pulmonary valve. Usually these newborns can be maintained on Prostaglandin E1 infusion, a stable source of Pulmonary blood flow (PBF) in the form of surgically created aorto-pulmonary shunt or a transcatheter PDA stenting procedure may be required if they are unable to be weaned even after 2-3 weeks. It is our practice to routinely stent the PDA in all the neonates with critical PS who have duct dependent circulation in order to ensure predictable pulmonary blood flow. PDA stenting should be done after stopping the PGE1 infusion and allowing the duct to constrict a little. This helps in preventing stent embolization. Another 10% may require repeat BPV within months of the initial procedure.

Incidence of moderate PR after BPV ranges from 5 to 24%. Moderate or severe pulmonary insufficiency is common if the procedure is done during neonatal period compared to of all other age groups. Moderate to severe normotensive PR is well tolerated for many years. However, long standing moderate to severe PR has deleterious effects on RV function and rhythm and may necessitate a pulmonary valve replacement (PVR) to minimize these risks.

Risk of procedure related death (0.24%) or major complications (0.35%) is very low. Complications, including transient bradycardia and hypotension during balloon inflation, transient or permanent right bundle branch block or atrioventricular block, balloon rupture, tricuspid valve chordae/papillary muscle rupture, and tears in the pulmonary artery have been reported, but rarely. All these complications are more common while dealing with a newborn having critical PS.

2. *Surgical Valvotomy*: It is reserved for only those with dysplastic valves with inadequate relief after BPV or those with multiple levels of obstruction.

Natural History: In the Second Natural History study, patients with catheter measured gradient ≤25 mm Hg had normal survival and no progression of their stenosis in 25 years of follow-up; patients with a gradient between 25-49 mm Hg had a 20% chance of ever needing an intervention; and the majority of patients with a gradient ≥50 mm Hg experienced progressive stenosis and required intervention.

Infective Endocarditis Prophylaxis (IE): IE prophylaxis is not recommended.

Exercise and Sports: Patients with mild PS do not need any exercise restriction. Those with moderate PS and normal biventricular function should avoid competitive and static sports. In patients with severe PS, the stenosis must be resolved before they can resume unrestricted physical activity.

SALIENT FEATURES

1. Valvar PS constitutes 7% of all CHDs accounting for 80-90% of all lesions with right ventricular out flow tract (RVOT) obstruction.

2. Majority of children with PS are diagnosed due to incidental detection of a murmur. Those with long standing moderate to severe stenosis present with exertional dyspnea and fatigue. Neonates with critical PS present with severe cyanosis at birth and may develop severe hypoxia and acidosis with PDA closure.
3. Echocardiography is the modality of choice for diagnosis as well as for decision-making about timing of intervention.
4. Balloon pulmonary valvuloplasty is the treatment of choice for moderate and severe PS.
5. Balloon diameter for valvuloplasty is chosen as 1.2–1.4 times the angiographically measured pulmonary annulus size.

BALLOON AORTIC VALVULOPLASTY

Introduction

Aortic stenosis can have varied anatomical spectrum, ranging from trileaflet calcified valve to severely dysplastic unicuspid valve. The outcomes of balloon aortic valvuloplasty (BAV) depends on the anatomic substrate. Dysplastic or unicuspid valves, often seen in neonates, are present in about 10% of infants and 3% of older children in whom the treatment is indicated. Tricuspid valves are seen in 25% of infants and in 40% of older patients who require treatment. Most of the stenotic aortic valves are bicuspid.[1]

There are two forms of bicuspid aortic valve: Balanced or 'anatomically bicuspid' and unbalanced or 'functionally bicuspid.' The anatomically bicuspid valve is composed of two equally sized cusps with two sinuses of Valsalva. The functionally bicuspid valve also opens as bicuspid, but it has three sinuses, two of them adjacent to a fused cusp which is formed by two unequal cusps conjoined by an unopened commissure [raphe]. In the balanced bicuspid valves as well as in tricuspid stenotic valves, the orifices are usually enlarged by a splitting of the functioning commissures, whereas in the unbalanced bicuspid valves, the fused cusp is often torn aside from the rudimental commissure.

Indications

Patient selection for BAV is challenging. The American Heart Association–American College of Cardiology task force guideline recommendations for therapy with BAV defines a narrow patient population. BAV is the treatment of choice for aortic stenosis in children and young adults upto the age of 21 years or less with aortic stenosis. In the younger population, valve stenosis severity is defined by gradient, because many of these patients will be growing and have a variable valve area. BAV in this group of patients is durable, and an expectation for good long-term results is extremely different than that seen in older adult patients with aortic valve stenosis.

INDICATIONS FOR BAV IN PATIENTS <21 YEARS AGE

Class I	Gradient >60 mm Hg Symptoms with peak gradient >50 mm Hg New electrocardiogram (ECG) changes at rest/exercise gradient >50 mm Hg
Class II	Gradient >50 mm Hg in patients who desire pregnancy or competitive sports
Class III	Gradient <50 mm Hg with no symptoms or ECG changes

Many a times, neonates with critical aortic stenosis present with low cardiac output and ventricular dysfunction. In such cases the gradients might be less and the severity underestimated. So, it is important to stress on anatomy and mobility of valve leaflets. They may also be associated with hypoplasia of left sided structures. Hence it is important to determine whether they are candidates for two-ventricle/uni-ventricle pathway prior to proceeding with a BAV.

Indications in adult patient are much different from pediatric population. As results with aortic valve replacement are well established, valvuloplasty is applied generally only when aortic valve replacement is either high risk or strategically better to defer (as in pregnancy).

INDICATIONS FOR BAV IN ADULTS

Class I	No indication
Class II a	Bridge to surgery in unstable, high-risk patients
Class II b	Palliation in patients with serious comorbid condition Prior to urgent non-cardiac surgery
Class III	Alternative to aortic valve replacement

With emergence of transcatheter aortic valve implantation (TAVI), the indications in adults are rapidly changing.

PRE-CATHETERIZATION PLANNING

Detailed history, examination, electrocardiogram, chest X-ray and 2D echo should be obtained. The 2D-echo should have information on aortic annulus size (Fig. 6), anatomy of aortic valve, peak/mean gradient across the valve, degree of aortic regurgitation, presence and severity of left ventricular hypertrophy, function of left ventricle and presence/absence of additional left-sided obstructive lesions.

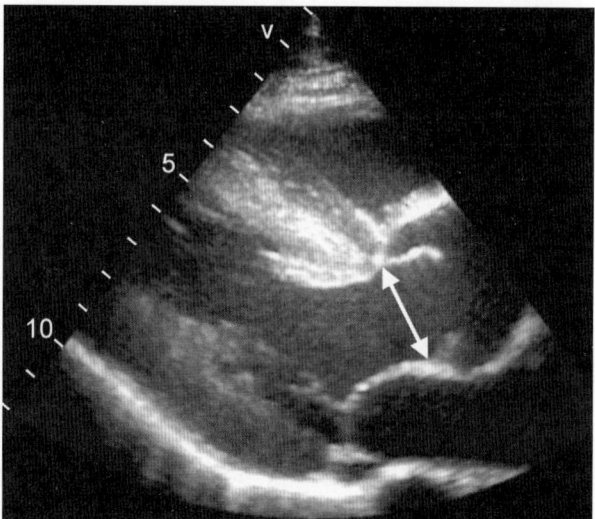

Fig. 6: Measuring aortic annulus on 2 D-Echo in para-sternal long axis view.

CONSENT

For all patients, the consent discussion should include the risk and consequence of aortic regurgitation, vascular complication, need of re-intervention, development of heart block tamponade and small possibility of fatality.

PROCEDURE

Anesthesia

In infants and sick children, the procedure is usually performed under general anesthesia.

Older children/adults who are hemodynamically stable can be done with conscious sedation.

Access

Arterial Access

Femoral arterial access. Usually 4 Fr in neonates, 5 Fr in infants, 6 Fr in children. Bigger size sheaths may occasionally be required but are associated with increased vascular complications. Some groups prefer a trans axillary or a trans carotid approach in neonates with critical AS

Venous Access

Venous Access for ventricular pacing/ante-grade crossing.

Catheters and Wires

Judkin's right coronary catheter and pigtail catheter.

Straight, soft tipped wire with stiff body. In neonates- 0.014" PTCA wire, while in older children 0.035" straight tip Terumo wire can be used for crossing the valve and exchanged for appropriate sized stiff wire to mount the balloon.

Balloon

Ideal balloon should be low-profile, non-compliant, rapidly inflating and deflating with appropriate diameter and length. The most commonly used balloons in pediatric patients are Tyshak II and Tyshak II mini balloons. In little older children or adolescents Optapro, Maxi LD, Conquest or even Atlas can be used. Due to the high profile, their use in small children should be avoided

Balloon Length

Balloon length is important for stability. Smaller balloons tend to melon seed during inflation while very long balloon can damage the mitral apparatus or sometimes the ascending aorta at its junction with the aortic arch. Roughly, the balloon length should be 2 cm in neonates/infants and 4 cm in older children/adults.

Balloon Diameter

The initial balloon size chosen should be 80–90% of the annulus size. The degree of aortic damage and regurgitation increases as the balloon- to-annulus ratio increases, very significantly so at 125%.[3] In newborns and infants, we do not prefer to go beyond 90% of the annulus in order to avoid moderate or severe AR. Our policy is to accept a residual stenosis rather than end up with significant regurgitation. However, in older children especially those who come back with are Aortic stenosis (AS) after initial BAV we gradually upsize the balloon even upto 125% of the annular size. In this subset of patients, 90% or even 100% balloon diameter is unable to increase the valve area or reduce the transvalvar gradient.

Balloon Pressure

In newborns, infants, children and adolescents, high pressure balloons are not required and the inflation can be performed with a hand held syringe. It is important to control balloon position rather than monitor the pressure on inflating device. In older patients with calcified valves, high pressure balloons may be needed.

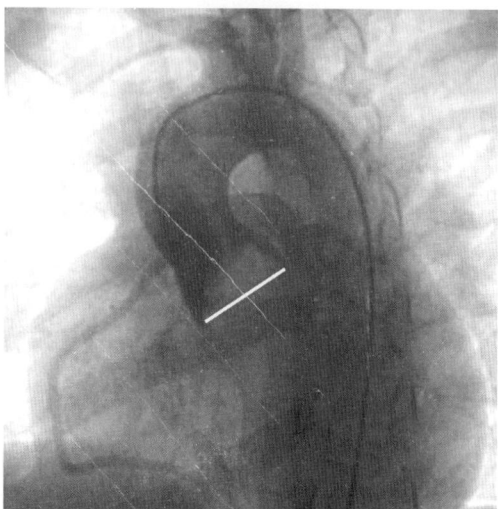

Fig. 7: Measuring aortic annulus in angiography.

Steps (Retrograde Approach)

After securing the femoral access, a Judkin's right coronary or similar angled catheter is advanced to ascending aorta. The baseline aortic pressure is measured. An aortography with contrast media injection into the aortic root in shallow LAO projection may be performed to measure the valve annulus, assess the position of the aortic valve orifice, and exclude or document aortic valve incompetence (Fig. 7). The aortic annulus diameter is measured between the leaflets' hinge points. Angiography is not mandatory and in our practice we almost never do it. The aortic annulus is measured precisely on 2DE in a systolic frame to decide on the size of the balloon to be used. The aortic valve is crossed with the catheter and straight tip Terumo wire. The catheter should be given a clockwise torque so that is faces leftward and posteriorly. After crossing the valve, the left ventricular pressure is measured, to get the baseline pressure gradient. The Terumo wire is exchanged for an appropriate size and length wire with a soft tip. The tip of the guide wire is given an additional secondary curve to prevent damage to ventricular myocardium and get stable wire position. It is important to visualize the wire position in LAO projection and assure that its free of mitral apparatus. An appropriate sized balloon is advanced over the wire and inflated across the valve, till the waist disappears (Fig. 8). Many a times the balloon is displaced due to the jet-effect and it becomes difficult to get a stable balloon position. This can be overcome by either using rapid RT pacing/intravenous adenosine or selecting a longer balloon. Adenosine injection does not give a predictable duration of asystole and hence our choice of the procedure for stabilizing the balloon is rapid right ventricular pacing. Usually a pacing

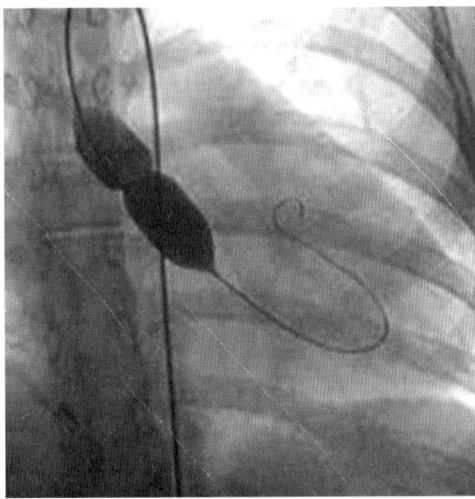

Fig. 8: Balloon dilation with waist in balloon.

rate of 180 to 200/min is adequate to drop the cardiac output significantly so as to achieve stable balloon position.

After getting a proper balloon inflation, the hemodynamic measurement is repeated and degree of aortic regurgitation reassessed. One millimeter higher size balloon is used if the result is unsatisfactory, however, the diameter of balloon should not exceed aortic annulus. The procedure is terminated if the gradients reduce > 50% of baseline or < 10 mm Hg residual gradient or more than mild aortic regurgitation develops.

Variations in Procedure

Double Balloon Technique

The aortic valve dilation can be performed by a simultaneous inflation of two balloons introduced into the valve from both the femoral arteries (Fig. 9). The advantages of this double-balloon technique are as follows:[4]

- In comparison to one big balloon, two smaller balloons usually require smaller sheaths and accordingly the risk of a femoral artery injury is decreased.
- The two balloons' apposition is never complete and blood can vent between them; this avoids a severe aortic pressure drop during the dilation.
- It is believed that, in bicuspid valves, the two balloons better comply with the valve anatomy and therefore are less likely to cause a cusp disruption than a single balloon.
- The double arterial access enables the most accurate measurement of the gradient and the valve area by simultaneous pressure recording in the left ventricle and the ascending aorta.

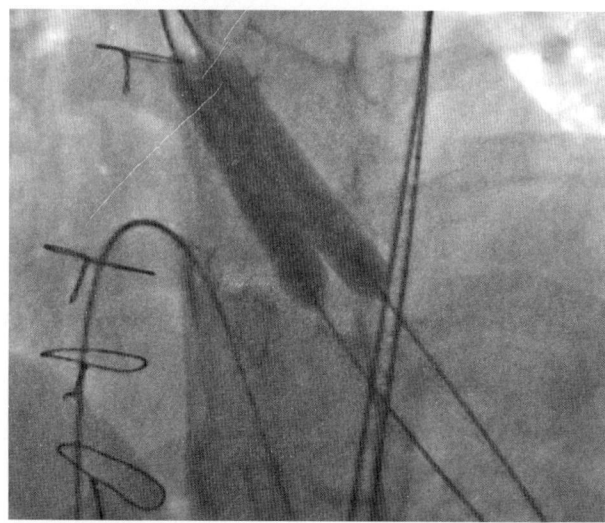

Fig. 9: Double balloon technique.

The disadvantages of double balloon technique are as follows:
- The valve needs to be crossed twice, hence increases the procedure time
- Requires additional personnel to stabilize the second balloon
- Cost of the hardware tends to get doubled.

  The effective diameters of two balloon is calculated as:
  [Diameter of balloon 1 + Diameter of balloon 2] $\times$ 0.8^5
  The target effective diameter should be 90% of aortic annulus.

ANTE-GRADE APPROACH

Occasionally it becomes difficult to cross the valve retrogradely. In such cases, if there is patent foramen ovale, the valve can be crossed from venous side by passing the wire and then the balloon from the right atrium to the left atrium to the left ventricle to the ascending aortae and then in the descending aorta. Care must be taken to prevent damage to mitral apparatus. In older children and adults, trans-septal puncture needs to be performed to enter the left side of heart. Crossing the stenotic aortic valve antegradely with the flow is extremely easy as compared to retrograde crossing of the valve.

Post-Procedure Care

After the valvuloplasty, the balloon catheter is replaced over the wire by a diagnostic catheter, the wire is removed, and the pullback gradient is measured. Exceptional care should be given to perfect hemostasis without causing arterial occlusion.

Complications

Occasionally left anterior hemi-block or even a complete left bundle branch block is produced by compression of the conductive tissue caused by the guide wire and/or the balloon, but it is almost always self-limiting.

Severe damage to the valve leaflets, myocardium, and the aortic wall can be prevented by avoiding oversized balloons and by keeping the inflated balloon stable across the aortic valve.

A vessel injury may result from balloon rupture.

The mitral valve may be injured by the balloon inflation if the exchange wire is accidentally threaded through the anterior leaflet chordae. One should pay a very close attention while inflating the balloon. Presence of more than one waist on the balloon should alarm the operator that the balloon may be traversing the Mitral valve (MV) chordate. The inflation should be immediately stopped, the balloon deflated and the wire repositioned.

SUMMARIZING

- Proper patient selection as per criteria. Results vary aortic stenosis per primary anatomy of the valve.
- Take a detailed informed consent
- Type of anesthesia depending on clinical condition
- Choosing the appropriate sized balloon is most important pre-requisite for good outcome
- Balloon diameter should be 80–90% of aortic annulus and should never exceed the aortic annulus
- Stability of balloon can be improved using rapid ventricular pacing/iv Adenosine/longer balloon
- Double balloon technique give better results in terms of aortic regurgitation but is more time consuming
- Occasionally antegrade approach may be needed if valve is not crossed retrogradely
- End-points of procedure: (a) residual gradient < 10 mm Hg or (b) > 50% drop in gradient or (c) Moderate or more aortic regurgitation
- Complications can be minimized by avoiding over-sized balloon and having good stability during inflation.

SUGGESTED READING

Behjati-Ardakani M, Forouzannia SK, Abdollahi MH, Sarebanhassanabadi M. Immediate, short, intermediate and long-term results of balloon valvuloplasty in congenital pulmonary valve stenosis. Acta Med Iran. 2013;51:324-8.

Holzer RJ, Gauvreau K, Kreutzer J, Trucco SM, Torres A, Shahanavaz S, Bergersen L. Safety and Efficacy of Balloon Pulmonary Valvuloplasty: A Multicenter Experience. Catheterization and Cardiovascular Interventions 2012;80:663-2.

Rigby ML. Severe aortic or pulmonary valve stenosis in premature infants. Early Hum Dev. 2012;88:291-4.

Taggart NW, Cetta F, Cabalka AK,Hagler DJ. Outcomes for Balloon Pulmonary Valvuloplasty in Adults: Comparison with a Concurrent Pediatric Cohort. Catheter Cardiovasc Interv 2013; 82:811-15.

REFERENCES

1. Reich O, Tax P, Marek J. et al. Long term results of percutaneous balloon valvoplasty of congenital aortic stenosis: independent predictors of outcome. Heart. 2004;90:70-6.
2. Task Force on Practice Guidelines (Committee on Management of Patients with Valvular Heart Disease). ACC/AHA guidelines for the management of patients with valvular heart disease. A report of the American College of Cardiology/American Heart Association. J Am Coll Cardiol. 1998;32:1486-588.
3. Sholler GF, Keane JF, Perry SB, et al. Balloon dilation of congenital aortic valve stenosis. Circulation 1988;78:351-60.
4. Mullins CE, Nihill MR, Vick GW. et al. Double balloon technique for dilation of valvular or vessel stenosis in congenital and acquired heart disease. J Am Coll Cardiol. 1987;10:107-14.
5. Yeager SB. Balloon selection for double balloon valvotomy. J Am Coll Cardiol. 1987;9:467-8.

19
Transcatheter Aortic Valve Replacement (TAVR)—Current Status

Ashwin B Mehta, Nihar Mehta

INTRODUCTION

The most common acquired valvular heart disease in adults in the developing world is aortic stenosis (AS), which has an increasing prevalence with age.[1] Symptomatic severe AS, if treated medically inevitably leads to functional deterioration, heart failure and death.[2] Although, surgical aortic valve replacement (SAVR) is the standard treatment with a Class 1 recommendation by ACC/AHA and ESC/EACTS guidelines in adults to alleviate symptoms and improve survival,[3,4] SAVR entails considerable risks for some patients with severe co-morbidities and in some anatomical subsets. About 30% of patients do not undergo the procedure.[5]

Since 2002, when the first transcatheter aortic valve replacement (TAVR) was performed by Dr Alain Cribier, this new technique has been used in many countries worldwide resulting in an additional option for these high-risk patients.[6,7] In the subgroup of patients who are inoperable or high risk, TAVR is now the standard of care and is a valid alternative to surgery. In patients with severe symptomatic AS a multidisciplinary team approach is recommended to assess the individual risk of the patient and choose between the options of SAVR and TAVR.

INDICATIONS OF AORTIC VALVE REPLACEMENT (SAVR OR TAVR)[3] (TABLE 1)

The following are the indications of AVR by SAVR or TAVR in patients with aortic stenosis.
- High gradient AS with symptoms on history or during exercise testing
- Symptomatic patients with a Low-flow low-gradient severe AS with a reduced left ventricular ejection fraction (LVEF)
- Symptomatic patients with a low-flow low-gradient severe AS who are normotensive and have a LVEF >50% if it is determined that the obstruction is the most likely cause of symptoms.

Table 1: Recommendations of AVR.[3]

Recommendations	Class of recommendation	Level of evidence
AVR is recommended for symptomatic patients with severe high-gradient as who have symptoms by history or on exercise testing (stage D1)	I	B
AVR is recommended for asymptomatic patients with severe AS (stage C2) and LVEF <50%	I	B
AVR is indicated for patients with severe AS (stage C or D) when undergoing other cardiac sugery	I	B
AVR is reasonable for asymptomatic patients with very severe AS (stage C1, aortic velocity ≥5.0 m/s) and low surgical risk.	IIa	B
AVR is reasonable in asymptomatic patients (stage C1) with severe AS and decreased exercise tolerance or an exercise fall in BP	IIa	B
AVR is reasonable in a symptomatic patients with low-flow/low-gradient severe AS with reduced LVEF (stage D2) with a low-dose dobutamine stress study that shows an aortic velocity >4.0 m/s (or mean pressure gradient ≥40 mm Hg) with a valve area ≤1.0 cm^2 at any dobutamine dose	IIa	B
AVR is reasonable in symptomatic patients who have low-flow/low-gradient severe AS (stage D3) who are normotensive and have an LVEF >50% if clinical, hemodynamic, and anatomic data support valve obstruction as the most likely cause of symptoms	IIa	C
AVR is reasonable for patients with moderate AS (stage B) (aortic velocity 3.0 to 3.9 m/s) who are undergoing other cardiac surgery	IIa	C
AVR may be considered for asymptomatic patients with severe AS (stage C1) and rapid disease progression and low surgical risk	IIb	C

For the strength of recommendations: Class I means the procedure/treatment should be performed/administered. Class IIa means it is reasonable to perform the procedure/administer treatment. Class IIb means the procedure/treatment may be considered. Class III means that the procedure or treatment is not useful/effective and may be harmful.

For the level of evidence: Level A means multiple populations evaluated; data derived from multiple randomized clinical trials or meta- analyses. Level B means limited populations evaluated; data derived from a single randomized trial or nonrandomized studies. Level C means very limited populations evaluated; only consensus opinion of experts, case studies, or standard of care.

(AS: Aortic stenosis; AVR: Aortic valve replacement by either surgical or transcatheter approach; BP: Blood pressure; LVEF: Left ventricular ejection fraction).

The following are indications for AVR by SAVR in patients with aortic stenosis:
- *Asymptomatic* patients with severe AS and LVEF <50%
- *Asymptomatic* patients with severe AS and decreased exercise tolerance or fall in BP during exercise.
- *Asymptomatic* severe AS undergoing other cardiac surgery
- *Asymptomatic* very Severe AS (velocity >5 m/s) and a low surgical risk

INDICATIONS FOR TAVR[4] (TABLE 2)

The indications for TAVR are evolving. TAVR can be used for native valve aortic valve stenosis or in bioprosthetic valve stenosis, regurgitation or a combination of both (the 'valve in valve' procedure).[8]
- *In native aortic valve stenosis*: In patients with calcific aortic stenosis who meet the indications for an aortic valve replacement, the surgical risk

Table 2: Recommendations for AS: Choice of SAVR or TAVR.

Recommendations	Class of recommendation	Level of evidence
Surgical AVR is recommended in patients who meet an indication for AVR with low or intermediate surgical risk	I	A
For patients in whom TAVR or high-risk surgical AVR is being considered, members of a Heart Valve Team should collaborate to provide optimal patient care	I	C
TAVR is recommended in patients who meet an indication for AVR for AS who have a prohibitive surgical risk and a predicted post-TAVR survival >12 mo	I	B
TAVR is a reasonable alternative to surgical AVR in patients who meet an indication for AVR and who have high surgical risk	IIa	B
Percutaneous aortic balloon dilation may be considered as a bridge to surgical or transcatheter AVR in severely symptomatic patients with severe AS	IIb	C
TAVR is not recommended in patients in whom existing comorbidities would preclude the expected benefit from correction of AS	III: No benefit	B

The above approach is similar to that in the 2014 AHA/ACC valve guideline.[3] However, recommendation for TAVR in intermediate-risk patients are based on studies published after these guidelines.
(AVR: Aortic valve replacement by either surgical or transcatheter approach; TAVR: Transcather aortic valve replacement; AS: Aortic stenosis; SAVR: Surgical aortic valve replacement).

and co-morbidities are estimated. The choice between SAVR and TAVR is based on these risks.

TAVR is preferred in the presence of certain technical and anatomical subsets, which lead to a high risk for SAVR. These are as follows:
- Porcelain aorta
- Prior significant mediastinal radiation
- Prior pericardiectomy with dense adhesions
- Prior sternal infection with complex reconstruction
- Patent left internal mammary graft lying beneath the sternum [as identified by computed tomography (CT) angiography].

- *Valve-in-valve TAVR*: In patients with a bioprosthetic aortic valve with symptomatic failure of the valve in the form of stenosis, regurgitation or both and a high surgical risk for SAVR.
- *Bicuspid aortic valve*: The anatomy of bicuspid aortic valves being asymmetrical with bulky leaflets predispose to suboptimal valve seating and deployment with a noncircular valve expansion. This increases the risk of paravalvular regurgitation and device migration. Whether newer valve designs will be able to account for these problems remains to be seen.

Prerequisites for TAVR

- To determine which patients are suitable candidates for TAVR, a multidisciplinary 'Heart-Valve Team', including cardiologists, interventionists, cardiac surgeons, anesthetist and other specialists if necessary, should assess every patient on an individual basis.
- The hospital should have cardiac surgery on-site.
- These high risk patients should have a life expectancy of more than 1 year after considering the co-morbidities
- They should be likely to have improvement in their quality of life.
- TAVR is recommended in patients who have a prohibitive surgical risk as deemed by the 'heart team'.[4]
- Among patients who have an intermediate or high risk but are still operable, TAVR may be performed if the heart team deemed that TAVR was favorable based on risk profile and anatomical suitability.

RISK ASSESSMENT

In patients with severe symptomatic calcific AS, the treatment decision between TAVR and SAVR is to be decided based on the risk assessment as well as the other co-morbidities and technical and surgical subsets (discussed above). The decision should be individualized by the Heart-Valve Team to optimize results.

The risk assessment is based on the Society of Thoracic Surgical – Predicted Risk of Mortality (STS-PROM) Risk Estimate (Table 3). Other scoring systems

Table 3: Risk assessment based on STS-PROM risk estimate, frailty, major organ system compromise and procedure specific impediment.[3]

	Low risk (must meet all criteria in this column)	Intermediate risk (any 1 criterion in this column)	High risk (any 1 criterion in this column)	Prohibitive risk (any 1 criterion in this column)
STS PROM*	<4% AND	4 to 8% OR	>8% OR	Predicted risk with surgery of death or major morbidity (all cause) >50% at 1 year OR
Frailty¶	None AND	1 Index (mild) OR	>2 Indices (moderate to severe) OR	
Major organ system compromise not to be improved postoperatively▲	None AND	1 Organ system OR	No more than 2 organ systems OR	>3 organ systems OR
Procedure-specific impediment•	None	procedure-specific impediment	Possible procedure-specific impediment	Severe procedure-specific impediment

*Use of the Society of Thoracic Surgeons Predicted Risk of Mortality (STS PROM) to predict risk in a given institution with reasonable reliability is appropriate only if institubonal outcomes are within one standard deviation of STS average observed/expected ratio for the procedure in question.

¶Seven frailty indices: Katz Activities of Daily Living (independence in feeding, bathing, dressing, transferring, toileting, and urinary continence) and independence in ambulation (no walking aid or assist required or 5-meter walk in <6 s). Other scoring systems can be applied to calculate no, mild-, or moderate-to-severe frailty.

▲Examples of major organ system compromise: Cardiac-severe LV systolic or diastolic dysfunction or RV dysfunction, fixed pulmonary hypertension; CKD stage 3 or worse; pulmonary dysfunction with FEVI <50% or $DLCO_2$ <50% of predicted; CNS dysfunction (dementia, Alzheimer's disease, Parkinson's disease, CVA with persistent physical limitation); GI dysfunction-Crohn`s disease, ulcerative colitis, nutritional impairment, or serum albumin <3.0; cancer-active malignancy; liver-any history of cirrhosis, variceal bleeding, or elevated INR in the absence of VKA therapy.

•Examples: Tracheostomy present, heavily calcified ascending aorta, chest malformation, arterial coronary graft adherent to posterior chest wall, or radiation damage.

(CKD: Chronic kidney disease; CNS: Central nervous system; CVA: Stroke; $DLCO_2$: Diffusion capacity for carbon dioxide; FEV1: Forced expiratory volume in 1 s; GI: Gastrointestinal; INR: International normalized ratio; LV: Left ventricular PROM: Predicted risk of mortality; RV: Right ventricular; STS: Society of Thoracic Surgeons; VKA: Vitamin K antagonist).

have also been used for risk assessment such as the logistic EuroSCORE (the European system for Cardiac Operative Risk Evaluation), Ambler Score and SURTAVI model.[9,10]

Based on the current evidence and the risk assessment, the following approach can be used for patients with severe symptomatic aortic stenosis
- *Prohibitive surgical risk*: With a predicted post–TAVR survival of more than 12 months, TAVR should be the procedure of choice compared to medical therapy.
- *Intermediate to high surgical risk (STS-PROM Score more than 4)*: Both, TAVR or SAVR can be viable options. The Heart-Valve Team should decide the optimal procedure based on individual patient factors, preferences, associated conditions like coronary disease, other valve lesions and other technical and anatomical subsets.
- *Low surgical risk (STS-PROM Score less than 4)*: SAVR should be the procedure of choice.

CONTRAINDICATIONS FOR TAVR (TABLE 4)

Types of TAVR Valves

Currently, two different TAVR devices are widely used:
1. Balloon-expandable Edwards SAPIEN, SAPIEN XT or SAPIEN 3 Transcatheter Heart Valve (Edwards Lifesciences, Irvine, CA, USA)
2. Self-expanding Medtronic CoreValve or EvolutR (Medtronic, Minneapolis, MN, USA)

Table 4: Absolute and relative contraindications for TAVR.

- Absolute contraindications
  - Absence of a Heart Valve Team or Cardiac surgery on-site
  - Appropriateness of TAVR, compared to SAVR, not confirmed by the Heart Team
- Clinical
  - Estimated life expectance <1 year
  - Improvement in quality of life by TAVR unlikely due to co-morbidities
  - Severe primary disease of other valves, contributing to symptoms, which can be treated by surgery only
- Anatomical
  - Inadequate annulus size–smaller than 18 mm (native valve) or 17 mm (bioprosthetic valve) or larger than 29 mm
  - Severe aortic regurgitation (>3+). (Not an exclusion when used to treat failed bioprosthetic valve for valve-in-valve procedure)
  - Active endocarditis
  - Increased risk of coronary ostial obstruction (small aortic sinuses, short distance between annulus and coronary ostium)
  - For transfemoral or subclavian approach: inadequate access (size, tortuosity, calcification)

Contd...

Contd...

- Relative contraindications
  - Bicuspid or Noncalcified valves
  - Untreated coronary artery disease
  - Acute myocardial Infarction within one month before procedure
  - Stroke or transient ischemic attack within 6 months of procedure
  - Left ventricular ejection fraction <20%
  - Hemodynamic instability requiring inotropes, mechanical ventilation or mechanical heart assistance within 30 days
  - Severe mitral regurgitation
  - Hypertrophic cardiomyopathy with or without obstruction
  - Severe pulmonary hypertension and right ventricular dysfunction
  - Intracardiac mass, thrombus or vegetation
  - Atheroma (>5 mm thick, protruding or ulcerated) ascending or arch of aorta
  - Thoracic or abdominal aortic aneurysm (>5 cm)
  - Narrowing (especially with calcification or irregularities) or tortuosity of abdominal or thoracic aorta
  - Any contraindication or hypersensitivity to anticoagulation
- Renal insufficiency or end-stage renal disease requiring chronic dialysis

(TAVR: Transcatheter aortic valve replacement; SAVR: Surgical aortic valve replacement).

- *Edwards Sapien XT and Sapien 3 Valve*
  Edwards SAPIEN XT valve is a trileaflet bovine pericardium valve mounted on a cobalt chromium frame. It is available in 20, 23, 26 and 29 mm sizes. It can be used via the retrograde route, transapical route or trans-aortic route (Fig. 1).
  SAPIEN 3 valve has a very low delivery profile and an outer skirt to prevent para-valvular regurgitation. It is available in 23, 26 and 29 mm sizes (Fig. 2 and Table 5).
- *Medtronic CoreValve and EvoluteR Valve*
  CoreValve is trileaflet valve made up of porcine pericardial tissue and mounted in self expanding nitinol frame. It is available in 26, 29 and 31 mm sizes. All valves initially required 24 or 25 French sheath for delivery of prosthesis but recent changes in the delivery systems have lead to a decrease to 18 French sheath for delivery. CoreValve can be used via the retrograde, transaortic or subclavian routes (Fig. 3).

  The EvoluteR has a lower delivery profile and a 14 French sheath can be used for delivery. Recapturing of the valve before releasing can be done up to three times in case of suboptimal positioning of the valve. (Tables 6 and 7).

Approaches for TAVR (Figs. 4A to E)

1. *Antegrade approach*:[6] Cribier initially used the antegrade approach. This involved percutaneous access to the femoral vein followed by a

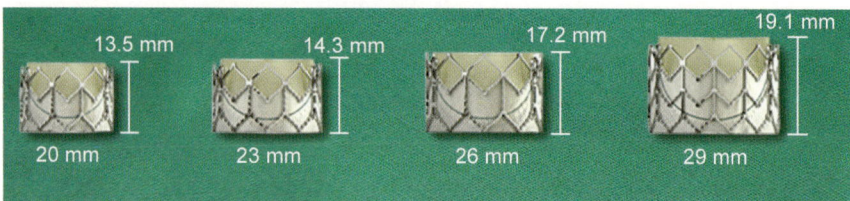

Fig. 1: SAPIEN XT Valve.

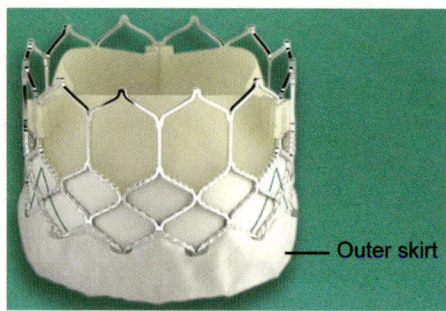

Fig. 2: SAPIEN 3 Valve.

Table 5: Specifications for the SAPIEN 3 Valve according to size.

	23 mm	26 mm	29 mm
Transfemoral sheath	14 F	14 F	16 F
Minimum access vessel diameter	5.5 mm	5.5 mm	6.0 mm
Native annulus size (TEE)	18–22 mm	21–25 mm	24–28 mm
Native annulus area	338–430 mm^2	430–546 mm^2	540–683 mm^2
Area derived diameter	20.7–23.4 mm	23.4–26.4 mm	26.2–29.5 mm

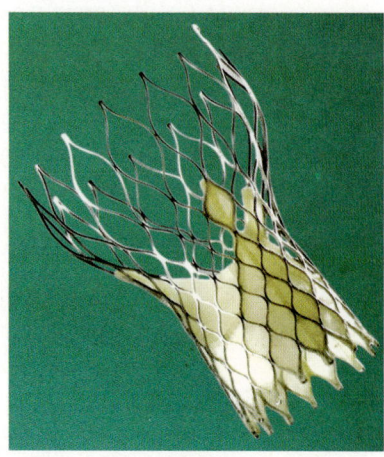

Fig. 3: Medtronic CoreValve.

Table 6: Specifications for the EvoluteR Valve according to size.

Size	23 mm	26 mm	29 mm
Annulus diameter	18–20 mm	20–23 mm	23–26 mm
Annulus perimeter*	56.5–2.8 mm	62.8–72.3 mm	72.3–81.7 mm
Sinus of Valsalva diameter (mean)	≥25 mm	≥27 mm	≥29 mm
Sinus of Valsalva height (mean)	≥15 mm	≥15 mm	≥15 mm

*Annulus perimeter = Annulus diameter × π

Table 7: Differences between SAPIEN Valve and CoreValve.

	Edward SAPIEN XT/SAPIEN 3 Valve	Corevalve/Evolute-R Valve
Expansion	Balloon expandable	Self-expandable
Frame	Stainless steel	Nitinol
Valve material	Bovine	Porcine
Sheath size	21–24/16–18/14 F	18/14 F
Annulus size	>18 mm, <25 mm	>20 mm, <27 mm
Area	1.7 cm^2	1.7–1.9 cm^2
Repositioning	No	Yes
Access site	Transfemoral, transapical	Transfemoral, subclavian, transaortic

trans-septal puncture. A wire was passed from the femoral vein and snared into the femoral artery to create a arteriovenous loop. The valve was crimped onto a balloon and introduced through the femoral vein, across the inter-atrial septum, across the mitral valve and finally across the aortic valve antegradely through the left ventricle. Since, this was technically challenging, the retrograde approach is preferred.

2. *Retrograde/transfemoral approach*:[10] This is the preferred approach currently. The femoral artery is punctured and a balloon aortic valvuloplasty is done through a 14 F sheath. The sheath can be changed to an 18, 19 or 22 F sheath and the valve is positioned across the aortic valve retrogradely through the arch and ascending aorta.

3. *Transapical approach*:[6] This involves a minimally invasive lateral thoracotomy, placement of an apical purse string suture, passing a stiff wire from the apex to the aortic arch, balloon aortic valvuloplasty during rapid ventricular pacing followed by deployment of the device.

4. *Subclavian/transaxillary approach*:[10,11] It is a percutaneous approach, used in patients with an unfavorable ilio-femoral anatomy.

5. *Transaortic approach*:[12,13] This involves a minimally invasive anterior thoracotomy allowing direct access to the aorta. It can be used in patients

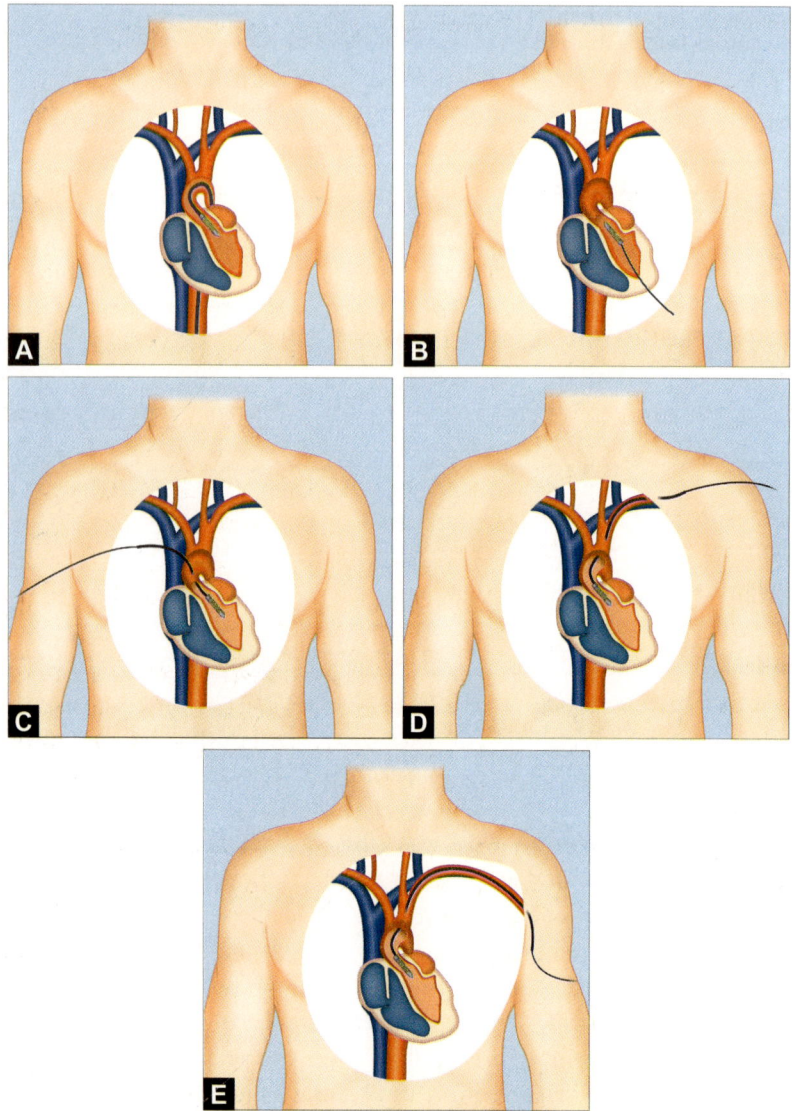

Figs. 4A to E: Approaches for TAVR: (A) Transfemoral approach; (B) Transapical approach. After left lateral minithoracotomy, the deliver catheter is advanced through the LV apex; (C) Transaortic approach. After right or mid ministernotomy, the delivery catheter is advanced directly through the ascending aorta; (D) Subclavian approach; (E) Transaxillary approach.[15]

with an unfavorable iliofemoral or subclavian anatomy as well due to factors like chest deformity, low ejection fraction or respiratory disease.

6. *Carotid approach*:[14] It has been proposed, however, in such cases, it is crucial to evaluate the cerebral arteries, carotid and vertebral arteries, and circle of Willis, to assess the risk of ischemic stroke.

PATIENT SPECIFIC SELECTION OF TAVR VALVE

For most patients undergoing TAVR, the Edward SAPIEN or Medtronic CoreValve are suitable. Certain patient related problems may influence the selection of the valves.
- *Annulus size*: All valves do not cover all annulus sizes. Depending on the patient's annulus size, the appropriate valve must be chosen.
- *Risk of annulus rupture*: Annulus rupture has been observed more commonly with a balloon expandable valve[16]. Therefore with patients with a high risk of annulus rupture like small and calcified annulus, a self expanding valve would be a better choice.
- *Risk of coronary obstruction*: Recapturable valves preferable in this subset of patients.
- *Valve-in-valve TAVR with a small bioprosthetic valve*: In this type, a supra-annular TAVR provides a greater effective orifice area.

CURRENT STATUS OF EVIDENCE

Several registries and randomized controlled trials have evaluated the outcomes of TAVR in patients with native aortic valve stenosis falling into different risk groups. Based on the evidence, the scope of TAVR has expanded from inoperable patients to patients with an intermediate or high risk.

PROHIBITIVE SURGICAL RISK (INOPERABLE) GROUP: TAVR VERSUS MEDICAL MANAGEMENT

Partner 1B Trial: The outcomes of TAVR were compared to medical management in inoperable patients with severe aortic stenosis using the Edward SAPIEN valve in the placement of aortic transcatheter valves (PARTNER) Trial Cohort B.[17,18] The mean age of the patients was 83 years and the mean STS-PROM Score was 11.7%. At one and two years, the mortality rate of TAVR was significantly reduced compared to the medically managed group. The New York Heart Associate (NYHA) functional class was also significantly better in the TAVR group. This trend continued at five years as well (Fig. 5 and Table 8).

With regards to the side effects, the stroke rate was higher in the TAVR group at 30 days, 1 year and 2 years but the risk of stroke was similar in both groups at 5 years. Thus there was no continuous risk of stroke in the TAVR group after the initial procedure. In the TAVR group, moderate or severe paravalvular regurgitation was seen in 12.4 and 8.8% at 30 days and one year respectively but the PVR improved in 42.6% at two years.

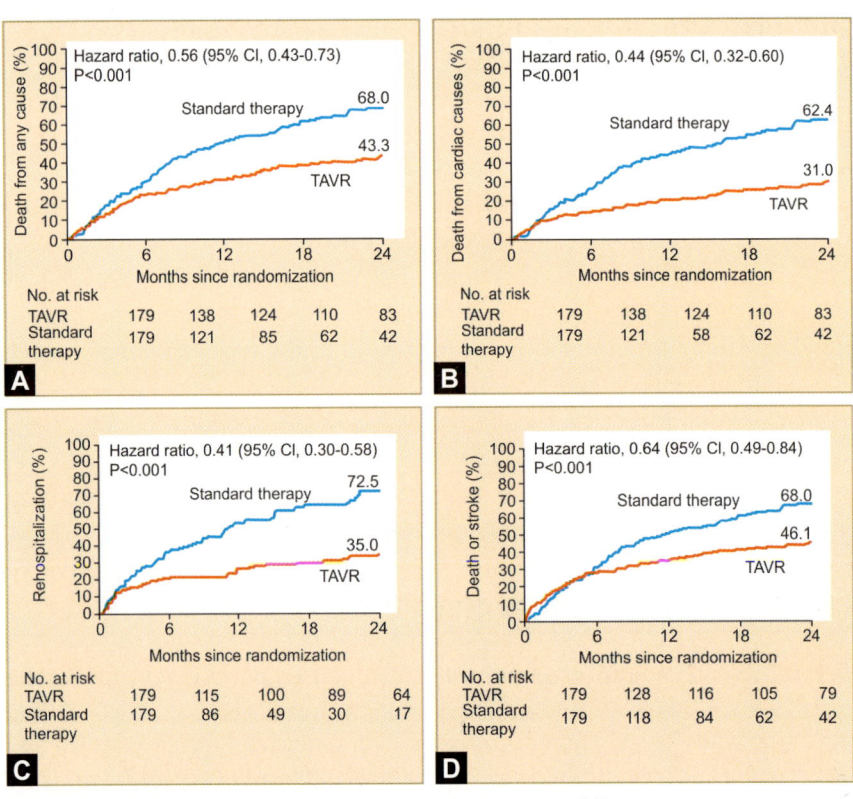

Figs. 5A to D: Two-year outcomes of the PARTNER IB Trial.[17]

THE COREVALVE PIVOTAL EXTREME RISK ILEOFEMORAL STUDY[19]

The CoreValve Pivotal Extreme Risk Ileofemoral Study evaluated the safety and efficacy of the CoreValve in severe aortic stenosis with a extremely high risk of surgery (mean STS-PROM Score of 10.3%). The outcomes showed the rate of all cause mortality or major stroke at 12 months was 26%. With regards to the side effects, the 30 days rate of life threatening bleeding was 12.7%, major vascular complications was 8.2% and need of permanent pacemaker was 21.6%. The rate of moderate or severe paravalvular regurgitation improved at 12 months from 10.7 to 4.2% (Fig. 6).

HIGH SURGICAL RISK GROUP: TAVR VERSUS SAVR

Partner 1A trial: The outcomes of TAVR (using the Edward SAPIEN valve) were compared to SAVR for patients with severe aortic stenosis with a high surgical risk in the PARTNER Trial Cohort A.[20,21] The mean age of the patients was 84 years and the mean STS-PROM Score was 11.7%. At 1, 2 and 5 years,

Table 8: One and two-year outcomes of the PARTNER IB TRIAL.[17]

Outcome	1 year			2 years		
	TAVR (N-179)	Standard therapy (N-179)	P Value	TAVR (N-179)	Standard therapy (N-179)	P value
All-cause mortality—no. (%)	55 (30.7)	89 (50.7)	<0.001	77 (43.3)	117 (68.0)	<0.001
Stroke—no. (%)	19 (11.2)	8 (5.5)	<0.001	22 (13.8)	8 (5.5)	0.01
Rehospitalization —no. (%)	43 (27.0)	79 (53.9)	<0.001	53 (35.0)	95 (72.5)	<0.001
Death or rehospitalization —no. (%)	79 (44.1)	126 (71.6)	<0.001	101 (56.7)	153 (87.9)	<0.001
Death or stroke —no. (%)	63 (35.2)	90 (51.3)	<0.002	82 (46.1)	117 (68.0)	<0.001
Cardiac death —no. (%)	35 (20.5)	75 (44.6)	<0.001	50 (31.0)	100 (62.4)	<0.001
NYHA class III or IV—no./total no. (%)	28/118 (23.7)	48/79 (60.8)	<0.001	16/95 (16.8)	23/40 (57.5)	<0.001
Myocardial infarction—no. (%)	1 (0.8)	1 (0.7)	0.9	2 (1.6)	2 (2.5)	0.69
Creatinine >3 mg/dL —no. (%)	2 (1.1)	5 (2.8)	0.4	2 (1.1)	5 (2.8)	0.45
Renal failure —no. (%)†	4 (2.3)	7 (4.7)	0.2	5 (3.2)	9 (7.6)	0.15
Major bleeding —no. (%)	41 (24.2)	21 (14.9)	0.04	48 (28.9)	25 (20.1)	0.09
Balloon aortic valvuloplasty —no. (%)	2 (1.1)	138 (82.3)	<0.001	4 (2.8)	140 (85.3)	<0.001
Aortic-valve replacement —no. (%)	0	10 (7.6)	0.002	1 (0.9)	11 (8.9)	0.005
Endocarditis —no. (%)	2 (1.4)	1 (0.8)	0.6	3 (2.3)	1 (0.8)	0.32
New pacemaker —no. (%)	8 (4.7)	14 (8.6)	0.15	10 (6.4)	14 (8.6)	0.47

* Percentages shown are Kaplan-Meier estimates, and P values are point-in-time analyses, with the exception of the percentages for creatinine >3 mg/dL (265 umol/liter) and for New York Heart Association (NYHA) class III or IV which are straight frequencies, with P values calculated with the use of Fisher's exact test. All events in this table were adjudicated by an independent clinic at events committee. TAVR denotes transcatheter aortic-valve replacement

†Renal failure was defined by the need for dialysis for any length of time.

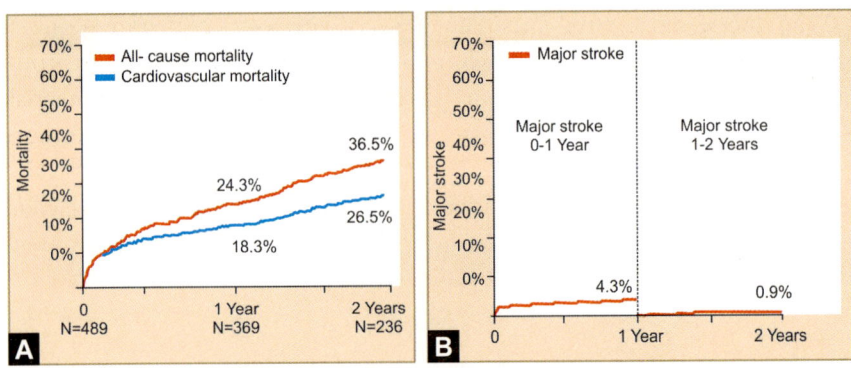

Figs. 6A and B: Outcomes of CoreValve Pivotal Extreme Risk Study.[19]

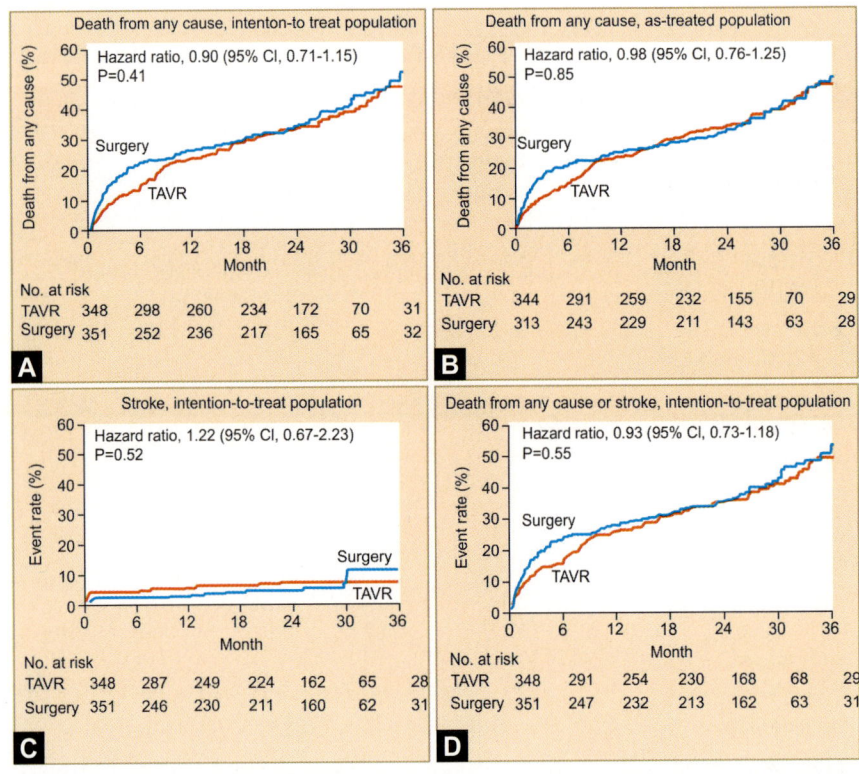

Figs. 7A to D: Outcomes of PARTNER IA TRIAL.[21]

the mortality rate of TAVR was comparable compared to the SAVR group. Improvement in the symptoms was more frequent in the TAVR group compared to the SAVR group at 1 year but was not statistically significant at 5 years (Fig. 7).

The rate of strokes and transient ischemic attacks was higher in the TAVR group at 30 days, one year and two years but were similar to the SAVR group at 5 years to which we can draw a similar conclusion of no continuous risk of stroke after the initial procedure. At 30 days, the TAVR group had more vascular complications where as the SAVR group had a higher incidence of atrial fibrillation and major bleeding. Moderate or severe paravalvular regurgitation was more in the TAVR group at 1, 2 and 5 years and was associated with an increased late mortality (Table 9).

Table 9: Outcomes of the PARTNER IA TRIAL.[21]

Outcome	1 year			2 years		
	Surgery (N=351)	TAVR (N=348)	P Value†	Surgery (N=351)	TAVR (N=348)	P Value†
	No. of patients (%)			No. of patients (%)		
Death						
From any cause	89 (26.8)	84 (24.3)	0.45	114 (35.0)	116 (33.9)	0.78
From cardiovascular causes	40 (13.0)	47 (14.3)	0.63	59 (20.5)	67 (21.4)	0.80
Repeat hospitalization‡	51 (17.7)	59 (18.6)	0.78	60 (21.7)	74 (24.7)	0.41
Death from any cause or repeat hospitalization‡	125 (37.7)	121 (34.9)	0.45	152 (46.5)	159 (46.6)	0.99
Stroke or TIA§						
All	13 (4.3)	28 (8.7)	0.03	18 (6.5)	34 (11.2)	0.05
Stroke	10 (3.2)	20 (6.0)	0.08	14 (4.9)	24 (7.7)	0.17
TIA	4 (1.5)	8 (2.6)	0.32	5 (2.0)	10 (3.6)	0.26
Death from any cause or stroke	95 (28.6)	95 (27.4)	0.74	119 (36.4)	127 (37.1)	0.85
Myocardial infarction	2 (0.6)	0	0.16	4 (1.5)	0	0.05
Major vascular complication◊	13 (3.8)	39 (11.3)	<0.001	13 (3.8)	40 (11.6)	<0.001
Major bleedingπ	88 (26.7)	52 (15.7)	<0.001	95 (29.5)	60 (19.0)	0.002
Endocarditis	3 (1.0)	2 (0.6)	0.63	3 (1.0)	4 (1.5)	0.61

Contd...

Contd...

Renal failure**	20 (6.5)	18 (5.4)	0.57	21 (6.9)	20 (6.2)	0.75
New pacemaker	16 (5.0)	21 (6.4)	0.44	19 (6.4)	23 (7.2)	0.69
SVD requiring surgical replacement	0	0		0	0	

*All percentages are Kaplan-Meier estimates at the specific time point and thus do not equal the number of patients divided by the total number in the study group.
†P valves are for between-group comparisons of the frequency of the event at each time point.
‡Repeat hospitalization were included in the analysis if they were for symptoms of heart failure, angina, or syncope due to aortic-valve disease that required aortic-valve intervention or intensified medical management.
§Stroke was defined as a neurologic deficit lasting more than 24 hours or lasting less than 24 hours with a brain-imaging study showing infarction.
◊Major vascular complications were defined as thoracic aortic dissection; access-site or access-related vascular injury leading to death, the need for substantial blood transfusion (> 3 units), or percutaneous or surgical intervention; and distal embolization (noncerebral) from a vascular source requiring surgery or amputation or resulting in irreversible end-organ damage.
¶Major bleeding was defined as any episode of major internal or external bleeding that caused death, hospitalization, or permanent injury or that necessitated the transfusion of at least 3 units of packed red cells or a pericardiocentesis procedure.
**Renal failure was defined as any condition requiring the initiation of any dialysis.
(SVD: Structural valve deterioration; TAVR: Transcatheter aorticvalve replacement; TIA: Transient ischemic attack).

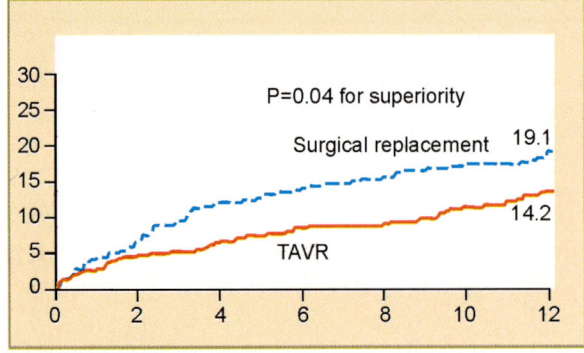

Fig. 8: One year outcome of the CoreValve Pivotal High Risk Study[22] showing superiority of TAVR over SAVR.

COREVALVE PIVOTAL HIGH RISK STUDY[22]

This study randomized high risk patients of severe aortic stenosis to TAVR using the CoreValve and SAVR. The mean ago of the patients was 83.2 years and the mean STS-PROM Score was 7.4%. The mortality at 1 year was lower in the TAVR group compared to the SAVR group (Fig. 8).

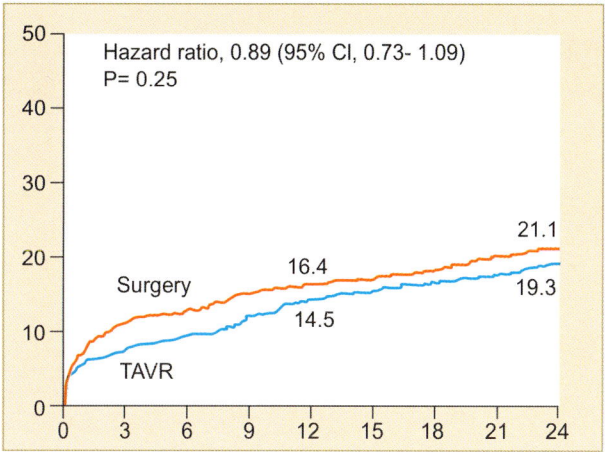

Fig. 9: Outcomes of PARTNER 2A Trial: Death from any cause or disabling stroke (%) at one year and two years.[23]

The TAVR group had a higher frequency of major vascular complications, cardiac perforation and permanent pacemaker implantation whereas the SAVR group had a higher frequency of life threatening bleeding, acute kidney injury and atrial fibrillation. There was no increase in the risk of stroke in the TAVR group compared to the SAVR group.

INTERMEDIATE SURGICAL RISK GROUP: TAVR VERSUS SAVR

PARTNER 2A TRIAL[23] was a randomized trial to compare TAVR using Edward SAPIEN Valve and SAVR in intermediate risk patients with severe aortic stenosis. The mean STS-PROM Score was 5.8%. The rate of death from any cause or disabling stroke was the same in the two groups at 1 year and 2 years (Fig. 9).

At 30 days, the TAVR group had a larger aortic valve area but also a higher frequency of major vascular complications. The SAVR group had a higher frequency of acute kidney injury, severe bleeding and atrial fibrillation. Moderate or severe paravalvular regurgitation was more in the TAVR group at 30 days and was associated with an increased late mortality at 2 years (Figs. 10A to C).

An observational study evaluated TAVR using the SAPIEN 3 valve in patients with severe aortic stenosis with an intermediate risk (mean STS-PROM Score of 5.2%). At one year, the all cause mortality of TAVR was 7.4%, disabling stroke was in seen 2% and moderate or severe paravalvular regurgitation was seen in 2%. TAVR was superior to SAVR for the composite end point of death from any cause, strokes and incidence of moderate or severe aortic regurgitation as well as for individual outcomes of death and stroke. SAVR caused less moderate or severe aortic regurgitation.[24]

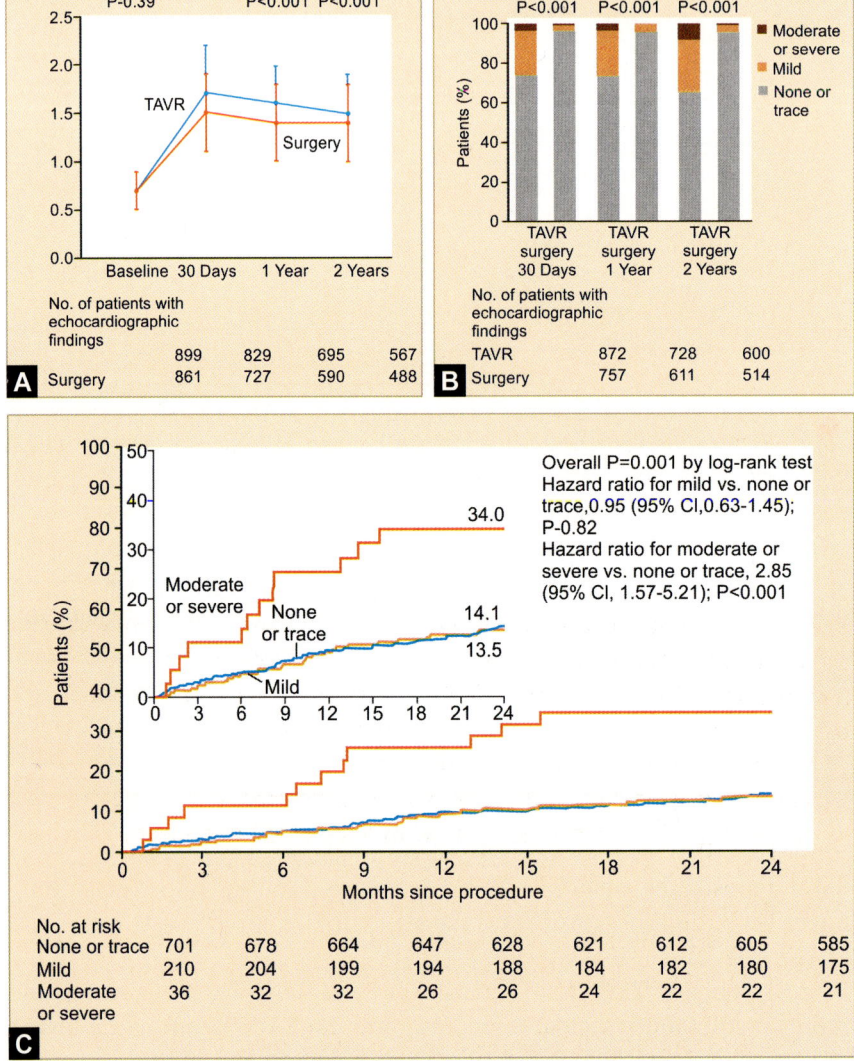

Figs. 10A to C: Echocardiographic outcomes of PARTNER 2A Trial:[23] (A) The change in aortic-valve area from baseline to 2 years, and (B) the percentage of patients with paravalvular aortic regurgitation at 30 days, 1 year, and 2 years after the procedure. (C) Time-to-event curves for death from any cause according to the severity of paravalvular aortic regurgitation. The inset shows the same data on an enlarged y axis.

CoreValve Surtavi Trial to compare the safety and efficacy of TAVR using the CoreValve with SAVR in patients with severe aortic stenosis with intermediate risk is ongoing.

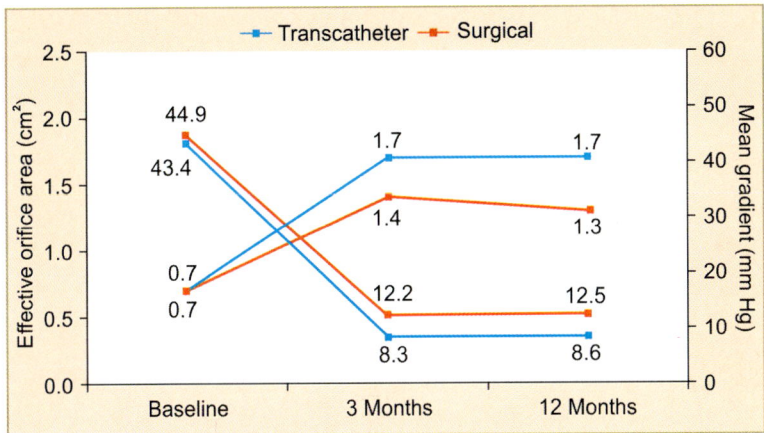

Fig. 11: Aortic valve hemodynamics measured as mean effective orifice area (in cm²) and mean aortic valve gradient (in mm Hg) according to implanted valve prosthesis at baseline, at 3 months, and at 1 year.[25]

LOW SURGICAL RISK GROUP: TAVR VERSUS SAVR

The Nordic Aortic Valve Intervention Trial (NOTION Trial)[25] evaluated the outcomes of patients with severe aortic stenosis with low or intermediate risk (average STS-PROM Score of 3%) receiving a TAVR using the CoreValve or undergoing SAVR. The composite primary outcome (death from any cause, stroke or myocardial infarction at one year) were similar in the TAVR and SAVR group (13.1% and 16.3% respectively). The TAVR group showed better valve hemodynamics at 1 year, with a lower effective orifice area compared to the SAVR group (Fig. 11). The TAVR group had a more frequent permanent pacemaker requirement, higher aortic regurgitation and lower NYHA functional class at 1 year. The SAVR group had more life threatening bleeding, cardiogenic shock, acute kidney injury and atrial fibrillation at one year (Table 10).

Although, data in this group is limited, the relative benefit of TAVR compared to SAVR is unlikely to be higher than the high-risk group. The long-term durability of the valve and paravalvular regurgitation are especially important since this subset of patients is likely to survive longer. Thus, current evidence favors SAVR in the low risk group of patients with severe aortic stenosis.

BALLOON-EXPANDABLE VERSUS SELF-EXPANDING VALVES IN TAVR

THE CHOICE TRIAL:[26] The Comparison of Transcatheter Heart Valves in High Risk Patients with Severe Aortic Stenosis (CHOICE) trial compared the

Table 10: Outcomes of the NOTION Trial[25]

	Index hospitalization* or 30 days			1 year		
	TAVR	SAVR	p Value	TAVR	SAVR	p Value
Major, life threatening disabling bleeding*	16 (11.3)	28 (20.9)	0.03			
Cardiogenic shock*	6 (4.2)	14 (10.4)	0.05			
Major vascular complication*	8 (5.6)	2 (1.5)	0.10			
Acute kidney injury stage II or III*	1 (0.7)	9 (6.7)	0.01			
All-cause death[†]	3 (2.1)	5 (3.7)	0.43	7.(4.9)	10 (7.5)	0.38
Cardiovascular death[†]	3 (2.1)	5 (3.7)	0.43	6 (4.3)	10 (7.5)	0.25
Neurological events[†]	4 (2.8)	4 (3.0)	0.94	7 (5.0)	8 (6.2)	0.68
Stroke[†]	2 (1.4)	4 (3.0)	0.37	4 (2.9)	6 (4.6)	0.44
Transient ischemic attack[†]	2 (1.4)	0 (0)	0.17	3 (2.1)	2 (1.6)	0.71
MI[†]		4 (2.8)	8 (6.0)	0.20	5 (3.5)	8 (6.0)	0.33
Valve endocarditis[†]	1 (0.7)	0 (0)	0.33	4 (2.9)	2 (1.6)	0.47
New-onset or worsening AF[†]	24 (16.9)	77 (57.8)	<0.001	30 (21.2)	79 (59.4)	<0.001
Permanent pacemaker implantation[†]	46 (34.1)	2 (1.6)	<0.001	51 (38.0)	3 (2.4)	<0.001

*Rate during index hospitalization; data reported as number of patients with events (percentage) in each treatment group; p values were calculator by Fisher exact test or chi-square test, as appropriate.
[†]Rates determined and 30 days and 1 year; data reported as number of subjects (Kaplan-Meier estimates) at the especific time point, and they do not equal the number of patients with events divided by the total number of patients in each treatment group; p value were calculated by the log-rank test for all data through 30 days or 1 year.

balloon-expandable Edward Sapien XT valve with the self-expanding Medtronic CoreValve.

The early outcomes of device success favored balloon-expandable valves (95.9%) as compared with self-expanding valves (77.5%). However, this difference was caused by a lower frequency of greater-than-mild aortic regurgitation and lower need for implanting more than one valve in the balloon-expandable group.

At 1 year, the rates of all-cause mortality (17.4 vs 12.8%), cardiovascular mortality (12.4 vs 9.4%), stroke (9.1 vs 3.4), and repeat hospitalization for heart failure (7.4 vs 12.8) were similar in both groups (Figs. 12A and B).

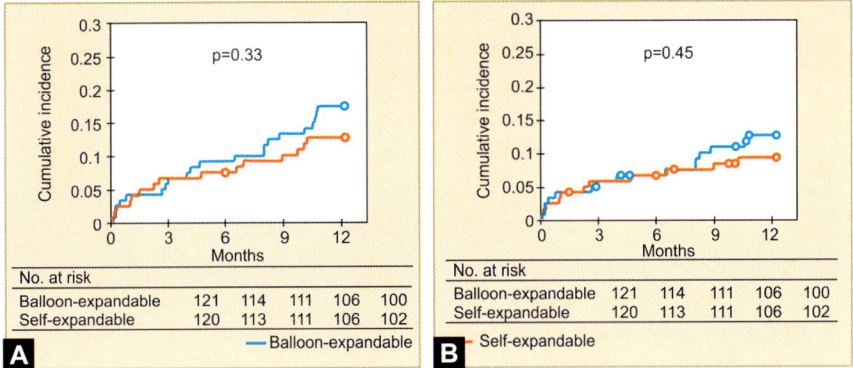

Figs. 12A and B: Outcomes of All cause mortality and cardiovascular mortality at one year in the CHOICE Trial[26]. (A) Cumulative incidence curves for all-cause mortality by device type. (B) Cumulative incidence curves for cardiovascular mortality by device type.

Permanent pacemaker placement was more frequent in the self-expanding group (37.6% vs 17.3%). Greater-than-mild paravalvular regurgitation was more frequently seen in the self-expandable group (1.1% vs 12.1%).

COMPLICATIONS OF TAVR

Common complications	Infrequent complications
Death	Annulus rupture
Bleeding	Myocardial injury
Coronary artery obstruction	Low cardiac output
Strokes or Transient ischemic attacks	Acute kidney injury
Post-TAVR aortic regurgitation	Prosthetic valve thrombosis
Vascular complications	Infective endocarditis
Conduction defects	Valve migration/Strut fracture

- *Bleeding*: Early and late (more than 30 days postprocedure) bleeding after TAVR is common. However, in the PARTNER 1A trial, the risk of periprocedural bleeding was higher in patients undergoing SAVR (Table 10).[21]

  Major bleeding post-TAVR has been reported in 17–24% in extreme risk cases, 11% in high risk cases and 7–10% in registries. The most frequent types of major bleeds were gastrointestinal (40.8%), neurological (15.5%), and traumatic fall-related (7.8%). Early and late bleeding complications are independently associated with increased mortality at 30 days and one year.[27,28]

- *Coronary artery obstruction*:[27,29] Coronary artery obstruction is an uncommon but potentially fatal complication of TAVR and occurs in about 0.7% of procedures with risk factors being low coronary artery ostia height

(<10 mm), small aortic sinuses, bulky asymmetric leaflet calcification, oversized prosthesis and high implantation. It is more common in women and with use of the balloon expandable valve.[29] To avoid this complication, evaluation before TAVR must include CT scan or transesophageal echocardiography to measure the distance from the aortic annulus to the coronary ostia, the sinus size and valve calcification. Coronary obstruction may be treated by percutaneous intervention or coronary artery bypass graft surgery.

Coronary artery obstruction is more frequent with valve-in-valve TAVR compared with native valve TAVR (3.5% vs 0.7%) due to proximity of the coronary ostia to the bioprosthetic leaflets and posts.[30]

- *Strokes/Transient ischemic attacks*:[31] The 30 days risk of strokes following TAVR is observational studies and clinical trials is 2–5%.[31] PARTNER Trial 1A and 1B showed that although the risk of stroke or transient ischemic attacks was higher than SAVR at 30 days, 1 year and 2 years, the risk was similar at 5 years which showed that there was no increased risk of stroke after the initial procedural risk.[17,21]

  Procedural and clinical factors that increase the risk of stroke are: manipulation of a wire or large catheter across the aortic arch, balloon aortic valvuloplasty, positioning the device, inadequate blood flow to the brain during rapid pacing and atrial fibrillation.

- *Post-TAVR aortic regurgitation*
  - *Paravalvular regurgitation (PVR)*: PVR is a common complication after TAVR, the incidence being 7–70% for mild PVR and 0–24% for moderate or severe PVR.[32] PVR is caused by incomplete apposition of the device with the aortic annulus due to calcific deposits that prevent adequate sealing or inadequate expansion of the device. The determinants of PVR are heavily calcified annulus, undersized prosthesis and improper valve positioning, inadequate balloon aortic valvotomy prior to deployment of a self-expanding valve. A meta-analysis found that moderate to severe PVR was associated with three times the 30 days mortality and 2.3 times the one year mortality after TAVR.[33]
  - *Central regurgitation*: It is usually caused by improper valve sizing or deployment.[31] It may be resolved by gentle probing of the leaflets with a wire. In case there is a severe central regurgitation, valve-in-valve deployment may be considered.
- *Vascular complications*: Vascular complications are common after TAVR with common vascular complications being
  - Arterial dissection,
  - Closure device failure,
  - Arterial closure device-induced stenosis, and
  - Hematoma at the puncture site.

- Artery avulsion ('artery on a stick'),
- Vessel perforation leading to retroperitoneal hematoma,
- Aortic dissection

    The increased incidence is due to large sized catheters used and high risk characteristics of the patients. The main determinants of vascular complications are small vessel diameter, severe atherosclerotic disease, calcified access arteries and tortuosity. Vascular complications are a predictor of increased late mortality after TAVR.[34]

- *Conduction disturbances*: Heart blocks are a common complications after TAVR, seen most commonly with the CoreValve than the Edward SAPIEN valve because of higher and long lasting radial force of the nitinol frame and deeper implantation site in the left ventricular outflow tract for the CoreValve. Left bundle branch block is the most common electrocardiogram (ECG) finding after TAVR. However, its long-term significance is unknown.

    The incidence of permanent pacemaker implantation after Edward SAPIEN valve is between 6.5% and 10% and after CoreValve is 25.8–37%. Risk factors for development of higher degree AV blocks are pre-existing right bundle branch block, complete AV block at the time of the procedure, small annulus diameter, improper implantation depth and the use of CoreValve device.[35]

- *Other complications*: Less common complications of TAVR are annulus rupture, myocardial injury, low cardiac output, acute kidney injury, prosthetic valve thrombosis, infective endocarditis, etc.

    Complications for native valve TAVR are similar to valve-in-valve TAVR with few exceptions. Annular rupture has not been reported in valve-in-valve TAVR. The rates of paravalvular regurgitation and permanent pacemaker requirement are lower in valve-in-valve TAVR. On the contrary, coronary artery obstruction is more frequent with valve-in-valve TAVR.[30]

INDIAN SCENARIO

Although, TAVR is an accepted and established interventional method of treatment of severe aortic stenosis in several countries, there are several roadblocks to its widespread use in India. The Indian patient tends to be more frail, with possibly smaller sizes of access arteries and smaller annulus sizes. Associated valvular diseases like rheumatic heart disease would play a role in case selection. TAVR has a long learning curve for the operator. It also involves significant costs, majority of which have to be born by patients. Additionally, in a country where the young are not optimally treated, the elderly population is likely to take a back seat.

A few centers in India do perform TAVRs but we are nowhere near having the experience of our western colleagues. In order for the TAVR program to be more successful, TAVRs should initially be done in large volume centers, with experience in structural heart disease. Collaboration between cardiologists, interventional cardiologists, cardiothoracic surgeons, radiologists and anesthetists is essential to ensure success and good outcomes.

CONCLUSION

The mainstay of treatment for severe symptomatic aortic stenosis is SAVR or TAVR so as to improve symptoms and survival. A multidisciplinary team should collaborate to decide the best treatment option for each individual patient. For patients with who are inoperable, TAVR is recommended rather than medical therapy. Even in patients who have an intermediate or high surgical risk, TAVR is as effective as surgery. More data is required on TAVR in low risk patients.

Although, SAVR and TAVR are equally effective, TAVR has a greater risk of paravalvular aortic regurgitation, permanent pacemaker implantation and major vascular complications, whereas SAVR has a greater risk of major bleeding, acute kidney injury and atrial fibrillation.

The devices used during TAVR are the Edward SAPIEN Valve and the Medtronic CoreValve. The CoreValve has a high incidence of permanent pacemaker requirement and paravalvular regurgitation, but the long term outcomes of both valves are similar.

With the expanding indications of TAVR and continuous improvement in the hardware resulting in a reduction in complication rates, this non-invasive approach to replacing a heart valve is likely to become in procedure of choice over surgery for severe aortic stenosis.

REFERENCES

1. Hoffman JIE. Incidence of congential heart disease. Postnatal incidence. Pediatr Cardiol 995;16:103-13
2. Ross J Jr, Braunwald E. Aortic stenosis. Circulation 1968;38:61-67.
3. Nishimura RA, Otto CM, Bonow RO, et al. 2014 AHA/ACC guideline for the management of patients with valvular heart disease: a report of the American College of Cardiology/American Heart Association Task Force on Practice Guidelines. J Am Coll Cardiol. 2014;63(22):e57.
4. Vahanian A, Alfieri O, Andreotti F, et al. Guidelines on the management of valvular heart disease (version 2012). The Joint Task Force on the Management of Valvular Heart Disease of the European Society of Cardiology (ESC) and the European Association for Cardio-Thoracic Surgery (EACTS). European Heart Journal (2012) 33, 2451-96.
5. Bach DS, Siao D, Girard SE, et al. Evaluation of patients with severe symptomatic aortic stenosis who do not undergo aortic valve replacement: the potential role

of subjectively overestimated operative risk. Circ Cardiovasc Qual Outcomes 2009;2:533-39.
6. Cribier A, Eltchaninoff H, Bash A, et al. Percutaneous transcatheter implantation of an aortic valve prosthesis for calcific aortic stenosis: first human case description. Circulation 2002;106:3006-08.
7. Généreux P, Head SJ, Wood DA, et al. Transcatheter aortic valve implantation 10-year anniversary: review of current evidence and clinical implications. European Heart Journal (2012) 33, 2388-2400
8. Dvir D, Webb JG, Bleiziffer S, et al. Transcatheter aortic valve implantation in failed bioprosthetic surgical valves. JAMA. 2014;312(2):162-170
9. Wenaweser P, Buellesfeld L, Gerckens U, et al. Percutaneous aortic valve replacement for severe aortic regurgitation in degenerated bioprosthesis: the first valve in valve procedure using the Corevalve Revalving system. Catheter Cardiovasc Interv 2007;70:760-64.
10. Hanzel GS, Harrity PJ, Schreiber TL, et al. Retrograde percutaneous aortic valve implantation for critical aortic stenosis. Catheter Cardiovasc Interv: 2005(64): 322-26.
11. Petronio AS, De Carlo M, Bedogni F, et al. Safety and efficacy of the subclavian approach for transcatheter aortic valve implantation with the CoreValve revalving system. Circ Cardiovasc Interv 2010;3:359-66.
12. Van Mieghem NM, Luthen C, Oei F, et al. Completely percutaneous transcatheter aortic valve implantation through transaxillary route: an evolving concept. EuroIntervention 2012;7:1340-42.
13. Bapat V, Khawaja MZ, Attia R, et al. Transaortic transcatheter aortic valve implantation using edwards sapien valve: a novel approach. Catheter Cardiovasc Interv 2012;79:733-40.
14. Modine T, Lemesle G, Azzaoui R, et al. Aortic valve implantation with the CoreValve ReValving System via left carotid artery access: first case report. J Thorac Cardiovasc Surg 2010;140:928-29.
15. Chandra P, Chauhan N, Kumar T. TAVI in 2013. CSI Cardiology Update 2013. Editor K. Venugopal
16. Park HB, Heo R, ó Hartaigh B, et al. Atherosclerotic plaque characteristics by CT angiography identify coronary lesions that cause ischemia: a direct comparison to fractional flow reserve. JACC Cardiovasc Imaging 2015; 8:1.
17. Makkar RR, Fontana GP, Jilaihawi H, et al. Transcatheter aortic-valve replacement for inoperable severe aortic stenosis. N Engl J Med 2012; 366:1696.
18. Kapadia SR, Leon MB, Makkar RR, et al. 5-year outcomes of transcatheter aortic valve replacement compared with standard treatment for patients with inoperable aortic stenosis (PARTNER 1): a randomised controlled trial. Lancet 2015; 385:2485.
19. Popma JJ, Adams DH, Reardon MJ, et al. Transcatheter Aortic Valve Replacement Using a Self-Expanding Bioprosthesis in Patients with Severe Aortic Stenosis at Extreme Risk for Surgery. J Am Coll Cardiol. 2014;63(19):1972-81
20. Kodali SK, Williams MR, Smith CR, et al. Two-year outcomes after transcatheter or surgical aortic-valve replacement. N Engl J Med 2012; 366:1686.
21. Mack MJ, Leon MB, Smith CR, et al. 5-year outcomes of transcatheter aortic valve replacement or surgical aortic valve replacement for high surgical risk patients with aortic stenosis (PARTNER 1): a randomised controlled trial. Lancet 2015; 385:2477.
22. Adams DH, Popma JJ, Reardon MJ, et al. Transcatheter aortic-valve replacement with a self-expanding prosthesis. N Engl J Med 2014; 370:1790.

23. Leon MB, Smith CR, Mack MJ, et al. Transcatheter or Surgical Aortic-Valve Replacement in Intermediate-Risk Patients. N Engl J Med 2016; 374:1609.
24. Thourani VH, Kodali S, Makkar RR, et al. Transcatheter aortic valve replacement versus surgical valve replacement in intermediate-risk patients: a propensity score analysis. Lancet 2016; 387:2218.
25. Thyregod HG, Steinbrüchel DA, Ihlemann N, et al. Transcatheter Versus Surgical Aortic Valve Replacement in Patients With Severe Aortic Valve Stenosis: 1-Year Results From the All-Comers NOTION Randomized Clinical Trial. J Am Coll Cardiol 2015; 65:2184
26. Abdel-Wahab M, Neumann FJ, Mehilli J, et al. 1-Year Outcomes After Transcatheter Aortic Valve Replacement With Balloon-Expandable Versus Self-Expandable Valves: Results From the CHOICE Randomized Clinical Trial. J Am Coll Cardiol 2015; 66:791.
27. Généreux P, Head SJ, Van Mieghem NM, et al. Clinical outcomes after transcatheter aortic valve replacement using valve academic research consortium definitions: a weighted meta-analysis of 3,519 patients from 16 studies. J Am Coll Cardiol 2012; 59:2317.
28. Tomey MI, Mehran R. Bleeding avoidance in transcatheter aortic valve replacement: a call to ACTion? JACC Cardiovasc Interv 2014; 7:152.
29. Ribeiro HB, Nombela-Franco L, Urena M, et al. Coronary obstruction following transcatheter aortic valve implantation: a systematic review. JACC Cardiovasc Interv 2013; 6:452.
30. Webb JG, Dvir D. Transcatheter aortic valve replacement for bioprosthetic aortic valve failure: the valve-in-valve procedure. Circulation 2013; 127:2542.
31. Holmes DR Jr, Mack MJ, Kaul S, et al. 2012 ACCF/AATS/SCAI/STS expert consensus document on transcatheter aortic valve replacement. J Am Coll Cardiol 2012; 59:1200.
32. Pibarot P, Hahn RT, Weissman NJ, et al. Assessment of paravalvular regurgitation following TAVR: a proposal of unifying grading scheme. JACC Cardiovasc Imaging 2015; 8:340.
33. Athappan G, Patvardhan E, Tuzcu EM, et al. Incidence, predictors, and outcomes of aortic regurgitation after transcatheter aortic valve replacement: meta-analysis and systematic review of literature. J Am Coll Cardiol 2013; 61:1585.
34. Czerwińska-Jelonkiewicz K1, Michałowska I, Witkowski A et al. Vascular complications after transcatheter aortic valve implantation (TAVI): risk and long-term results. J Thromb Thrombolysis. 2014;37(4):490-8.
35. Erkapic D, De Rosa S, Kelava A, et al. Risk for Permanent Pacemaker After Transcatheter Aortic Valve Implantation. A Comprehensive Analysis of the Literature. J Cardiovasc Electrophysiol. 2012;23(4):391-97.

20
Transcatheter Closure of Congenital Heart Defects

Prafulla Kerkar, Dhiraj Kumar

INTRODUCTION

More than 40 years have elapsed since the first attempts at transcatheter closure (TCC) by Porstmann et al.[1] for patent ductus arteriosus (PDA) and King et al.[2] for atrial septal defect (ASD). Ever since then, TCC interventions have captured the attention of interventional cardiologists all around the world. Subsequently many refinements have taken place in the devices, delivery sheaths and techniques. This chapter will review contemporary practices and procedural aspects of TCC of congenital heart defects (CHDs), especially those encountered in adolescents and adults.

The common defects amenable to TCC include ASD, ventricular septal defect (VSD) and PDA; and the rare defects like ruptured sinus of Valsalva aneurysm (SOVA) and coronary artery fistula (CAF).

ATRIAL SEPTAL DEFECT

Atrial septal defect is the most common CHD diagnosed in adults. Although many devices are available for TCC, Amplatzer septal occluder (ASO) (St. Jude Medical) or Amplatzer-like devices (Lifetech, Vascular concepts and Occlutech) are more commonly used. All these are double disk devices with a self-centering mechanism and made of nitinol which has super elastic properties and molecular memory allowing stretchability and use of small sheath for its delivery. Transcatheter closure is possible only for the secundum type of ASD that has sufficient rims (>5 mm) all around. Irrespective of the patient's symptoms, TCC is indicated if echocardiographically there is evidence of right-sided volume overload.[3] Contraindications include: Ostium primum and sinus venosus type of ASD, deficient superior or inferior vena cava (IVC), mitral or free atrial rims (<5 mm), abnormal pulmonary venous drainage and pulmonary hypertension with pulmonary vascular resistance (PVR) more than 8 woods units.

Precatheterization planning: Detailed transthoracic echocardiography (TTE) to delineate type, size and number of ASD is required followed by transesophageal echocardiography (TEE) (which is a must, at least, pre-procedure if not intra-procedure) to show the rims and their adequacy in 0° for mitral and free atrial, in 45° for aortic and posterior and 90-120° (bicaval view) for IVC and SVC rims. A deficient aortic rim <5 mm is not necessarily a contraindication.

Procedure steps: A right femoral vein is accessed with 7-8 F short sheath. Arterial access may be taken in case the patient has a marginal condition or if the procedure is performed under general anesthesia. The entire procedure is guided by TEE (although some use TTE for patients with good echocardiographic windows) and fluoroscopy. TEE is used to size the defect in all views and maximum defect size is taken for device selection (Fig. 1A). In adults device is oversized by 4-6 mm and in children device no more than 2 mm of defect size.

Heparin to achieve an activated clotting time (ACT) of >200 seconds at the time of device deployment is given and Cefazolin 1 g is used as the antibiotic of choice.

A Judkins right (JR) coronary catheter or a multipurpose catheter is parked in the SVC and pulled down with a clockwise turn to enter the left atrium (LA) and then either the left or right superior pulmonary vein, which can be confirmed by TEE. Ensure that the catheter is not in a wedged position to avoid sucking in of air into the left circulation. After flushing the catheter and ensuring a good back bleed, the catheter is exchanged for a super-stiff exchange length Amplatz guidewire. Balloon sizing of the device is used rarely when rims are flimsy or when multiple defects are suspected.

For balloon sizing, an Amplatzer sizing balloon, (St Jude Medical) available in two sizes (24 and 34 mm) is advanced over the guidewire and inflated till the color flow across the ASD ceases. The indented waist of the balloon is then measured using TEE and also fluoroscopically by angulating X-ray beam (usually left anterior oblique) perpendicular to balloon (such that the markers on the balloon are separated and discrete). The size is measured after calibration and the balloon is deflated and withdrawn.

An appropriate sized device is prepared and the delivery system is advanced over the guidewire to left upper pulmonary vein. Dilator is removed and extreme care is taken to make sure that the sheath does not contain any air by continuously flushing the side port of the sheath. The device is the screwed to the tip of delivery cable, immersed in normal saline or blood and drawn into the loader underwater and flushed with the attached Y-connector to expel air bubbles from it. The cable with the ASO device is advanced to the distal tip of the sheath, taking special care not to rotate during advancement (lest it unscrews the device). After deploying the LA disk close to the pulmonary vein, the entire assembly is pulled back as one unit until the LA disk is seated on the left side of the interatrial septum (IAS) (Fig. 1B) Keeping a gentle tug on the system, the right atrium (RA) disk is then deployed on the right side of the septum by unsheathing it whilst stepping on the delivery cable (Fig. 1C). All this is done on simultaneous fluoroscopy and TEE guidance (Fig. 1D), ensuring that all rims are captured and there is no residual shunt by the side of the device. Residual intradevice shunting is typically seen on TEE. After ensuring capture of all rims and no encroachment on the AV valves (no new or increase in regurgitation), the device is released by unscrewing the delivery cable). Before release fluoroscopy in the hepato-clavicular [left anterior oblique (LAO) 30/30] projection shows the device in profile where the well-separated disks are appreciated. Wiggling the device to ensure good seating is no longer necessary.

Preventing LA disk prolapse into RA during deployment can be challenging and it can be overcome by i) changing the mode of delivery, i.e. either from the right superior pulmonary vein or from roof of the LA or even by pulmonary vein entrapment of the LA disk, ii) changing the delivery system, i.e. using the Hausdorf sheath (Cook) or beveling the tip of the delivery sheath and iii) by using additional support either a dilator or a balloon[4,5]

Major complications following TCC of ASD are rare.[6] These include:
1. *Device embolization and malposition is rare (2.6%)*:[6] It can be retrieved using a snare and and upsized delivery sheath (2F sizes more).
2. *Arrhythmia*: Supraventricular ectopy and non-sustained supraventricular arrhythmias.

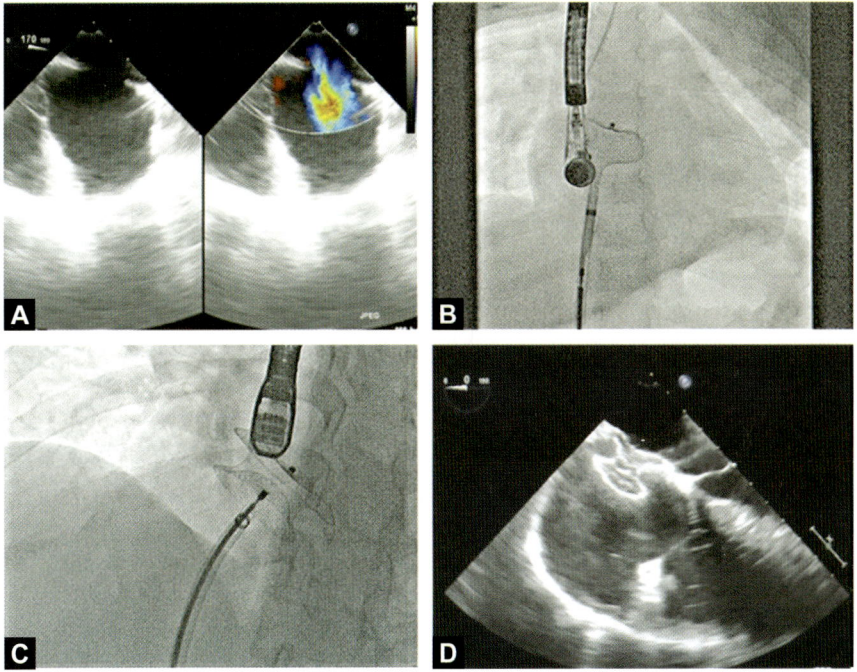

Figs. 1A to D: TCC of ASD: (A) TEE of ASD showing good margins. (B) LA disk seated in left side of IAS. (C) Before release both disks deployed across IAS. (D) Post device TEE showing well-captured margins.

3. *Cardiac erosions (up to 0.3%)*: A recent report suggested that deficiency of any rim, especially aortic rim, device >5 mm larger than ASD diameter, and weight: device size ratio were associated with erosion.[7] Pre-discharge pericardial effusion may be the warning sign of cardiac erosion.
4. *Cobra head formation*: Left disk opened in left atrial appendage (LAA) or pulmonary vein can lead to cobra head formation.

VENTRICULAR SEPTAL DEFECT

A VSD can occur as a congenital defect or can be acquired in the setting of an acute myocardial infarction (AMI) too. Congenital VSDs are the most common form of CHDs. The most common type, the perimembranous, accounts for 80% of all VSDs, the other 20% are muscular and are further subdivided as inlet, trabecular and infundibular.

Large, non-restrictive VSDs cause a large left to right shunt and congestive heart failure in first few weeks of life to infancy and if left untreated lead to development of pulmonary arterial hypertension (PAH) and increased PVR with Eisenmenger's physiology when the shunt reverses to a predominant right to left shunt and leads to inoperability. Small, restrictive VSDs cause loud murmurs and hence detected early. However, they do not require closure. Closure of symptomatic, non-restrictive VSDs is indicated in infancy. Most such VSDs are not amenable to TCC due to limitations of the bulky hardware for small babies.

Surgical closure (mostly pericardial patch) can be performed with low operative mortality (1–2%) and good long-term results, and remains the treatment of choice.[8] In patients with increased risk factors for surgery, multiple previous cardiac surgical interventions, or VSDs that are poorly accessible for surgical closure, TCC can be considered. In muscular VSDs that are located centrally in the interventricular septum, TCC can be considered as an alternative to surgical closure.[9] In perimembranous VSD it has been shown to be feasible, however, whether the risk of complete atrioventricular (AV) block and entrapment of tricuspid valve (TV) tissue leading to tricuspid regurgitation (TR), or the risk of aortic regurgitation (AR) that has been observed in children, are relevant in adults remains to be seen.

Currently as per American College of Cardiology/American Heart Association (ACC/AHA) guidelines 2008,[3] TCC of VSD is only a Class IIb indication that too if it is sufficiently far away from aorta and tricuspid valve.

Congenital VSDs in Adults

Large, nonrestrictive VSDs in adults are invariably Eisenmengerised and do not require closure. If a small VSD persists into adolescence or adulthood, closure, however, is needed if there is i) left ventricular volume overload (LVVO), ii) history of infective endocarditis or iii) development of AR.[3]

As an alternative to surgical closure which is the gold standard, TCC of VSD can be considered in patients with muscular defects, especially if the VSD is away from the TV and aortic valve (AV). Patients with residual defects after surgical closure or patients with iatrogenic defects after aortic valve replacement (AVR) or myomectomy[10] could be offered TCC too. Peri-membranous VSDs are today increasingly closed with the amplatzer duct occluder (ADO) rather than the Amplatzer perimembranous VSD occluder due to a high incidence (about 5–6%) of complete heart block with the latter.[11]

Post-MI Ventricular Septal Rupture (VSR)

Post-MI VSR is one of most dreaded complications of AMI with an extremely poor prognosis of untreated patients (90% mortality). Since operative mortality is also high (about 50%),[12] TCC of post-myocardial infarction ventricular septal rupture (post-MI VSR) is an attractive option. Patient selection and timing of VSR closure are important determinants of the outcome. The procedure can be complicated by the unstable hemodynamics and the friable nature of the VSRs, which are large and irregular with necrosis of the surrounding tissue, making stable device positioning problematic. Even with successful device implantation, the mortality could be in the range of 35–40%. Hence proper family counseling is important.

Procedure

Transcatheter VSD closure is technically more demanding than TCC of ASD. However, success rates are as high as 90%. Closing post-MI VSR is even more challenging. Figure 3 shows the steps using the Amplatzer muscular occluder. After prior TTE (Figs. 2A to D) evaluation for the size, number and location of the VSD ensuring good margins from the AV (at least 2 mm) and TV, the procedure is performed under general anesthesia with fluoroscopic and TEE guidance. Femoral arterial and venous accesses are obtained for perimembranous and high muscular VSDs. However, for VSDs located in the mid-muscular, posterior or apical septum, a right internal jugular vein (RIJV) access is obtained. Left ventriculography is performed to define the location, size and number of VSDs. A deep LAO cranial (60/20) is preferred for perimembranous VSDs whereas a shallow LAO cranial (35/35) (Fig. 2B) is used for mid-muscular VSDs. The VSD is sized both on TEE and angiography and a device 2 mm larger is selected (for post-MI VSR at least 6 mm larger). The VSD is crossed from the left ventricular side using a JR catheter and an angled tip glide wire (Terumo Inc. Japan). This is exchanged for an exchange length Noodle wire (St. Jude Medical) that is exteriorized with a Goose-Neck Snare (ev3, Amplatzer) out of the venous side (jugular for mid and apical muscular VSDs, femoral for perimembranous and high muscular VSDs) (Figs. 2C and D), creating a stable arteriovenous (AV) loop.

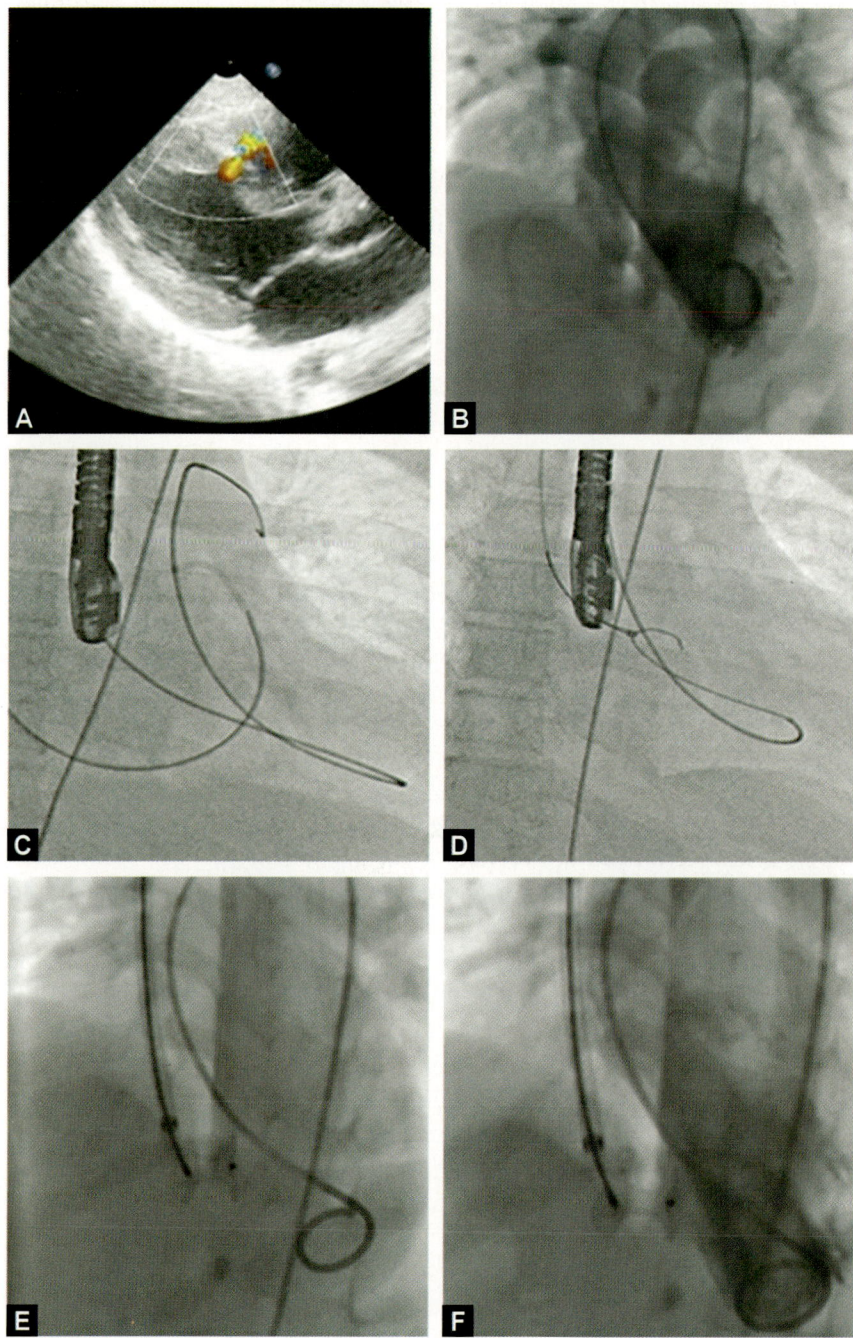

Figs. 2A to F: TCC of midmuscular VSD: (A) CD echo showing turbulent flow across the VSD. (B) LV angiogram in LAO 35° Cranial 35° view showing midmuscular VSD. (C and D) Creation of AV loop. Noodle wire across VSD being snared from LPA to right internal jugular vein (RIJV) using Gooseneck snare. (E) Device across VSD before release. (F) Control LV angiogram before release showing well-seated device across VSD.

The delivery sheath is advanced over this wire into the LV. The placement of the VSD occluder is similar to the ASO with sequential deployment of the left-side disk, followed by the waist and the right-sided disc (Fig. 2E) Before release, a stable position of the device and is confirmed by echocardiography and/or angiography (Fig. 2F). Also the normal functioning of the surrounding valves is confirmed, mainly by echocardiography.

Potential major complications include device embolization, arrhythmias, hemolysis (especially after post-MI VSR closure), valvar regurgitation, high degree heart blocks and pericardial effusion. Initial complication rates were about 10%, but in more recent studies these are down to 2–3%.[13]

PATENT DUCTUS ARTERIOSUS

Isolated PDA is common congenital heart disease with approximate prevalence of 10%. Many children present with high output cardiac failure symptoms the rest are detected incidentally due to the presence of a continuous murmur. The PDA is a vascular structure that connects the left pulmonary artery near its origin to the descending aorta just after the left subclavian artery; it is an essential fetal structure that closes spontaneously in about 90% of full-term infants during the first 48 hours of life. Persistent patency of the PDA beyond a few weeks is considered abnormal and is mainly encountered in neonates with ventilatory or circulatory abnormalities or in premature infants. Formally speaking, PDA is considered a form of congenital heart disease, defined as a persistent patency beyond the third month of life in term infants; it can be associated with various other congenital heart diseases. In the adult PDA is usually an isolated lesion.

Indications and Contraindications[3]

1. PDA should be closed in patients with signs of LV volume overload[2] (Class of Recommendation I, Level of evidence (LOE): C).
2. PDA should be closed in patients with PAH but PAP < 2/3 of systemic pressure or PVR < 2/3 of SVR (COR I, LOE C).
3. TCC is the method of choice where technically suitable (COR I LOE C)
4. TCC is indicated in a patient with prior history of endocarditis (COR I, LOE C) ACC/AHA 2008)
5. PDA closure should be considered in patients with PAH and PAP > 2/3 of systemic pressure or PVR > 2/3 of SVR but still net L–R shunt (Qp:Qs > 1.5) or when testing (preferably with nitric oxide) or treatment demonstrates pulmonary vascular reactivity (Class IIa, LOE C)
6. TCC should be considered in small PDAs with continuous murmur (normal LV and PAP) (Class IIa LOE C).

Devices used in PDA closure include Amplatzer duct occluder (ADO) I, ADO II and ADO II AS (St. Jude Medical) Amplatzer-like devices from

Lifetech and Vascular Concepts. Rarely double disk devices like muscular VSD device are used for hypertensive large PDAs.[14,15] Gianturco coils (Cook Inc.), both free and controlled-release used in the past for small to medium-sized ducts are nowadays used infrequently due to high incidence of residual shunting and the procedure being technically more demanding.

The ADO consists of an aortic retention disk and a plug that is 4 mm smaller in diameter than the retention disk. The largest ADO (16/14 mm) can be used to close PDAs measuring 11 to 12 mm. For larger PDAs Amplatzer-like devices (Lifetech) or VSD devices or even ASOs have been used.[16] The Amplatzer Vascular Plug II (AVP II) has been used for long tubular ducts in small babies.[17]

Precatheterization planning: The decision about TCC of the PDA is made in the echo room. The TTE is essential to determine the morphology and size (narrowest diameter, invariably at the PA end) of the PDA (Fig. 3A), the presence of gradients, direction of flow, left ventricular volume and function the presence and grade of pulmonary hypertension, and the presence of additional structural abnormalities like coarctation of aorta and VSD, However, angiography in the lateral projection remains the gold-standard for delineating the exact morphology and size of the PDA and its ampulla at the aortic end as also the size of the juxta-ductal aorta.

Procedural details: General anesthesia is used only for small children. Both arterial access and venous access are taken.

After hemodynamic study, a descending aortogram is performed just below the level of the PDA in lateral projection. If the PDA is not defined clearly then an RAO 30 degree (Fig. 3B) is used to image the PDA. The tracheal air column serves as a useful fluoroscopic landmark during TCC and its relation to the opening of the PDA and the ampulla should be memorized.

Device sizing: An ADO I device that is at least 2 mm larger than the narrowest PDA diameter should be chosen. However for larger ducts device may be upsized by 4 mm. The delivery sheath is placed from the venous side into the descending aorta over an exchange length wire after crossing the PDA using a JR catheter and a straight tipped regular wire. The device is deployed similar to other Amplatzer devices. Control angiography is performed to verify the device position prior to release (Fig. 3C). In very small children a PA angiogram through the delivery sheath in PA caudal projection may done to look for device impingement on LPA. If the device position is not optimal, it can be captured and the steps repeated. Small intra-device residual shunting is common. It usually disappears in 24-48 hours. Post procedure echocardiography to look for device position (Fig. 3D), left ventricular function, gradients across left pulmonary artery and descending thoracic aorta (acquired coarctation).

Complications are unusual and include rare embolization and hemolysis.[18]

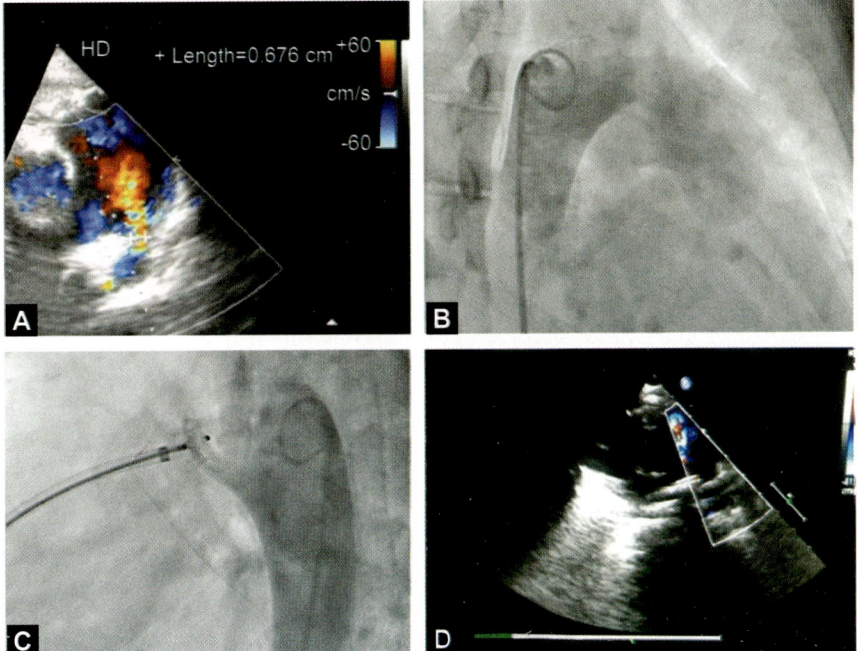

Figs. 3A to D: TCC of PDA: (A) CD echo in high parasternal short axis view showing turbulent flow across a large PDA. (B) Descending aortogram in RAO 30° shows a large PDA. (C) Before release angiogram in lateral view shows an appropriately deployed device. (D) Post procedure CD echocardiography shows device in situ.

RUPTURED SINUS OF VALSALVA ANEURYSM

Ruptured SOVA, a rare but well-recognized clinical entity, more commonly seen in Asians, mostly presents in adolescence and young adulthood, with about 80% of cases being symptomatic. The SOVA ruptures invariably into right-sided heart chambers causing an acute or subacute left to right shunt. Initially a surgical repair was the only option but ever since Cullen in 1994 demonstrated the feasibility of TCC,[19] there have been several case reports and case series of TCC of ruptured SOVA[20-25] the largest series being reported from India.[26,27] Today for suitable ruptured SOVAs without associated defects requiring surgical correction, TCC has become the procedure of choice.[28] Important exclusion criteria for TCC include associated VSD and significant AR, aortic end larger than 12 mm, any suspicion of infective endocarditis and multiple rupture sites.

Procedure

After a detailed TTE and TEE assessment (Figs. 4A to D), the procedure is performed under general anesthesia with fluoroscopic and TEE guidance.

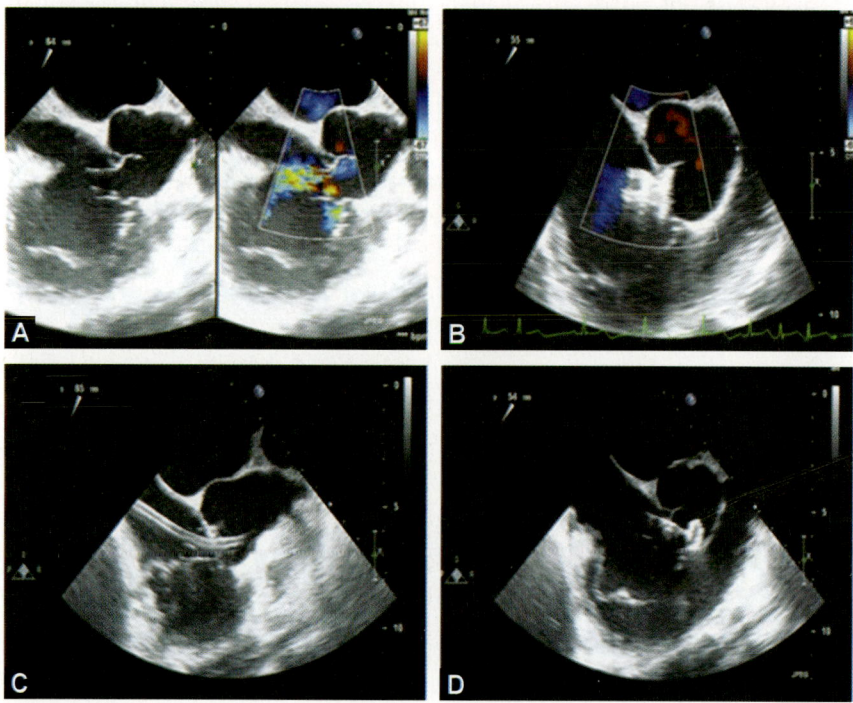

Figs. 4A to D: TCC of ruptured SOVA. Intraprocedural TEE in short axis view showing (A) windsock like SOVA from RCC to RA, (B) post deployment device in situ with no flow, (C) sheath across ruptured SOVA and (D) opened aortic disk and attached delivery system in ascending aorta being pulled toward the defect.

The technique is very similar to TCC of perimembranous VSD, given that the defect is above the aortic valve instead of beneath it. It entails crossing the defect from the left side and exteriorizing the exchange wire from the venous side to form a stable arteriovenous loop, over which the delivery sheath is brought from the venous side into the ascending aorta (Fig. 4). Given that the SOVA is broad at the aortic end, the ADO is most suitable device. During device deployment, it is imperative to gently seat the aortic disk of the ADO at the aortic end of the defect avoiding slippage into the aneurysmal sac so as to completely close the aneurysm and not merely the rupture site to avoid recurrence. For pre and control ascending aortography, the LAO with cranial tilt projection is preferred for SOVA draining into RA and right ventricular (RV) inflow and the right anterior oblique view for SOVA rupturing into RV or RVOT. The ruptured SOVA is measured at its aortic end as well as at the rupture site both on TEE (Fig. 4) and angiography. The larger of the two measurements is considered for device selection. The size of the ADO selected is such that its aortic segment is 2–4 mm larger than this diameter. Prior to release, the surrounding valves and coronaries are interrogated confirming no encroachment. A mild increase in or new AR occurrence is not worrisome as this could be related to afterload mismatch due to sudden disconnection of the low resistance pulmonary circulation.

In our own experience, the success rate was 90% in a large series of 20 patients.[26] Acute complications encountered were residual shunting in five patients (small in four, moderate with self-abating hemolysis in one) and trivial procedure-related AR in four patients. On a median follow-up of 24 months (1-60 months), the residual shunting disappeared in three out of five and procedure-related AR vanished in two out of four. There was no AR progression, recurrence, or infective endocarditis or device embolization.

Associated defects like ASD and coarctation of aorta have been corrected by the transcatheter technique either sequentially or simultaneously.[22,23]

Potential complications of the procedure include failure to deploy due to flimsy margins and large size of the defect, device embolization, residual shunting and hemolysis, iatrogenic AR, and coronary encroachment, which is extremely rare.

CORONARY ARTERIAL FISTULA

Coronary artery fistula is a direct connection between a coronary artery and the lumen of a cardiac chamber coronary sinus, superior vena cava, pulmonary artery or vein, without an intervening capillary network. It is a rare congenital anomaly constituting 0.3% of all congenital heart disease and around 0.13-0.22% of all angiographies.[29,30]

Indications of closure[31,32] include (i) Large left to right shunt (ii) Heart failure and growth impairment, (iii) Myocardial steal: Clinical, stress ECG or myocardial perfusion scan, (iv) Aneurysmal fistula: Risk of rupture or thrombosis (v) Progressive enlargement of fistula on FU and (vi) Postsurgical residual shunt.

Precatheterization evaluation is done with Color Doppler echocardiography that is helpful in determining the origin, course, drainage, and magnitude of the shunt, LV function and evidence of pulmonary hypertension if any. CT Coronary angiography is very useful as it gives a high resolution, in-depth anatomical information about the measurements of the fistula, presence of side branches and their relation to the exit.

Procedure

Transcatheter closure of CAF can be challenging due to the excessive tortuosity and aneurysmal and high flow nature of CAF. The selection of the approach whether antegrade or retrograde depends upon (i) age and size of the patient, (ii) catheter size that can be used in the given patient, (iii) the size of the vessel to be occluded and (iv) the magnitude of the proximal tortuosity of the vessel for the catheter to reach the occlusion site. Proximal fistulas are easier to close than distal fistulas. Generally a femoral arterial

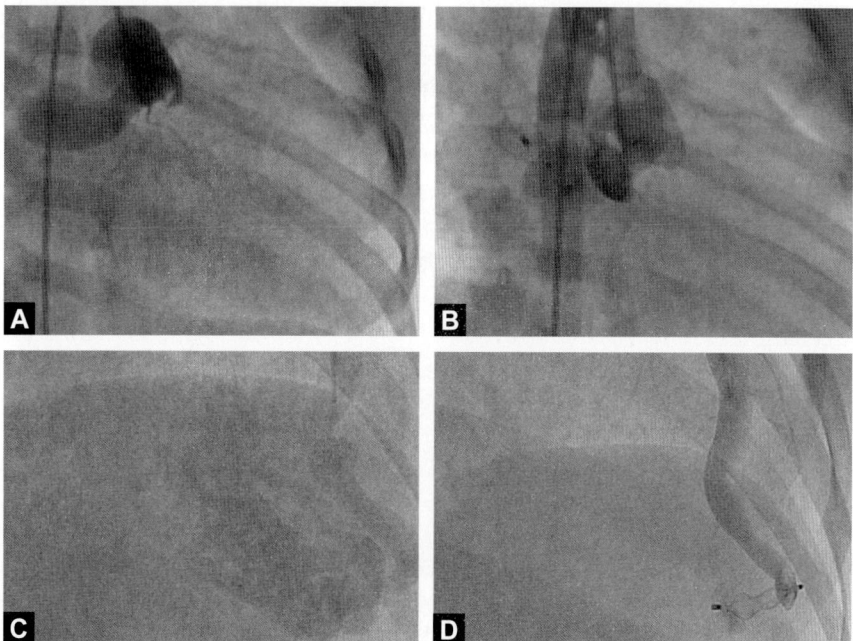

Figs. 5A to D: (A and B) TCC of proximal CAF from Left circumflex to RA. Pre (A) and Post (B) angiograms showing large proximal fistula closed with AVP at the proximal narrow point close to the origin and with ADO at the exit point into RA. (C and D) TCC of a distal CAF from LAD to RV apex. Pre (C) and post (D) angiograms showing distal CAF from LAD to RV apex closed with AVP II distally. Note the dilated and tortuous LAD with many at-risk septal and diagonal branches along its course.

and a femoral venous access are obtained. For LAD fistulas draining into middle of the RV, a jugular venous route is preferred. An extra arterial access may be required for control angiography if retrograde approach is preferred. Once access is secured, all patients receive an intravenous heparin bolus (60 to 100 U/kg). After obtaining hemodynamic data, the coronary arteries are engaged selectively using various diagnostic coronary guides and catheters. Hand injection of contrast allows visualization of coronary anatomy, and location of fistulae including origin and drainage sites. Balloon occlusion angiography may be necessary to better delineate the important coronary artery branches in the vicinity of the occlusion point as also to test occlude the fistula and watch for clinical and ECG changes. It is preferable occlude the fistula as close to its origin as possible but sparing important branches (Figs. 5A to D). To access the fistula, guides, microcatheters, and coronary guide wires are used. Multiple different closure devices are used including coils, detachable balloon and glue. The Amplatzer duct occluders and plugs (St. Jude Medical) are most useful. Devices are selected based on the size and other characteristics of the fistulae. Coils are primarily used in small fistulae, whereas the Amplatzer devices are used to occlude larger fistulas.

Devices are deployed either via the femoral artery (retrograde approach) or via the femoral or jugular vein {anterograde approach using an arteriovenous wire loop (via femoral artery and femoral vein or jugular vein) when necessary. Selective coronary angiography is performed immediately after device deployment to assess presence of residual flow.

Potential complications include thrombus formation and slow flow (especially in distal fistula˚ with aneurysmal dilatation of the main vessel, air embolism, coronary artery dissection and spasm, arrhythmias and embolization. Following TCC of CAF a regular follow-up is necessary to look for long-term effects. In our own experience[33] with angiographic follow-up, TCC of proximal CAF is safe and effective, however the large size, distal type of CAF may be at high-risk for coronary events post closure and requires review of indication and close follow-up.

RETRIEVAL OF EMBOLIZED DEVICES

The catheterization laboratory should be well equipped with retrieval devices like the Goose Neck Snare (ev3) Alligator forceps (Cook), Biopsy forceps (Cook) and bailout sheaths (St. Jude Medical). Anecdotally devices do embolize (Figs. 6A to C). The operator should have basic understanding

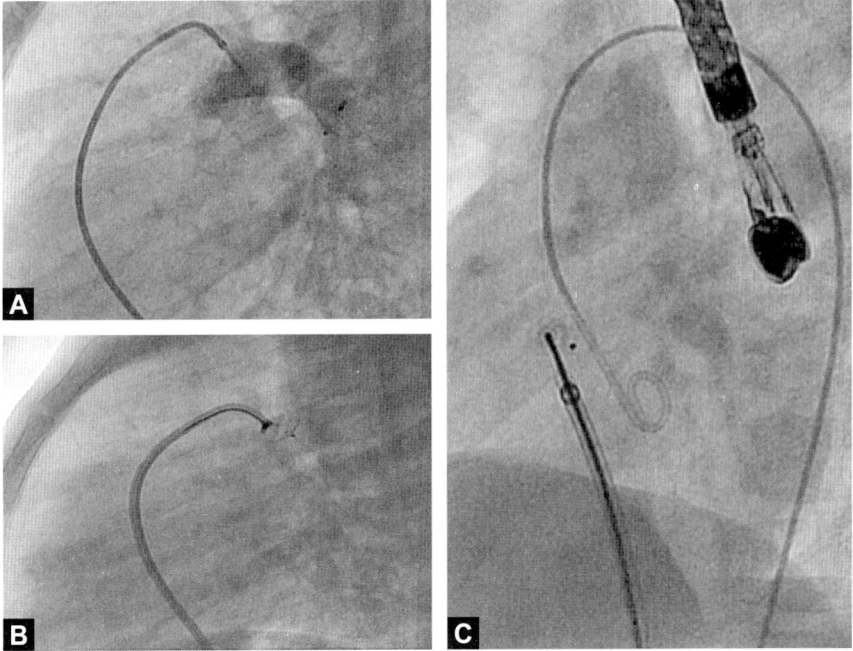

Figs. 6A to C: Device retrieval of ADO II during TCC of perimembranous VSD. (A) Pulmonary artery angiogram showing ADO II embolized into LPA. (B) ADO II snared with gooseneck snare. (C) Before release, well seated ADO I across VSD.

of how to use these devices before embarking upon TCC of congenital heart defects. Moreover, surgical stand-by should be available.

CONCLUSION

Currently, TCC of congenital heart defects has evolved into an established procedure with remarkable efficacy and safety. In fact it has become a preferred procedure over surgery. Today, surgery should be reserved only for the large defects with insufficient margins. The advent of Amplatzer series of devices has revolutionized this field. However, the interventional cardiologist should not go overboard to close very small defects without significant left to right shunt, lest their approach should be castigated as Holistic!

REFERENCES

1. Porstmann W, Wierny L, Warnke H. The closure of the patent ductus arteriosus without thoracotomy. (Preliminary report). Thoraxchir Vask Chir. 1967;15:199-203.
2. King TD, Thompson SL, Steiner C, Mills NL. Secundum atrial septal defect. Nonoperative closure during cardiac catheterization. JAMA 1976;235:2506-09.
3. Warnes, et al. ACC/AHA 2008 Guidelines for Adults With CHD; Circulation 2008;118:e714-e833.
4. Wahab HA, Bairam AR, Cao QL, Hijazi ZM. Novel technique to prevent prolapse of the Amplatzer septal occluder through large atrial septal defect; Catheter Cardiovasc Interven. 2003;60;543-5.
5. Dalvi BV, Pinto RJ, Gupta A. New technique for device closure of large atrial septal defects. Catheter Cardiovasc Interv. 2005;64:102-7.
6. Spence MS, Qureshi SA. Complications of transcatheter closure of atrial septal defects. Heart. 2005;91(12):1512-14.
7. McElhinney DB, Quartermain M, Kenny D, et al. Relative Risk Factors for Cardiac Erosion Following Transcatheter Closure of Atrial Septal Defects: a case-control study. Circulation. 2016;3;133(18):1738-46.
8. Hijazi ZM. Device closure of ventricular septal defects; Catheter Cardiovasc. Interv. 2003;60:107-114.
9. Tofeig M, Patel RG, Walsh KP. Transcatheter closure of a mid-muscular ventricular septal defect with an Amplatzer VSD occlusion device. Heart. 1999;81:438-40.
10. Singh V, et al. Retrograde transcutaneous closure of Ventricular Septal defect after myomectomy of HOCM. Texas Heart Institute J. 40. pp. 471-73.
11. Butera G, Carminati M, Chessa M, et al. Transcatheter closure of perimembranous ventricular septal defects: early and long-term Results. J Am College Cardiol. 2007;50(12):1189-95.
12. Crenshaw BS, Granger CB, Birnbaum Y, et al. GUSTO-I (Global Utilization of Streptokinase TPA for Occluded Coronary Arteries) Trial Investigators. Circulation. 2000;101:27-32.
13. Holzer R, Balzer D, Cao QL, et al. Device closure of Muscular Ventricular Septal with amplatzer Muscular VSD occluder; Immediate and midterm results of a US Registry. J Am College Cardiol. 2004;43:1257-63.
14. Niu MC, Mallory GB, Justino H, et al. Treatment of severe pulmonary hypertension in the setting of the large patent ductus arteriosus. Pediatrics. 2013;131(5):1643-9.

15. Bhalgat PS, Pinto R, Dalvi BV. Transcatheter closure of large patent ductus arteriosus with severe pulmonary arterial hypertension: Short and intermediate term results. Ann Pediatr Card. 2012;5:135-40.
16. Spies, C., Ujivari, F. and Schräder, R. (2005), Transcatheter closure of a 22 mm patent ductus arteriosus with an Amplatzer atrial septal occluder. Cathet Cardiovasc Interv. 2005;64:352–55.
17. Garay FJ, Aguirre D, Cárdenas L, et al. Use of the amplatzer vascular plug II device to occlude different types of patent ductus arteriosus in pediatric patients; J Interv Cardiol. 2015 Apr;28(2):198-204.
18. El-Said HG, Bratincsak A, Foerster SR, et al. Safety of percutaneous patent ductus arteriosus closure: an unselected multicenter population experience. J Am Heart Assoc. 2013;2(6):e000424.
19. Cullen S, Somerville J, Redington A. Transcatheter closure of ruptured aneurysm of sinus of valsalva. Br Heart J. 1994;71:479-80.
20. Kerkar PG. Ruptured sinus of valsalva aneurysm: Yet another hole to plug! Ann Pediatr Card. 2009;2(1):83-4.
21. Kerkar P, Suvarna T, Burkule N, Panda R. Transcatheter closure of ruptured sinus of Valsalva aneurysm using the Amplatzer duct occluder in a critically ill post-CABG patient. J Invasive Cardiol. 2007;19:E169-71.
22. Mehta N ;Mishra N,Kerkar P ; Percutaneous closure of ruptured sinus of valsalva aneurysm and atrial septal defect. J Invasive Cardiol. 2010;22:e82-5.
23. Pahwa JS, Verma G, Phadke MS, et al. Simultaneous trans-catheter closure of ruptured sinus of valsalva aneurysm and stent implantation for aortic coarctation. Indian Heart J. 2015; 67 (Suppl 3):S81-4.
24. Chang CW, Chiu SN, Wu ET, et al. Transcatheter closure of a ruptured sinus of Valsalva aneurysm. Circ J. 2006;70:1043-7.
25. Zhao SH, Yan CW, Zhu XY, et al. Transcatheter occlusion of the ruptured sinus of Valsalva aneurysm with an Amplatzer duct occluder. Int J Cardiol. 2008;129:81-5.
26. Kerkar P, Lanjewar C, Mishra N, et al. Transcatheter closure of ruptured sinus of Valsalva aneurysm using the Amplatzer occluder: immediate result and mid term follow-up. Eur Heart J. 2010;31:2881-7.
27. Mahimarangaiah J, Subramanian A, Srinivasa KH, Usha MK. Transcatheter closure of ruptured sinus of valsalva: different techniques and mid-term follow-up. Catheter Cardiovasc Interv. 2016;87(3):516-22.
28. Kerkar PG, Pawha JS, Bhargava R. Ruptured Sinus of Valsalva: No longer a surgical domain; Chapter 54; Cardiol. Society of India Update. 2016;383-8.
29. Hobbs RE, Millit HD, Raghavan PV, et al. Coronary artery fistulae: a 10-year review. Cleve Clin Q. 1982;49:191-7.
30. Yamanaka O, Hobbs RE. Coronary artery anomalies in 126,595 patients undergoing coronary arteriography. Catheter Cardiovasc Diagn. 1990;21:28-40.
31. Armsby LR, Keane JF, Sherwood MC, et al. Management of coronary artery fistulae. Patient selection and results of transcatheter closure. J Am Coll Cardiol. 2002;39:1026-32.
32. Latson LA. Coronary artery fistulas: how to manage them. Catheter Cardiovasc Interv. 2007;70:110-6.
33. Phatarpekar A, Mate S, Lanjewar C, et al. To assess the immediate and mid-term outcomes of transcatheter closure (TCC) in patients with coronary cameral fistula. Category Adult congenital; B073;SCAI 2016; Abstracts

21
Interventions in Hypertrophic Cardiomyopathy

Samin K Sharma, Mithun J Varghese, Annapoorna Kini

Since the time Donald Teare described a series of autopsies of patients with asymmetric hypertrophy of left ventricle,[1] hypertrophic cardiomyopathy (HCM) transformed from an enigmatic disease with no cure, to one of the most well researched cardiac disorder with multiple management options. More than two thirds of patients with HCM develop dynamic obstruction of the left ventricular outflow tract (LVOT), defined as gradient >30 mm Hg either at rest or under physiologic provocation.[2] Relieving mechanical obstruction by surgical myectomy was the only available treatment for limiting symptoms of HCM till the mid-nineties; this however dramatically transformed with the introduction of alcohol septal ablation (ASA) by Ulrich Sigwart.[3] Since then this procedure has grown exponentially and has become the primary modality of treatment of obstructive symptoms of HCM in India as well abroad. In this review we will look into interventional treatment options of HCM with special emphasis on septal ablation.

EPIDEMIOLOGY AND PATHOPHYSIOLOGY

Hypertrophic cardiomyopathy is the most common inherited cardiac illness of truly global distribution, with cases reported from >50 countries in all continents.[4] Although no formal population studies from India are available, extrapolation of data from the west suggest that a staggering 2.5 million people are affected with this malady in India alone. As the available data is based on probands with clinically expressed disease, even this is likely to be an under-estimation of the true prevalence of HCM.

Dynamic obstruction of the left ventricle due to the subaortic hypertrophy along with systolic anterior motion (SAM) of anterior mitral leaflet (AML) is widely recognized as the pathophysiological basis of symptoms in HCM. Basal septal hypertrophy and narrowing of the LVOT leads to localized acceleration of the blood with resultant forward drag of the AML due to Venturi effect. Elongated AML with redundant tip, a recently identified phenotypic feature of HCM, may also contribute to the LVOT obstruction in a subset of these patients.[5] This mitral-septal dynamics causes pressure difference across the LVOT, which further pulls the AML toward the basal septum, thus establishing an amplifying loop of LVOT obstruction till the end of systole. This leads to diastolic dysfunction, mitral regurgitation (MR) of varying severity and even reduction in cardiac output in severe cases leading to increased left ventricular end-diastolic pressures. Further, thickening of coronary walls along with reduced coronary flow reserve may cause myocardial ischemia even with patent epicardial vessels. The symptoms of HCM such as dyspnea, chest pain and syncope are the result of a combination these features.

ALCOHOL SEPTAL ABLATION

The notion of percutaneous myectomy first originated from the observation that large anterior myocardial infarctions can lead to disappearance of clinical and echocardiographic features of subaortic obstruction in HCM.[6] Sigwart and Grbic made the seminal observation that temporary balloon occlusion of the first septal artery favorably changes the degree of LVOT obstruction in HCM.[7] This steered them to propose percutaneous creation of a small myocardial infarction by injecting alcohol into the septal braches as a treatment option for HCM and finally led its successful clinical application in 1994 and later to its widespread clinical adoption. Multiple acronyms have been used for this technique which include, but not limited to, Ethanol septal ablation (ESA), nonsurgical myocardial reduction (NMSR), percutaneous transluminal septal myocardial ablation (PTSMA) and transcoronary ablation of septal hypertrophy (TASH).

Criteria for Patient Selection and Anatomical Considerations (Table 1)

It is essential to be sure of the diagnosis of HCM and rule out other similar pathologies that is responsive to alternative treatment, before embarking on a destructive procedure such as ASA. The patient selection criteria for ASA essentially parallel that of septal myectomy with the additional anatomical considerations. The American heart association and the recent European guidelines recommend septal reduction therapy in patients with significant symptoms (NYHA class III or IV) despite maximum tolerated medical therapy and a resting or maximum provoked LVOT gradient >50 mm Hg (Class I). Recurrent syncope during exertion due to LVOT obstruction is also a valid indication for need for invasive treatment (Class IIa).[8,9]

The thickness of the basal septum is an important echocardiographic criterion for patient selection. ESC guidelines recommend 17 mm in diastole as the minimum thickness for consideration of septal reduction therapy. At the other end of the spectrum, ASA should not be considered in patients with septal thickness >30 mm due to the lack of proven benefit. Anatomical

Table 1: Criteria for selecting patients for ASA.

Essential criteria

1	Significant symptoms (NYHA III or IV) due to LVOT obstruction refractory to medical therapy. It may be dyspnea, angina or disabling syncope/presyncope
2	Resting or provocable gradient >50 mm Hg
3	Septal thickness >17 mm
4	Suitable coronary anatomy with septal branch supplying the area of septal-mitral contact

Other considerations

1	High surgical risk
2	Absence of associated valvular pathology which will benefit from open surgery
3	Absence of associated severe coronary artery disease which will benefit from coronary artery bypass surgery
4	Patient preference after discussing pros and cons of myectomy and ASA

suitability also depends on the availability of septal branches supplying the hypertrophied basal ventricular septum which are amenable to alcohol injection. Angelini recently proposed a key anatomic-functional entity, 'First septal unit' (FSU) defined as first septal coronary branch and the hypertrophied septum dependent on it, at the level of septal-mitral contact.[10] This important zone is the primary target for septal ablation in order to obtain optimal result with ASA. The FSU is most commonly associated with the first or the second septal branch of left anterior descending (LAD) artery. Infrequently, this may be arising from a diagonal, ramus intermedius, left circumflex, left main or even the right coronary artery. Occasionally, more than one septal branch needs to be treated for getting the desired result. Identification and targeting the correct septal branch supplying the FSU is critical to a successful ASA.

Procedure

Alcohol septal ablation (ASA) is usually performed under local anesthesia with additional intravenous analgesics to provide pain free procedure. A baseline transthoracic echocardiogram is performed in cath-room for postprocedural comparison. A temporary transvenous pacing wire is secured in the right ventricular apex and is kept for 48 hours after the procedure. We prefer to place the pacing wire through a neck venous access to avoid complications related to longstanding femoral venous lines. Two arterial accesses are ideally needed for the procedure which may be either both femoral arteries, radial arteries or a combination of both. Procedure is performed with simultaneous monitoring of the left ventricular apical pressure through an end-hole catheter and central aortic pressure through the guide catheter. An extra-stimulus or Valsalva maneuver is often used to unmask provoked gradient.

Procedure is performed using intravenous heparin so as to avoid thromboembolic complications. Initially, the coronary artery is engaged with a 6F guide catheter and a selective coronary angiogram is done to identify the septal branches suitable for ASA. A standard floppy tip 0.014 inch guidewire is used for wiring the target septal branch presumed to supply the septal area of interest. The wire is usually preloaded in a short (10-12 mm) over the wire balloon, which is then introduced into this septal branch and the balloon is inflated. The balloon should be chosen such that its diameter is at least equal to the diameter of the septal branch at the level where it is inflated. A short balloon is preferred as it allows more selective ablation without projecting into the main vessel. After balloon inflation, angiography is performed to confirm complete occlusion of septal artery. Myocardial contrast echocardiography (MCE) for accurate localization of the FSU is the standard of care and should be performed in all cases of ASA. We use either Definity (Lantheus Medical imaging, MA, USA) or Optison (GE Healthcare, NJ, USA) diluted with saline at 1: 3 to 5 ratio for MCE. Approximately 1 to 2 mL of diluted echocardiographic contrast is injected through the central lumen of the inflated over the wire balloon after removing the guide wire. Simultaneous transthoracic echocardiogram will identify the myocardium supplied by this septal branch. Opacification of other cardiac structures including papillary muscle and left ventricular free wall has to be reliably excluded. MCE alters the interventional strategy in 15% of procedures by either changing the target vessel or abandoning the procedure.[11] Once the target area of myocardium is confirmed, 1-3 mL of 96% alcohol is injected slowly through central lumen of inflated balloon under continuous fluoroscopic monitoring. It is imperative to inject very slowly and steadily over a period of 5 minutes to avoid over-spilling of alcohol into the LAD. After completion of the injection, the balloon should be kept inflated for further 5 minutes. The entire assembly of balloon and wire are then slowly withdrawn back into the guide catheter.

In case of successful ablation, a reduction in LVOT gradient due to myocardial stunning is obtained immediately by echocardiogram. In general, we aim to attain resting LVOT gradient of <20 mm Hg and post ventricular ectopic gradient <40 mm Hg. In a minority of cases, incomplete gradient reduction may warrant targeting additional septal branches to obtain optimal outcome. An angiogram is always performed at the end, to ensure occlusion of the septal branch and patency of LAD. Invasive hemodynamic study is done to confirm adequate reduction in LVOT gradient.

Better understanding of the pathophysiology and improved echocardiographic localization of the culprit septal branch has led to reduction in the amount of alcohol used for the procedure in the past decade. Studies have shown no significant difference in hemodynamic benefit between low dose (1-2 mL) versus standard dose of alcohol (3-5 mL), albeit higher risk of conduction disturbance with latter.[12,13] Currently in our cathlab, we use a cumulative dose of <3 mL of alcohol in majority of cases with excellent hemodynamic results.

After the Procedure

Our practice is to monitor the patient for 48 hours after the procedure with a temporary pacing wire in the telemetry. At the end of this period, the pacing wire is removed, if there is no requirement of pacing. Using scoring systems at the end of 48 hours monitoring can help in predicting the need for permanent pacemaker (PPM) and thus aids in early decision making (Table 2).[14] A transthoracic echocardiogram is performed 24 hours after the procedure, to confirm the immediate success of the procedure. It is essential to monitor the typical rise and fall of cardiac enzymes after ASA, ideally once in 8 hours. The discharge from the hospital is done once conduction issues are resolved and when cardiac enzyme starts down-trending after the initial rise.

Pathophysiologic Mechanism of Response to ASA

The underlying mechanism behind the efficacy of ASA is by the thinning of the basal left ventricular septum due to occlusion of the septal branch. This typically follows a triphasic response pattern.[15]

1. *Immediate 'Flaccid Aknesia' phase*: The immediate gradient reduction during the procedure is due to the stunning of the myocardium due to ischemia.

Table 2: Scoring system for predicting permanent pacemaker need (modified from Faber et al).[14]

Parameter	Cut-off value	Points
Baseline LVOT gradient by echo (mm Hg)	>70	+2
Baseline minimal heart rate (per minute)	< 50	+2
Baseline PQ interval (ms)	>160	+2
Complete heart block during ASA	yes	+2
Complete heart block in CCU after procedure	yes	+2
Recovery of AV conduction in <12 hours	yes	-2
No recovery after 12 hours	yes	+1
No recovery after 24 hours	yes	+2
No recovery after 48 hours	yes	+3
Maximum QRS width in first 48 hours (ms)	>155	+3
Peak AST time after procedure (hours)	>16	+1

2. *Early 'Edematous Halo' phase*: There is a gradual increase in gradient during the first 10 days after the procedure due to the development of peri-infarction edema.
3. *Late 'Dense Scar' phase*: Infarct created by ASA forms a scar which gradually thins out leading to a permanent reduction LVOT gradient. This phase usually lasts for 3-12 months. The long-term effects of ASA can be reliably assessed only after a minimum of 3 months after the procedure.

Complications

Despite various refinements in technique, conduction disturbances including high grade AV block remain the most common complication of ASA. Right bundle branch block (RBBB) is very common after the procedure and is reported to occur in 35-60% of patients. Other EKG changes after ASA include first degree AV block in 52% of patients and left bundle branch block in 6%.[16] High grade AV block requiring PPM is reported to be between 9% and 17% in various studies.[17-19] This rate is significantly lower at 6.5% in experienced centers in the North American Registry.[18] Multivariate predictors of need for PPM after septal ablation include baseline LBBB (OR - 39), presence of first degree AV block in baseline ECG (OR - 14), bolus injection of ethanol (OR - 51), ablation of more than 2 septal branches (OR - 4.6) and female gender (OR - 4.3).[20] Pooled analysis of various studies reports other rare complications associated with ASA including in hospital ventricular fibrillation or ventricular tachycardia (1.5-3%), dissection or thrombus in LAD (0.7-1.8%) and pericardial effusion (0.5-1.4%).[17-18] Procedure related mortality is described to be 0 to 4% in various studies. Large North American and European multicenter registries however pens in-hospital death at 0.3% to 0.6%.[18,19]

The deliberate creation of scar tissue during septal ablation raises concern regarding late proarrhythmic effects and sudden cardiac death (SCD) risk. Although a few small case series have suggested potentially increased arrhythmic events, large studies have not supported these concerns. In a prospective study of patients of HCM with implanted cardioverter defibrillator (ICD), the annual rate of device discharges for treatment of arrhythmia was lower among patients who had undergone ASA than among those implanted for primary SCD prevention, thus proving lack of proarrhythmic effects of this procedure.[21]

Outcome Data

In a systematic review of 42 published studies of alcohol ablation between 1996 and 2005, Alam et al. analyzed outcomes 2959 patients who underwent ASA.[16] The procedural success reported in the series was 89% with 6.6% requiring multiple septal ablation and <2% requiring surgical myectomy.

They found sustained LVOT gradient reduction both at rest (65–15 mm Hg) and at provocation (125–31 mm Hg) due to reduction in septal thickness (20.9–13.9 mm) after an average follow-up of 1 year. This was associated significant improvement in NYHA class and exercise capacity (both p <0.01).

Recent data on longer term outcome of ASA from the large Euro-ASA registry involving 1275 patients further underscores the efficacy and safety of this procedure.[19] At a median clinical follow-up of 3.9 years, the LVOT gradient reduced from 67 ± 36 mm Hg to 16 ± 21 mm Hg and NYHA class improved from 2.9 ± 0.5 to 1.6 ± 0.7 (both p <0.001). Nearly 90% patients reported improvement of symptoms by at least 1 NYHA class. Overall 171 (13%) patients died during 7057 patient years of follow-up. This corresponds to an all-cause mortality rate of 2.42 deaths per 100 patient-years, indicating excellent safety.

The Debate: Surgical Myectomy versus ASA

Both surgical myectomy and ASA are effective procedures for treatment of symptomatic LVOT obstruction in patients with HCM. The advantages of the former include sustained near complete relief of obstruction, lesser requirement of permanent pacing and lesser potential for arrhythmogenicity. Surgery also provides more options for treatment of other associated abnormalities such as mitral valve disease. This has to be weighed against the need for thoracotomy requiring longer times to recuperate which in turn drives up the cost of the procedure as well. In resource poor settings such as in India, the required surgical expertise may be another issue against surgical myectomy. In view of marked heterogeneity in HCM and low event rate, a high quality randomized trial comparing both these procedures is unlikely in foreseeable future; hence we have to rely on observational data for comparison.[22] Meta-analysis of observational studies comparing ASA and myectomy showed no difference in short-term or long-term mortality between the two procedures.[23,24] Both the procedures showed similar improvements in functional class, occurrence of ventricular arrhythmia and the need for reinterventions. As expected, the conduction disturbances including need for pacemaker were higher in the ASA group. Although both the procedures resulted in reduction in gradient, there was small but significant higher residual gradient with ASA in comparison to myectomy.

Despite tremendous improvements in safety and efficacy of ASA, guidelines continue to recommend surgical myectomy as the treatment of choice for obstructive symptoms of HCM; ASA is recommended only as an alternative in patients with higher surgical risk.[8,9] In this day of personalized medicine, however, preferences of the patient remains paramount and very often they prefer a percutaneous option. This continues to drive much higher rates of ASA compared to surgery across the world, including India.

ALTERNATIVE APPROACHES FOR SEPTAL ABLATION

Various other techniques have been tried instead of alcohol for septal ablation in patients with HCM, in order to reduce the adverse effects of injecting alcohol into the coronary artery. Alternative options tried include coils,[25] cyanoacrylate glue,[26] gelatin particles,[27] polyvinyl alcohol particles[28] and angioplasty wires.[29] As these techniques rely on inducing myocardial ischemia rather than direct myocardial damage as in alcohol ablation, their long-term efficacy is limited by development of collaterals. Due to lack of longer term outcome data, none of these methods have been widely adopted.

Despite advances in ASA techniques, a subset of patients of HCM with obstruction is not eligible for this treatment due restrictions of coronary anatomy. In such patients, direct endocardial radiofrequency (RF) ablation of the obstructing septum offers a percutaneous alternative to surgical myectomy. As first reported by Lawrenz,[30] this may be attempted from either right or left ventricular aspect; the latter is more preferred due to higher technical success. Use of electroanatomical mapping and intracardiac echo aids in precise application of RF energy. Recent systematic review of this procedure concluded that this is a viable alternative for the treatment of patients who are otherwise not candidates for either ASA or open surgery. Although the learning curve is steep and the long term efficacy unknown, the procedure was associated with reliable improvement in symptoms and acceptable rates of complications.[31]

PERCUTANEOUS TREATMENT OF MITRAL VALVE FOR OBSTRUCTIVE HCM

In addition to outflow tract obstruction, concomitant mitral valve abnormalities including MR resulting from SAM are common in HCM. This usually calls for surgery as the choice of treatment due to its ability to treat both obstruction and valve regurgitation. Recent advent of Mitraclip (Abbott Vascular, IL, USA) however provides a percutaneous option for treating both these evils simultaneously. Schafer et al treated three such patients with both LVOT obstruction and severe MR due to SAM with Mitraclip procedure of A2-P2 segments of mitral valve.[32] This resulted in successful immediate reduction of LVOT gradients along with considerable reduction in MR. At 6 weeks follow-up, patients had remarkable improvement in symptoms with persistent echocardiographic benefits. Although long-term efficacy of this modality is currently unknown, it may offer percutaneous treatment option for SAM related severe MR and LVOT obstruction.

CONCLUSION

Even though surgical myectomy continues to be the gold standard for the treatment of symptoms of obstructive HCM, ASA has emerged as an excellent percutaneous alternative. Despite the higher need for pacemaker implantation, ASA provides exceptional hemodynamic and clinical benefit at medium term follow-up. Since adequately powered randomized trials comparing the two are unlikely, large multicenter prospective registries with long-term data are the only way to provide a definitive answer to the vexing "which is better?" query. Till then, availability of surgical expertise, the cost of the procedure and the preference of a well-informed patient will decide what the best choice is. Meanwhile newer treatments such as endocardial RF ablation and Mitraclip therapy may provide percutaneous alternatives for patients who are not candidates for either ASA or surgical myectomy.

Low risk (Cumulative score < 8)—Can be discharged from monitoring
Intermediate risk (Cumulative score 8-12)—Need prolonged monitoring
High risk (Cumulative score > 12)—Need early PPM.

REFERENCES

1. Teare D. Asymmetrical hypertrophy of the heart in young adults. Br Heart J. 1958;20(1):1-8.
2. Maron MS, Olivotto I, Zenovich AG, et al. Hypertrophic cardiomyopathy is predominantly a disease of left ventricular outflow tract obstruction. Circulation. 2006;114(21):2232-9.
3. Sigwart U. Nonsurgical myocardial reduction for hypertrophic obstructive cardiomyopathy. Lancet Lond Engl. 1995;346(8969):211-4.
4. Maron BJ, Ommen SR, Semsarian C, et al. Hypertrophic cardiomyopathy: present and future, with translation into contemporary cardiovascular medicine. J Am Coll Cardiol. 2014;64(1):83-99.
5. Maron MS, Olivotto I, Harrigan C, et al. Mitral valve abnormalities identified by cardiovascular magnetic resonance represent a primary phenotypic expression of hypertrophic cardiomyopathy. Circulation. 2011;124(1):40-7.
6. Come PC, Riley MF. Hypertrophic cardiomyopathy. Disappearance of auscultatory, carotid pulse, and echocardiographic manifestations of obstruction following myocardial infarction. Chest. 1982;82(4):451-4.
7. Sigwart U, Grbic M, Payot M, et al. Ventricular wall motion during balloon occlusion. In: Ventricular Wall Motion. New York: 1983. pp. 206-10.
8. Gersh BJ, Maron BJ, Bonow RO, et al. ACCF/AHA guideline for the diagnosis and treatment of hypertrophic cardiomyopathy: executive summary: a report of the American College of Cardiology Foundation/American Heart Association Task Force on Practice Guidelines. Circulation. 2011;124(24):2761-96.
9. Authors/Task Force members, Elliott PM, Anastasakis A, et al. ESC Guidelines on diagnosis and management of hypertrophic cardiomyopathy: the Task Force for the Diagnosis and Management of Hypertrophic Cardiomyopathy of the European Society of Cardiology (ESC). Eur Heart J. 2014;35(39):2733-79.

10. Angelini P. The "1st septal unit" in hypertrophic obstructive cardiomyopathy: a newly recognized anatomofunctional entity, identified during recent alcohol septal ablation experience. Tex Heart Inst J. 2007;34(3):336-46.
11. Faber L, Ziemssen P, Seggewiss H. Targeting percutaneous transluminal septal ablation for hypertrophic obstructive cardiomyopathy by intraprocedural echocardiographic monitoring. J Am Soc Echocardiogr Off Publ Am Soc Echocardiogr. 2000;13(12):1074-9.
12. Veselka J, Duchonová R, Páleníckova J, et al. Impact of ethanol dosing on the long-term outcome of alcohol septal ablation for obstructive hypertrophic cardiomyopathy: a single-center prospective, and randomized study. Circ J Off J Jpn Circ Soc 2006;70(12):1550-2.
13. Veselka J, Tomašov P, Zemánek D. Long-term effects of varying alcohol dosing in percutaneous septal ablation for obstructive hypertrophic cardiomyopathy: a randomized study with a follow-up up to 11 years. Can J Cardiol. 2011;27(6):763-7.
14. Faber L, Welge D, Fassbender D, et al. Percutaneous septal ablation for symptomatic hypertrophic obstructive cardiomyopathy: managing the risk of procedure-related AV conduction disturbances. Int J Cardiol. 2007;119(2):163-7.
15. Yoerger DM, Picard MH, Palacios IF, et al. Time course of pressure gradient response after first alcohol septal ablation for obstructive hypertrophic cardiomyopathy. Am J Cardiol. 2006;97(10):1511-4.
16. Alam M, Dokainish H, Lakkis N. Alcohol septal ablation for hypertrophic obstructive cardiomyopathy: a systematic review of published studies. J Intervent Cardiol. 2006;19(4):319-27.
17. Jensen MK, Almaas VM, Jacobsson L, et al. Long-term outcome of percutaneous transluminal septal myocardial ablation in hypertrophic obstructive cardiomyopathy: a Scandinavian multicenter study. Circ Cardiovasc Interv. 2011;4(3):256-65.
18. Nagueh SF, Groves BM, Schwartz L, et al. Alcohol septal ablation for the treatment of hypertrophic obstructive cardiomyopathy. A multicenter North American registry. J Am Coll Cardiol. 2011;58(22):2322-8.
19. Veselka J, Jensen MK, Liebregts M, et al. Long-term clinical outcome after alcohol septal ablation for obstructive hypertrophic cardiomyopathy: results from the Euro-ASA registry. Eur Heart J. 2016;37(19):1517-23.
20. Chang SM, Nagueh SF, Spencer WH, Lakkis NM. Complete heart block: determinants and clinical impact in patients with hypertrophic obstructive cardiomyopathy undergoing nonsurgical septal reduction therapy. J Am Coll Cardiol. 2003;42(2):296-300.
21. Cuoco FA, Spencer WH, Fernandes VL, et al. Implantable cardioverter-defibrillator therapy for primary prevention of sudden death after alcohol septal ablation of hypertrophic cardiomyopathy. J Am Coll Cardiol. 2008;52(21):1718-23.
22. Olivotto I, Ommen SR, Maron MS, Cecchi F, Maron BJ. Surgical myectomy versus alcohol septal ablation for obstructive hypertrophic cardiomyopathy. Will there ever be a randomized trial? J Am Coll Cardiol. 2007;50(9):831-4.
23. Agarwal S, Tuzcu EM, Desai MY, et al. Updated meta-analysis of septal alcohol ablation versus myectomy for hypertrophic cardiomyopathy. J Am Coll Cardiol. 2010;55(8):823-34.
24. Singh K, Qutub M, Carson K, et al. A meta analysis of current status of alcohol septal ablation and surgical myectomy for obstructive hypertrophic cardiomyopathy. Catheter Cardiovasc Interv Off J Soc Card Angiogr Interv. 2016;88(1):107-15.

25. Durand E, Mousseaux E, Coste P, et al. Non-surgical septal myocardial reduction by coil embolization for hypertrophic obstructive cardiomyopathy: early and 6 months follow-up. Eur Heart J. 2008;29(3):348-55.
26. Oto A, Aytemir K, Deniz A. New approach to septal ablation: glue (cyanoacrylate) septal ablation. Catheter Cardiovasc Interv Off J Soc Card Angiogr Interv. 2007;69(7):1021-5.
27. Llamas-Esperón GA, Sandoval-Navarrete S. Percutaneous septal ablation with absorbable gelatin sponge in hypertrophic obstructive cardiomyopathy. Catheter Cardiovasc Interv Off J Soc Card Angiogr Interv. 2007;69(2):231-5.
28. Gross CM, Schulz-Menger J, Krämer J, et al. Percutaneous transluminal septal artery ablation using polyvinyl alcohol foam particles for septal hypertrophy in patients with hypertrophic obstructive cardiomyopathy: acute and 3-year outcomes. J Endovasc Ther Off J Int Soc Endovasc Spec. 2004;11(6):705-11.
29. Trehan V, Mukhopadhyay S, Rangasetty UC. Percutaneous transseptal myocardial ablation with wire (PTSAW): a new technique. J Invasive Cardiol. 2004;16(4):204-6.
30. Lawrenz T, Borchert B, Leuner C, et al. Endocardial radiofrequency ablation for hypertrophic obstructive cardiomyopathy: acute results and 6 months' follow-up in 19 patients. J Am Coll Cardiol. 2011;57(5):572-6.
31. Poon SS, Cooper RM, Gupta D. Endocardial radiofrequency septal ablation - A new option for non-surgical septal reduction in patients with hypertrophic obstructive cardiomyopathy (HOCM)?: A systematic review of clinical studies. Int J Cardiol. 2016;222:772-4.
32. Schäfer U, Frerker C, Thielsen T, et al. Targeting systolic anterior motion and left ventricular outflow tract obstruction in hypertrophic obstructed cardiomyopathy with a MitraClip. EuroIntervention J Eur Collab Work Group Interv Cardiol Eur Soc Cardiol. 2015;11(8):942-7.

22 Interventions in Pulmonary Embolism

Bharat Shivdasani, Rahul Chhabria

INTRODUCTION

Venous thromboembolism (VTE) is a terminology which includes deep vein thrombosis (DVT) and pulmonary embolism (PE). VTE is one of the leading causes of morbidity and mortality with an overall annual incidence of 100–200 per 100 000 inhabitants.[1] VTE can lead to mortality in acute phase or it can lead to complications in chronic phase,[2] but it is also often preventable. Acute PE has a 30 days mortality of around 9 to 11% and 3 months mortality around 8.6 to 17%.[3]

CLASSIFICATION OF PULMONARY EMBOLISM

Based on various parameters acute PE has been classified by European Society of Cardiology (ESC) 2014 guidelines[4] into low, intermediate and high-risk (Table 1).

Table 1: Classification of PE based on various clinical parameters.

	Shock or hypotension	Signs of RV dysfunction on imaging	Cardiac biomarkers (Troponins or BNP)
High-risk	+	+	+
Intermediate	–	+	+
Low	–	–	–

It is very important to classify the patients with Acute PE as the management is dependent upon the risk. High-risk patients require urgent interventions.

MANAGEMENT OF PE

Treatment Options

Flowchart 1: Treatment options in acute PE according to the risk category.

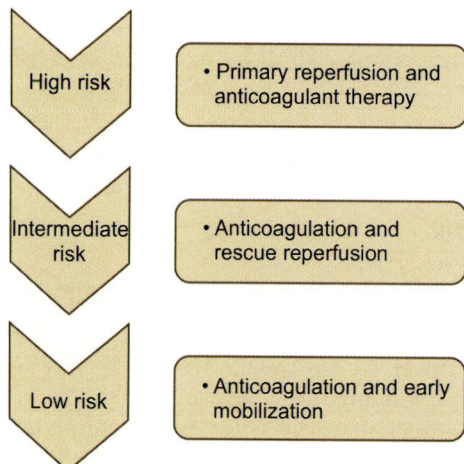

Treatment Algorithm

Flowchart 2: Algorithm of management of Acute PE.

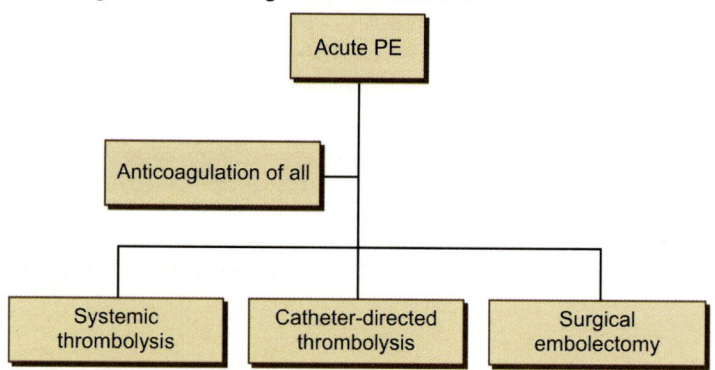

Anticoagulation

In all patients with acute PE, anticoagulation is recommended. It reduces morbidity and mortality is these patients. As per the 2014 ESC guidelines, the duration of anticoagulation should be at least 3 months. However, in selected cases the duration is extended, especially in patients with unprovoked VTE. The risk of bleeding should be weighed in these cases. During this period the therapy includes administration of parental anticoagulation [Unfractionated heparin (UFH), low molecular weight heparin (LMWH) or fondaparinux] which is overlapped with a vitamin K antagonist (VKA) or a new oral anticoagulant (NOAC).

Parenteral Anticoagulation

In patients with high or intermediate clinical probability for PE, parenteral anticoagulation should be initiated whilst awaiting the results of diagnostic tests. LMWH or fondaparinux are preferred over UFH for initial anticoagulation in PE, as they carry a lower risk of inducing major bleeding and heparin-induced thrombocytopenia (HIT).[5] On the other hand, UFH is recommended for patients in whom primary reperfusion is considered, as well as for those with serious renal impairment (creatinine clearance, 30 mL/min), or severe obesity. These recommendations are based on the short half-life of UFH, the ease of monitoring its anticoagulant effects, and its rapid reversal by protamine.[6]

The LMWHs approved for the treatment of acute PE are as follows (Table 2):

Table 2: Doses of approved LMWH for PE.

Drug	Dose
Enoxaparin	1.0 mg/kg every 12 hours
Dalteparin	100 IU/Kg every 12 hours
Fondaparinux	5 mg (body weight <50 kg); 7.5 mg (Weight 50–100 kg); 10 mg (Weight >100 kg) Once daily

Other approved LMWH include Tinzaparin (175 U/kg OD) and Nadroparinc (86 IU/kg BD), however these drugs not available in India.

Oral Anticoagulants

Vitamin K antagonists should be initiated as soon as possible. For years together VKA's have been gold standard oral anticoagulant. It should be overlapped with parental anticoagulant for at least 5 days, till the target INR (2-3) has been achieved. The problems with warfarin include need for repeated monitoring, narrow therapeutic range, and multiple drug and food interactions. The addition of pharmacogenetic testing have failed to show any added advantages for achieving target INR.

New oral anticoagutants are alternative to VKA's for maintaining anticoagulation in patients with acute PE (Table 3). Trials have shown non-inferiority to warfarin for treating acute PE with decrease in bleeding complications as compared to warfarin. These drugs have advantages of less drug and food interactions, eliminating the need for frequent blood tests and more safety as compared to warfarin. However, the problems with NOACs include problems with reversal in case of bleeding, and the cost.

Table 3: Doses of NOACs used for treating acute PE.

S. No.	Drug	Initial Dose	Maintenance Dose	Special Precautions
1.	Dabigatran	150 mg BD	150 mg BD	Crt Cl < 30
2.	Rivaroxaban	15 mg BD for 21 days	20 mg OD	Crt Cl <30; Severe liver disease
3.	Apixaban	10 mg BD for 7 days	5 mg BD	Crt Cl <15; Severe liver disease
4.	Edoxaban	60 mg OD	60 mg OD	Crt Cl <50, Weight <60 kg, Severe Liver Disease

At present drugs approved for treatment include dabigatran, rivaroxaban, and apixaban, and Edoxaban.

Systemic Thrombolysis

Thrombolytic therapy restores RV function rapidly by restoring pulmonary perfusion more rapidly as compared to anticoagulation with heparin alone.[7] It also leads to early resolution of pulmonary resolution and rapid reduction in pulmonary artery resistance and pressure.

Indications of Thrombolysis

1. Hemodynamic Instability related to PE who have symptom onset for less than 14 days.
2. In patients with intermediate risk, i.e. patients with acute PE with no shock but presence of either RV dysfunction or positive biomarkers [troponin or brain natriuretic peptide (BNP)].

Approved thrombolytic regimens for PE as per ESC (Table 4):

Table 4: Doses of thrombolytic agents approved by ESC for treating acute PE.

Drug	Dose
Streptokinase	250 000 IU as a loading dose over 30 minutes, followed by 100000 IU/h over 12–24 hours
Urokinase	4400 IU/kg as a loading dose over 10 min, followed by 4400 IU/kg per hour over 12–24 hours
rTPA	100 mg over 2 hours; or 0.6 mg/kg over 15 minutes (maximum dose 50 mg)

Tenecteplase and Reteplase have been studied in trials and showed better results as compared to placebo and have shown better outcomes. Dose of tenecteplase is weight based bolus dose and dose of Retelplase is fixed—10 Units and 10 Units bolus. These agents are not approved yet for treatment but they are used on practical level. The advantage of these agents is that they have high fibrin specificity and have rapid and easy administration.

Contraindications for Thrombolysis (Table 5)

Table 5: Contraindications of thrombolysis.

Absolute Contraindications	Relative Contraindications
Hemorrhagic stroke or stroke of unknown origin at any time	Transient ischemic attack in the preceding 6 months
Ischemic stroke in the preceding 6 months	Oral anticoagulant therapy
Central nervous system damage or neoplasms	Pregnancy, or within 1 week postpartum
Recent major trauma/surgery/head injury in the preceding 3 weeks	Non-compressible puncture site
Gastrointestinal bleeding within the last month	Traumatic resuscitation
Known bleeding risk	Refractory hypertension (systolic blood pressure >180 mm Hg)
	Advanced liver disease
	Infective endocarditis
	Active peptic ulcer

A meta-analysis of 15 trials including a total of 2000 patients showed that fibrinolysis reduced overall mortality (odds ratio [OR]: 0.59; 95% CI: 0.36 to 0.96) and achieved a significant reduction in the combined endpoint of death or treatment escalation (OR: 0.34; 95% CI: 0.22 to 0.53), PE-related mortality (OR: 0.29; 95% CI: 0.14 to 0.60), and PE recurrence (OR: 0.50; 95%CI: 0.27 to 0.94). At the same time, however, major hemorrhage (OR: 2.91; 95% CI: 1.95 to 4.36) and fatal or intracranial bleeding (OR: 3.18; 95% CI: 1.25 to 8.11) were significantly more frequent among patients receiving thrombolysis.[8]

Percutaneous Catheter-Directed Interventions

The high-risk of major bleeding with systemic thrombolysis includes Intracranial hemorrhage (approx. 1%) has dampened enthusiasm for this potential life-saving therapy. Catheter directed interventions holds promise that it has good efficacy with lower major side effects.[9] The doses of thrombolytic therapy used in interventional therapy reduces to one fourth of dose used in systemic thrombolysis thereby reducing the major side effects.

The main objective of interventional treatment is removal of obstructing thrombi from the main pulmonary arteries, and rapid recovery of RV function, improve symptoms and survival. These interventions are indicated in patients with massive PE or high-risk PE with contraindications to systemic thrombolysis or with recurrent PE or patients not responding to thrombolysis.

Various percutaneous catheter directed treatment options include (Table 6). Table 7 shows a step by step approach in general for catheter directed procedures.

Table 6: Various catheter-based treatment options for PE.

S. No.	Catheter-Directed Treatment
1.	Catheter-Directed Thrombolysis
2.	Mechanical Thrombus Fragmentation
3.	Suction Thrombectomy
4.	Rotational Thrombectomy
5.	Rheolytic Thrombectomy
6.	Pharmacomechanical Thrombolysis

Table 7: Step–by-step approach to a catheter-directed treatment.

S. No.	Suggested Step-by-Step Approach for Catheter Interventions in Acute PE
1.	Obtain venous access at the common femoral vein using a standard sheath
2.	Use 8 F long sheath (45 cm)
3.	Administer 80 Units/Kg IV UFH
4.	Perform right heart catheterization and obtain hemodynamic data from RA, RV and PA
5.	Perform selective angiography using 20° LAO view for LPA and 20° RAO for RPA. Catheter trip should be paced proximal to occlusion site which is confirmed by a non-dampened pressure tracing.
6.	Cross the embolic occlusion using a standard diagnostic catheter and an angle-tipped exchange-length hydrophilic 0.035-inch guide wire (e.g., Terumo Glidewire with torque device).
7.	Introduce the desired catheter over the wire.

1. Conventional Catheter-Directed Thrombolysis (CDT)

This method includes administration of thrombolytic therapy through a catheter placed in the pulmonary artery and infusion of drug in a much lower dose as compared to systemic dose.

Various drug regimens have been tried for this method. For example rTPA at a dose of 2-5 mg bolus followed by 0.5-2.0 mg per hour as a continuous infusion. Since the total dose of thrombolytic therapy comes down to approximately one fourth of systemic dose, the bleeding risk reduces significantly. This method can be used alone or it can be combined with other mechanical interventions.

Various regimes used for different drugs. Dose of Tenecteplase is 1 to 5 mg bolus followed by 0.125 to 0.25 mg/hr of continuous infusion.

Dose of Reteplase used is 2 to 5 Units bolus followed by 0.25 to 0.5 Units/hr continuous infusion.
- Fountain Catheter with multiple holes at the end can used for infusing the thrombolytic agent.

2. **Mechanical Thrombus Fragmentation**

   Mechanical thrombus fragmentation is achieved by mechanically disrupting the thrombus into smaller fragments by manual rotation of a pigtail catheter or with a peripheral balloon. It has advantage that it does not increase bleeding risk but it has a disadvantage of risk of macro-embolization which can lead to hemodynamic deterioration when fragments from a large non-obstructive thrombus embolize.[10] This method can also be combined with other mechanical or pharmacomechanical approaches.

3. **Suction Thrombectomy**

   Suction of thrombi can be achieved by large lumen catheters (8–9 F), with which manual aspiration can be done with an aspiration syringe. Conventional sheaths cannot be used to aspirate such large thrombi as it can get trapped in the hemostatic valves present. It requires dedicated aspiration sheath with a detachable hemostatic valve, permitting percutaneous removal of thrombus without the need for surgical cut down.

4. **Rotational Thrombectomy**

   Aspirex catheter system can be used for rotational thrombectomy. The central part of the Aspirex catheter is a protected, high-speed rotational coil that creates negative pressure through an L-shaped aspiration port at the catheter tip, resulting in maceration and aspiration of the thrombus.[20] This technique can also be combined with other mechanical or pharmacomechanical interventions.

5. **Rheolytic Thrombectomy**

   This method includes an Angiojet device with a high-pressure saline jet which generates a pressure gradient by Bernoulli's principle, enabling the removal of thrombus fragments.[11] It has an advantage that simultaneous local injection of thrombolytic therapy can be administered by the power pulse spray technique. Common side effects include Bradycardia, heart block or asystole due to release of bradykinin, adenosine, or potassium secondary to hemolysis.

6. **Pharmacomechanical Thrombolysis (PMT)**

   PMT is defined as the combination of CDT with a mechanical catheter intervention technique. This combination therapy may be particularly useful in hemodynamically unstable patients who require rapid removal of obstruction and improvement of hemodynamic. Another PMT approach is the Power Pulse spray technique for intraclot delivery of low doses of thrombolytic agents, facilitating rheolytic thrombectomy with the AngioJet device.

A review on percutaneous interventional treatment was done which included 35 non-randomized studies covering 594 patients.[11] It measured Clinical success which was defined as stabilization of hemodynamic parameters, resolution of hypoxia, and survival to discharge. The clinical success was achieved in 87% of cases. The contribution of the mechanical catheter intervention per se to clinical success is unclear because 67% of patients also received adjunctive local thrombolysis. Publication bias probably resulted in underreporting of major complications (reportedly affecting 2% of interventions), which may include death from worsening RV failure, distal embolization, pulmonary artery perforation with lung hemorrhage, systemic bleeding complications, pericardial tamponade, heart block or bradycardia, hemolysis, contrast-induced nephropathy, and puncture-related complications. While anticoagulation with heparin alone has little effect on improvement of RV size and performance within the first 24–48 hours, the extent of early RV recovery after low-dose catheter directed thrombolysis appears comparable to that after standard dose systemic thrombolysis.[12]

Venous Filters

Venous filters are filter inserted in the Inferior vena cava (IVC) which prevents the further embolization of clots from lower limb veins to the pulmonary circulation.

Common indications for venous filters include:
1. Absolute contraindications to anticoagulation;
2. Complication to anticoagulation; and
3. Recurrent PE despite therapeutic levels of anticoagulation.

Venous filters are usually placed in the infra-renal portion of the IVC. If thrombus is identified in the renal veins, suprarenal placement may be indicated.

Types

Interior vena cava filter can be permanent or non-permanent. Non-permanent IVC filters are further classified as temporary or retrievable devices. Temporary filters must be removed within few days, while retrievable filters can be left in place for longer periods.[13] When non-permanent filters are used, it is recommended that they be removed as soon as it is safe to use anticoagulants. Despite this, they are often left in situ for longer periods, with a late complication rate of at least 10%; this includes filter migration, tilting or deformation, penetration of the cava wall by filter limbs, fracturing of the filter and embolization of fragments, and thrombosis of the device (Table 8).[14]

Table 8: Various types of IVC filters.

			Non-retrievable				
Type	Titanium Greenfield	Over-the-Wire Greenfield	Vena Tech LP	Vena Tech LGM	Simon Nitinol Filter (SNF)	TrapEase	Gianturco-Roehm Bird's Nest
Diagram							
Maximum IVC diameter (mm)	28	28	28	28	28	30	40
Manufacturer	Boston Scientific	Boston Scientific	B. Braun Medical	B. Braun Medical	Bard	Cordis (J&J)	Cook
Required sheath size	12F	12F	9F	12F	9F	6F	12F
Insertion sites	Jugular femoral	Jugular femoral	Jugular femoral	Jugular femoral/single system	Jugular femoral, subclavian, antecubital	Jugular, femoral, antecubital	Jugular, femoral
Material	Titanium	316 stainless	Phynox	Phynox	Nitinol (NiTi)	Elgiloy	304 stainless steel

Contd...

Contd...

Type	Retrievable						
	Denali	OptEase	Gunther Tulip	Cook Celect	Option	ALN Filter	Crux Filter
Diagram							
Maximum IVC diameter (mm)	28	30	30	30	30	32	28
Manufacturer	Bard	Cordis (J&J)	Cook	Cook	Argon Medical	ALN International	Crux Biomedical
Required sheath size	8.5F	6F	8.5F	7F (IJ), 8.5 (F)	6.5F	7F	9F
Insertion sites	Jugular, subclavian, femoral	Jugular, femoral, antecubital	Jugular femoral	Jugular femoral UniSet	Jugular, femoral	Jugular, femoral, basilic	Jugular femoral
Material	Nickel-titanium alloy	Elgiloy	Conichrome	Conichrome	Nitinol (NiTi)	316 stainless steel	Nitinol (NiTi)

Procedure

Once the access is obtained via femoral or jugular route, a guide-wire is used to access the vena cava. A catheter is then advanced over the wire. When using the jugular approach the catheter should be advanced till common iliac vein. A venogram is then taken to delineate the anatomy and decide the position of placement of filter. Venogram also shows if any clot is present in the vena cava. The diameter of the IVC should also be measured to ensure it does not exceed the upper limit for the planned filter. Measurement should be done in 2 views as IVS is frequently oval than round.

With a standard anatomy the filter should be positioned with the tip of the filter just at the inflow of the renal veins, which minimizes the accumulation of thrombus above the filter in the event of filter thrombosis. Suprarenal placement is indicated in renal vein thrombosis, gonadal vein thrombosis, IVC thrombus extending above the renal veins, and thrombus in the infrarenal IVC that does not provide sufficient room for the filter to be placed above the thrombus and below the renal veins.

Observational studies have shown that insertion of a venous filter might reduce PE-related mortality rates in the acute phase. However this benefit comes at a cost of increased risk of recurrent VTE. Complications of IVC filters include insertion site thrombosis, recurrent DVT, post-thrombotic syndrome and occlusion of filter.[15]

Surgical Embolectomy

Surgical embolectomy was first performed way back in 1924 several decades before invent of medical treatment for PE. Over decades the treatment option has remerged for patients with high-risk PE. It involves direct surgical removal of large visual thrombus from the main pulmonary arteries and immediate relieve of obstruction and improvement of hemodynamic. It is presently indicated in patients with high-risk PE as a treatment option especially with high bleeding risk, selected cases of intermediate risk PE and patients where thrombolysis of catheter therapy has failed.

The surgical mortality of the procedure is about 6%.[15] Preoperative thrombolysis increases the risk of bleeding, but it is not an absolute contraindication to surgical embolectomy. Over the long-term, the post-operative survival rate, World Health Organization functional class, and quality of life were favorable in Published series.[16] However, extraction is limited to directly visible clots.

Future Perspective

Ultrasound-Assisted Catheter-Directed Thrombolysis

Ultrasound assisted thrombolysis is a form of pharmacomechanical thrombolysis. It is a combination of catheter directed thrombolysis with a catheter

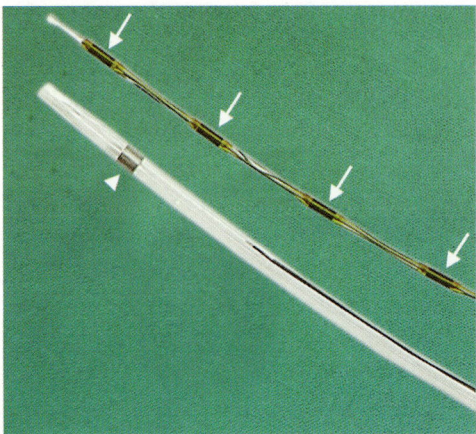

Fig. 1: Tip of the ultrasound-assisted thrombolysis catheter, EkoSonic® Endovascular System (EKOS Corporation, Bothell, WA, USA). The catheter is composed of a 5.2-Fr multi-sidehole drug infusion catheter (treatment zone marker delineated with an arrowhead) and a microsonic core wire containing the ultrasound elements (marked with small arrows).

system that employs ultrasound energy. Studies have shown that ultrasound exposure causes a reversible disaggregation of uncrosslinked fibrin fibers, an effect that may create additional binding sites and facilitate the thrombolysis effect. In addition, ultrasound pressure waves may increase thrombus penetration of thrombolytic drugs by acoustic streaming. One such available device approved by US-FDA is Ekosonic endovascular system. It combines a multi-sidehole drug infusion catheter with a multi-element ultrasound core wire (Fig. 1). The thrombolytic drug is delivered through the infusion catheter while the ultrasound core delivers high-frequency (2.2 GHz), low energy (0.5 W per transducer) intravascular ultrasound along the entire treatment zone. Initial Studies have shown promising results, however randomized trials are ongoing.

REFERENCES

1. Heit JA. The epidemiology of venous thromboembolism in the community. Arterioscler Thromb Vasc Biol 2008;28(3):370-72.
2. Klok FA, van Kralingen KW, van Dijk AP, Heyning FH, Vliegen HW, Kaptein AA, Huisman MV. Quality of life in long-term survivors of acute pulmonary embolism. Chest 2010;138(6):1432-40.
3. Laporte S, Mismetti P, De´cousus H, Uresandi F, Otero R, Lobo JL, Monreal M. Clinical predictors for fatal pulmonary embolism in 15,520 patients with venous thromboembolism: findings from the Registro Informatizado de la Enfermedad TromboEmbolica venosa (RIETE) Registry. Circulation 2008;117(13):1711-16.

4. Stavros Konstantinides et al 2014 ESC Guidelines on the diagnosis and management of acute pulmonary embolism. Europ Heart J. doi:10.1093/eurheartj/ehu283
5. Stein PD, Hull RD, Matta F, Yaekoub AY, Liang J. Incidence of thrombocytopenia inc hospitalized patients with venous thromboembolism. Am J Med 2009;122(10):c919-30.
6. Raschke RA, Gollihare B, Peirce JC. The effectiveness of implementing the weight based heparin nomogram as a practice guideline. Arch Intern Med. 1996; 156(15):1645-49.
7. Dalla-Volta S, Palla A, Santolicandro A, et al. PAIMS 2: alteplase combined with heparin versus heparin in the treatment of acute pulmonary embolism. Plasminogen activator Italian multicenter study 2. J Am Coll Cardiol. 1992;20 (3):520-26.
8. Marti C, John G, Konstantinides S, et al. Systemic thrombolytic therapy for acute pulmonary embolism: a systematic review and meta-analysis. Eur Heart J. 2015;36:605-14.
9. Engelberger RP, Kucher N. Catheter-based reperfusion treatment of pulmonary embolism. Circulation. 2011.124:2139.
10. Brady AJ, Crake T, Oakley CM. Percutaneous catheter fragmentation and distal dispersion of proximal pulmonary embolus. Lancet. 1991;338:1186-89
11. Drasler WJ, Jenson ML, Wilson GJ, et al. Rheolytic catheter for percutaneous removal of thrombus. Radiology. 1992;182:263-67.
12. Becattini C, Agnelli G, Salvi A, et al. Bolus tenecteplase for right ventricle dysfunction in hemodynamically stable patients with pulmonary embolism. Thromb Res. 2010;125(3):e82-e86
13. Zhu X, TamMD, Bartholomew J, et al. Retrievability and device-related complications of the G2 filter: a retrospective study of 139 filter retrievals. J Vasc Interv Radiol. 2011;22(6):806-12.
14. Muriel A, Jime´nez D, Aujesky D, et al. RIETE Investigators. Survival effects of inferior vena cava filter in patients with acute symptomatic venous thromboembolism and a significant bleeding risk. J Am Coll Cardiol. 2014;63(16):1675-83.
15. Aymard T, Kadner A, Widmer A, et al. Massive pulmonary embolism: surgical embolectomy versus thrombolytic therapy: should surgical indications be revisited? Eur J Cardiothorac Surg. 2013;43(1):90-94.
16. Vohra HA, Whistance RN, Mattam K, et al. Early and late clinical outcomes of pulmonary embolectomy for acute massive pulmonary embolism. Ann Thorac Surg. 2010;90(6):1747-52.

23
Recent Advances in Cardiac Electrophysiology

Andhalkar Bhagyashree, Amit Vora

Last few decades have seen tremendous strides in the field of cardiac electrophysiology and it continues to be a rapidly evolving field with technological advances and unifying concepts. This article predominantly focuses on the recent progress in ablation procedures for various tachyarrhythmias. It will encompass advancement in mapping techniques, ablation energy, diagnostic and therapeutic catheters. Finally, current understanding of the mechanism and ablation strategy for atrial fibrillation (AF), ventricular tachycardia (VT), and various scar related arrhythmias will be discussed.

MAPPING TECHNIQUES (TABLE 1)

The advent of three-dimensional (3D) electro-anatomical mapping system nearly two decades ago revolutionized the understanding of AF, VT and other scar related tachycardias and guided effective ablation strategy. This technique essentially is a nonfluoroscopic catheter localization and a 3D display of activation sequences and electrogram voltage mapping. This could be integrated with noninvasive images of heart obtained by CT or MRI. Over the years, significant refinements have been made in this technology wherein, accuracy, shorter acquisition time and effective ablation with limited fluoroscopy and radiation exposure have been achieved.

Table 1: Mapping systems.

CARTO 3	3D activation, propagation and voltage mapping for AF and VT
EnSite velocity	Multiple catheters of various vendors can be imaged during 3D mapping
Rhythmia	Quick, automated acquisition of thousands of points for 3D map creation
ECVue	256 lead ECG superimposed on CT for entire heart activation in one beat
FIRM Rotor mapping	Map AF rotors

The two mapping systems available so far were the CARTO system (Biosense-Webster) and the EnSite Velocity (St. Jude) system. The recent entrants in this field are Rhythmia (Boston), FIRM and ECVue.

CARTO: It uses the catheter with magnetic sensor and reference sensor along with an external ultra-low magnetic emitter and processing unit to yield locations in three dimension. The recorded electrogram leads to formation of the electro-anatomical maps and tagging the points help in ablation. The latest generation CARTO 3 (Fig. 1), has improved upon its earlier versions by allowing to visualize multiple catheters; the fast anatomical mapping (FAM) technology helps in creating the chamber geometry and activation sequence quickly by simultaneously acquiring data points while the catheter is moving. Advanced technology helps to compensate for the patient and cardiac motion. The ablation catheter has a sensor which works only for 24 hours after the catheter is opened.

EnSite velocity is the latest 3D mapping system by St. Jude. It is an open platform, using three low amplitude high frequency current fields in three axes over the patients thorax to compute the positions of electrode in the thorax relative to a reference electrode that can be placed in the heart or on patients thorax. The greatest advantage of this system is that multiple catheters – diagnostic and therapeutic, of any vendor can be used. It provides visibility of patient rhythm in the fewest possible cardiac cycles when using contact mapping and can be integrated with most ablation generators and recording systems and also with the remote navigation systems and rotational angiography.

Rhythmia system is designed to intelligently automate map creation, increasing speed and improving the density of mapping. The system also

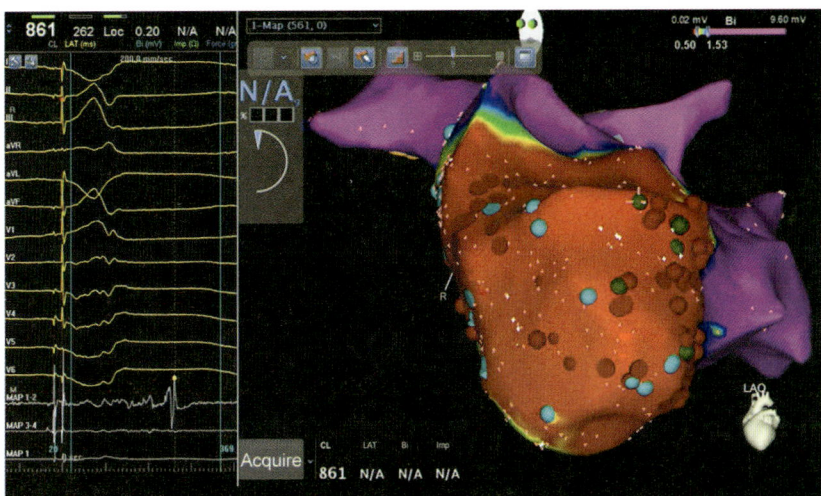

Fig. 1: The ablation and scar isolation in a patient with ventricular tachycardia.

features vMap, a validation map, which is designed to rapidly confirm the endpoints of the ablation treatment. Continuous mapping of thousands of data sets is its unique feature. This eliminates the need for manual annotation.

ECVue is another 3D electrocardiographic mapping system by CardioInsight. It is noninvasive and uses a 256-lead electrocardiogram (ECG) vest, which is worn during a computed tomography (CT) scan. A 3D reconstruction of the heart model is used, on which the electrical activity is superimposed from this vest. The imaging is created in one heartbeat and produces a colored map of the entire heart. This method of mapping would help to visualize rotors and also guide cardiac resynchronization therapy (CRT) lead implants.

Focal Impulse and Rotor Modulation (FIRM), is yet another electroanatomic mapping technique (RhythmView, Topera), especially to visualize the rotation of electrical activation in cardiac tissue, which is believed to be the cause of AF. Small studies like CONFIRM and PRECISE, have looked at whether FIRM ablation can effectively treat AF. Although preliminary results appear promising, they do not seem to be reproducible and the concept needs to be validated in larger patient population.

ABLATION ENERGY

Since its introduction in early 90's, radiofrequency ablation is the standard treatment for various supraventricular and VT. But there are limitations associated with its use like risk of steam ops, perforation due to high energy delivery or in-effective ablation because of insufficient energy delivery to ensure durable, large, transmural lesions. This difficulties can be tackled with the help of various newer technologies like alternative energy sources, contact force sensing catheters, stabilizing sheaths, higher radiofrequency (RF) induced heating by use of different agents. The various alternative energy sources that have been proposed are cryoenergy, microwave, laser, high intensity focused ultrasound and more recently electroporation for ablation. Cryoablation is the most promising for quick pulmonary vein isolation (PVI) for AF and ablation around the atrioventricular (AV) node to prevent complete heart block.

Cryoablation for tachycardia's like atrioventricular nodal reentry tachycardia (AVNRT), Para-Hisian accessory pathways and junctional tachycardia's has been suggested to be superior to RF energy, preventing AV blocks requiring permanent pacemaker implantation, especially in children. "Ice mapping", with reversibility of the AV block was proposed as an advantage for arrhythmias around the AV node. However a retrospective analysis confirms equal efficacy, safety and long-term outcomes of both sources of energy.[1]

Cryoablation for AF using the Arctic Front Advance, by Medtronics has already received the food and drug administration (FDA) approval and there are recent trials to suggest its safety and efficacy. The FIRE and ICE investigators published, Cryoballoon (CB) versus RF energy for PVI in patients with paroxysmal AF. The study established the non-inferiority of CB and also the safety as compared to RF ablation.[2] Future technological advances in both forms (cryo and RF) of ablation therapy are likely to impact their outcomes.

CATHETERS (TABLE 2)

Open irrigated catheters allows a more deeper and transmural lesions to achieve a long-term success with low recurrence for AF and VT ablations. However a low contact force can lead to ineffective lesions, and an excessive force may cause perforations. The latest trend in transcatheter ablation technology has been the development of force sensing catheters to apply enough force, resulting in adequate lesions, to improving outcomes. Biosense Webster and Endosense are the two companies manufacturing these catheters. A 1-year safety and efficacy (SMART-AF)[3] results of the Thermocool Smart-touch catheter (Biosense Webster) was presented for symptomatic, drug refractory, paroxysmal AF. The system enables electrophysiologists to directly measure contact force. An increased percent of time in contact force range correlated with increased freedom from arrhythmia recurrence. 84.4% patients were arrhythmia-free at 12 months when the force was within the targeted range >82% of the time. Endosense presented data from its EFFICAS I prospective multicenter study, which led to the development of guidelines for target and minimum contact force, as well as minimum force time integral (FTI), during the catheter ablation treatment of paroxysmal AF. The newly created guidelines call for a contact force target of 20 gm (and minimum CF of 10 gm) and minimum FTI of 400 gm per individual ablation lesion. The results of EFFICAS I demonstrated the importance of CF in the long-term effectiveness of catheter ablation for treating paroxysmal AF.

Table 2: Advancement in catheter technology.	
Diagnostic catheters	Variable curve PV mapping catheter
	Multi-electrode Basket catheters
Therapeutic catheters	8 mm tip RF ablation
	Irrigated tip catheter (bi-directional variable curves)
	Contact force catheter
	CRYO-Balloon
	Multi-electrode ablation catheter

Multi-electrode ablation with phased RF-energy is feasible and initial data on efficacy and safety are promising for PVI. The procedure and fluoroscopy time may be shortened. However this technology needs to undergo the rigor of clinical trials before it can be accepted as mainstream technology.

Variable curve LASSO, bi-directional different curve ablation catheters have helped to compensate for the variable chamber and pulmonary vein size to effectively map and ablate. Steerable sheaths help in circumventing the problem of catheter movement due to respiration and cardiac motion. Stabilizing the catheter during RF ablation for AF reduces the procedure time and improves success and freedom from AF recurrences.

High frequency jet ventilation[4] is another attempt in achieving catheter stability. General anesthesia and muscle relaxants eliminate the respiratory movement, minimizing catheter dislodgement and destabilization at the catheter-tissue interface. High frequency jet ventilation helps to maintain the oxygenation. Proper case selection and technique must be ensured.

High rate pacing[4] is an innovative approach in reducing the motion variation and improve catheter stability. High right atrium (RA) or coronary sinus (CS) pacing is performed to minimize cardiac motion.

ATRIAL FIBRILLATION ABLATION

Ablation strategy for AF continue to be varying from operator to operator and various attempts have been made to optimize the lesions necessary for an effective long-term success. In patients with paroxysmal AF, PVI is performed either by segmental ablation using the LASSO catheter or circumferential ablation encircling the pulmonary veins. Antral PVI methods are extremely effective for paroxysmal AF ablation and are preferred. This technique is likely to eliminate arrhythmogenic sites within pulmonary veins (PVs) and their antrum by debulking of left atrium by about 25 to 30%; ablation of anchor points or 'Rotors' which are near antrum; ablation of the ganglionated plexi and possibly ablation of the ligament of Marshall. The wide area circumferential ablation necessarily requires 3D anatomic mapping.

The Substrate and Trigger Ablation for Reduction of Atrial Fibrillation trial Part II (STAR AF II) compared the strategy of PVI alone vs. PVI plus complex fractionated abnormal electrograms ablation vs. PVI plus left atrial linear ablation lines in patients with persistent AF. The lesions in addition to PVI did not yield better outcomes, and freedom from AF recurrence without anti-arrhythmic drugs is only 41% at 1 year.[5] This clearly suggested further refinements are necessary and in this regards using contact force irrigation ablation catheter might fill the gap.

Many centers use adenosine to assess the completeness of PVI ablation, however this endpoint remains to be established conclusively. Electrical

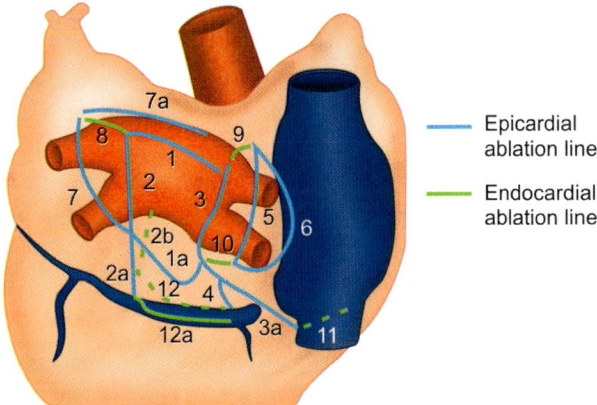

Fig. 2: Convergent lesion sets using endo and epicardial ablation for atrial fibrillation.

isolation of the left atrial appendage by ablation and targeting the ganglionated plexus is being evaluated for AF ablation.

Convergent procedure integrate the epicardial approach with the routine endocardial approach for the ablation of the long standing AF by PVI, coronary sinus ablation, creation of cavotricuspid isthmus & posterior left atrial exclusion (Fig. 2). Through subxiphoid route sheath is introduced in pericardial space & then mapping of the epicardial surface is done. Care should be taken to avoid injury to epicardial coronary vessels & angiography can help to localize these vessels.

VENTRICULAR TACHYCARDIA ABLATION

To achieve long-term success in ischemic-scar related VT ablation, there is an on-going debate regarding targeting the clinical VT morphology using the activation and entrainment mapping technique versus the substrate mapping. This was prospectively answered in the VISTA study,[6] comprising of 118 patients with well-tolerated, ischemic VT. At 1-year follow-up, the substrate ablation strategy resulted in a significant reduction in VT recurrence (16% vs. 48%); lower use of antiarrhythmic drugs (12% vs. 58%); and a lower incidence of the combined endpoint of death or re-hospitalization (21% vs. 47%). Extensive ablation targeting abnormal late and complex fractionated signals within the scar during sinus rhythm appears to be more effective exposing the limitations of entrainment mapping. In clinical practice it seems prudent to do substrate mapping and then targeting the VTs if still inducible by the activation map and entrainment techniques.

Survival advantage with ablation of VT in structural heart disease remains questionable. A multicenter, retrospective study of ablation outcomes in 2,061 patients,[7] implied that those without VT recurrences had better survival. The 12-month incidence of death or heart transplant was 15% in patients undergoing successful VT ablation.

Epicardial ablation for VTs in non-ischemic dilated cardiomyopathy was first performed by Sousa et al. and now is practiced world over. The VT focus in ischemic heart disease and scar is often subendocardial and amenable by standard endocardial ablation approach. However in the non-ischemic dilated cardiomyopathy, the scar can be subepicardial and not accessible by the endocardial route. Overall about 17% of VTs require epicardial approach for ablation.[8] Most often it is used after a failed endocardial attempt. However the understanding of the epicardial focus is improving and some high volume centers begin with pericardial access to begin with. A long Tuhoy needle is used to access the pericardial space, often using contrast and tenting the parietal pericardium. Activation map and endocardial mapping is simultaneously done and it is also important to identify no coronary artery is close during epicardial ablation.

REMOTE NAVIGATION SYSTEMS

During the ablation procedure, a stable and reproducible catheter movements are very important to increase the success rate and prevent the catheter related complications. To deal with these limitations the remote navigation systems are developed to allow manipulation of the catheters in precise and reproducible manner and from a distant control room. Two navigation systems are available in clinical practice.

The Niobe magnetic navigation system[9]—in this system two large permanent magnets are used to create low intensity magnetic field in patients chest. The catheters having permanent magnet in there distal portions are then navigated in cardiac chambers by changing the orientation of magnetic fields by use of joystick in the control room with highly precise control of the catheter. For the use of this system the catheterization laboratory should be equipped with the steel plates and specialized equipment to prevent magnetic field interference with other equipment.

The Sensei robotic navigation system[9]—uses the steerable sheaths with catheter placed within it, which are then manipulated within the heart via a pull wire mechanism by robotic arm fixed at fluoroscopy table. With use of 3D joystick broad range of motion in virtually all planes, can be achieved from central computer workstation. This system is transportable and does not require construction of specialized room. Although all electro-anatomical systems may be used, but NAVX is most commonly used along with it.

The recent advances and publications in clinical electrophysiology[10] in the past few years have considerably impacted the outcomes of heart rhythm disorders. From improvements in mapping systems to innovations in catheter technology and the remote navigation, the future of ablation is exciting. Crystallizing the concepts of arrhythmia origin and mechanism should help standardize the ablation procedural steps; these should be reproducible amongst electrophysiologists across the globe to have a meaningful impact on patients with arrhythmias. The advancement of technology adds to the cost of the procedure, which needs to be countered by accepting the most effective tools usable and applicable to the vast majority of the patients world-wide.

REFERENCES

1. Schwagten B, Knops P, Janse P. et al. Long-term follow-up after catheter. Ablation for atrioventricular nodal reentrant tachycardia: a comparison of cryothermal and radiofrequency energy in a large series of patients. J Interv Card Electrophysiol. 2011;30:55-61.
2. Kuck KH, Brugada J, Fürnkranz A. et al. Cryoballoon or radiofrequency ablation for paroxysmal atrial fibrillation. N Engl J Med. 2016;374:2235-45.
3. Natale A, Reddy VY, Monir G, et al. Paroxysmal AF catheter ablation with a contact force sensing catheter: results of the prospective, multicenter SMART-AF trial. J Am Coll Cardiol. 2014;64:647-56.
4. Rafael A, Heist EK. Techniques to optimize catheter contact force during ablation of atrial fibrillation. Innovat Card Rhythm Manag. 2015;6:1990-95.
5. Verma A, Jiang CY, Betts TR, et al. The STAR AF II investigators. Approaches to catheter ablation for persistent atrial fibrillation. New Engl J Med. 2015;372:1812–22.
6. Luigi Di Biase, Burkhardt JD, Lakkireddy D. et al. Ablation of stable VTs versus substrate ablation in ischemic cardiomyopathy - The VISTA randomized multicenter trial. J Am Coll Cardiol. 2015;66:2872-82.
7. Tung R, Vaseghi M, Frankel DS, et al. Freedom from recurrent ventricular tachycardia after catheter ablation is associated with improved survival in patients with structural heart disease: an International VT Ablation Center Collaborative Group study. Heart Rhythm. 2015;12:1997-2007.
8. Maccabelli G, Mizuno H, Bella PD. Epicardial ablation for ventricular tachycardia. Indian Pacing Electrophysiol J. 2012;12(6):250-68.
9. Lien NB, Jose ML, Eli GS. Remote navigation for ablation procedures – a new step forward in the treatment of cardiac arrhythmias. Europ Cardiol. 2010;6(3):50-6.
10. Wilber DJ, Singh JP. Advances in clinical electrophysiology 2015 in review. JACC: Clinical Electrophysiology. 2016;2(1):124-7.

24 Newer Devices in Electrophysiology: Leadless Pacemakers and Subcutaneous ICD

Ameya Udyavar

INTRODUCTION

There has been substantial improvement in devices like pacemakers and defibrillators in the last 50 years. These devices have reduced in size, improved in circuitry and battery longevity and use automatic algorithms to optimize their utility and longevity. However, the implant procedure entails risk like hemothorax or pneumothorax due to subclavian artery or lung injury respectively. During long-term follow-up, there could be issues like subclavian vein thrombosis/occlusion, lead fractures and generator infections. To overcome these problems, the last few years have seen development of leadless pacemakers or subcutaneous leads to avoid complications associated with the lead, which happen to be the weakest link in this procedure.

The leadless pacemakers and subcutaneous implantable cardioverter defibrillators (ICDs) have proven their efficacy in clinical trials and are now commercially available in India. However they are advised only for a particular subset of patients. In this chapter we will be discussing about the devices available in India, the device hardware and the steps necessary to implant these devices. The article will end with the current indications and brief overview about their clinical trial data.

LEADLESS PACEMAKER

With advancement of technology, the pacemakers have been miniaturized with the lead and the generator accommodated in a single unit. This obviates the need for pacing leads and their introduction through the veins and its concurrent complications.

Though the idea of using a leadless system was tested in a canine 40 years ago,[1] its was only after another 20 years it was found feasible in preclinical testing.[2] Currently 2 types of leadless pacemakers are commercially available for clinical use. These are:
1. The Nanostim leadless pacemaker from St. Jude Medical.

Chapter 24: Newer Devices in Electrophysiology   337

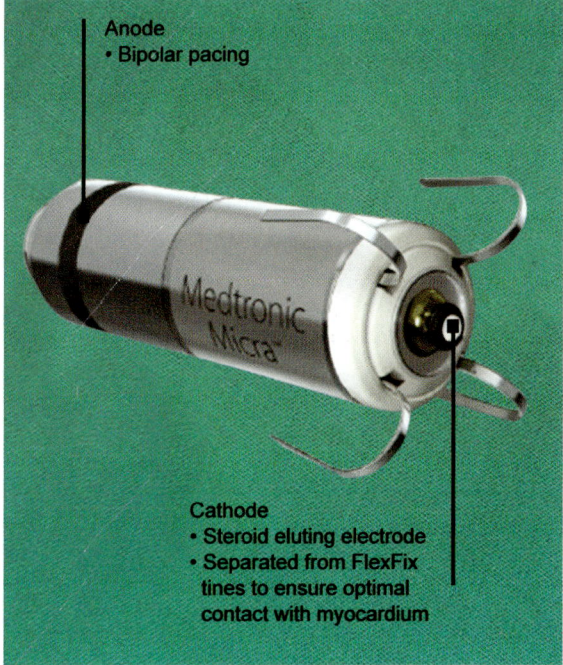

Fig. 1: The leadless pacemaker (Micra) from Medtronic.
Courtesy: Medtronic.

2. Micra Transcatheter Pacing system from Medtronic (Fig. 1). Both are leadless pacemakers with the battery, circuit and the pace/sense lead encased in a single unit. The Micra device is the one, which is currently available in India and has already been implanted in few patients in last few months. Currently these devices are single chamber pacemakers and can pace/sense only in one chamber. This restricts their utility to patients who need VVI pacing. Its expected that with further advancements they will be available for use in both chambers in the years to come.

MICRA TRANSCATHETER PACING SYSTEM (TPS)

The Micra Transcatheter Pacing system is composed of an introducer, a delivery system and a leadless pacemaker.
1. **Leadless pacemaker** (Fig. 1)
   The Micra pacemaker is a capsule like device measuring 26 mm with an outer diameter of 6.7 mm (20.1 Fr). The volume is 0.8 cc with a mass of 1.75 g. The electrodes are made of titanium nitride and are 18 mm apart.[3] The cathode electrode at the tip (which is in contact with the muscle after deployment) is steroid eluting. The fixation mechanism is by 4 Nitinol FlexFix tines (Fig. 1). These tines are in the delivery sheath

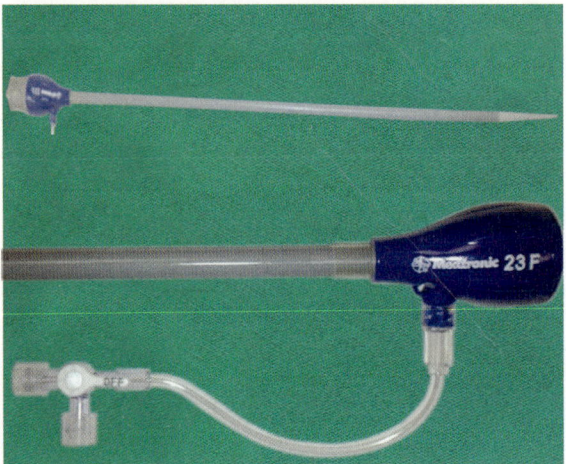

Fig. 2: The introducer with the dilator.
Courtesy: Medtronic.

before deployment and are released once the device is pushed out of the sheath to be anchored in the trabeculae. The device is attached/tethered to the delivery system and then cut once the device is deployed. The battery is made of Lithium-hybrid carbon monofluoride/silver vanadium oxide. The device is magnetic resonance imaging compatible and has an estimated longevity of 10-12 years. The device has rate responsive feature, which gets activated by an accelerometer sensor.

2. **The introducer with dilator** (Fig. 2)
   The introducer sheath is a large bore sheath with an internal diameter of 7.8 mm (23F) and outer diameter of 27F. It is hydrophilic coated and has length of 73 mm with a working length of 55.7 cm. The sheath has a stopcock for aspiration and flushing and a radiopaque marker on end of the introducer for location identification. The Dilator has a working length of 70 cm with a guide wire compatibility of 0.034 inches.

3. **The Delivery system** (Figs. 3 and 4).
   The Micra delivery system consists of the following parts:
   a. A delivery catheter designed to deliver and position the device for implant in the right ventricle by accessing this chamber through the femoral vein. The delivery catheter has a steerable, flexible shaft with a distal end that contains a device cup to hold the device and a recapture cone to retrieve it. It has an outer diameter of 23F (which is compatible with the Micra Introducer) and has an effective length of 105 cm. Additionally, it can function as a retrieval catheter post tether removal.
   b. A handle with controls to navigate the delivery catheter and deploy the device. The handle also provides a tether designed as an aid to

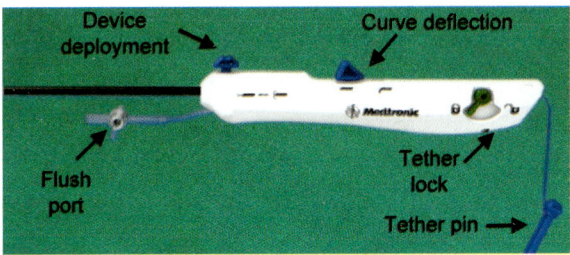

Fig. 3: Micra delivery system handle.
Courtesy: Medtronic.

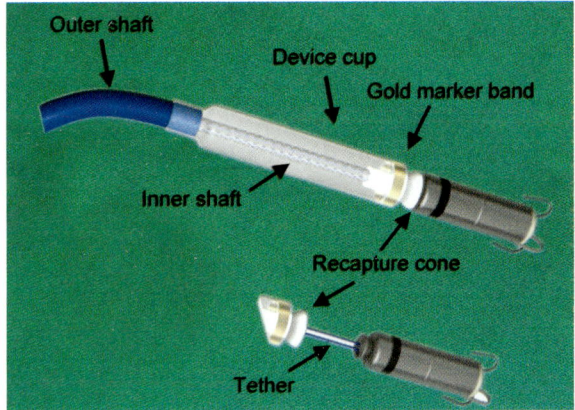

Fig. 4: The distal end of the Micra delivery system.
Courtesy: Medtronic.

test the device fixation and to recapture and reposition the device for proper fixation during the implant procedure.

IMPLANT PROCEDURE (FIG. 5)

The steps of the Micra pacemaker implant are as follows:[4,5]
1. **Venous access and insertion of the introducer**
   Femoral vein access is achieved and confirmed by fluoroscopy and a 6F/10F sheath is passed into the femoral vein. A stiff guide wire (Amplatz Super Stiff guidewire is passed up to the right atrium. The sheath is then removed and exchanged for the Micra introducer. The 23F introducer sheath is flushed with normal saline, which is attached to the stop cork at the distal end. The sheath is continuously flushed to avoid clot formation and prevent air embolism in the sheath while withdrawing the dilator. The introducer is passed up to the right atrium and then the dilator withdrawn.

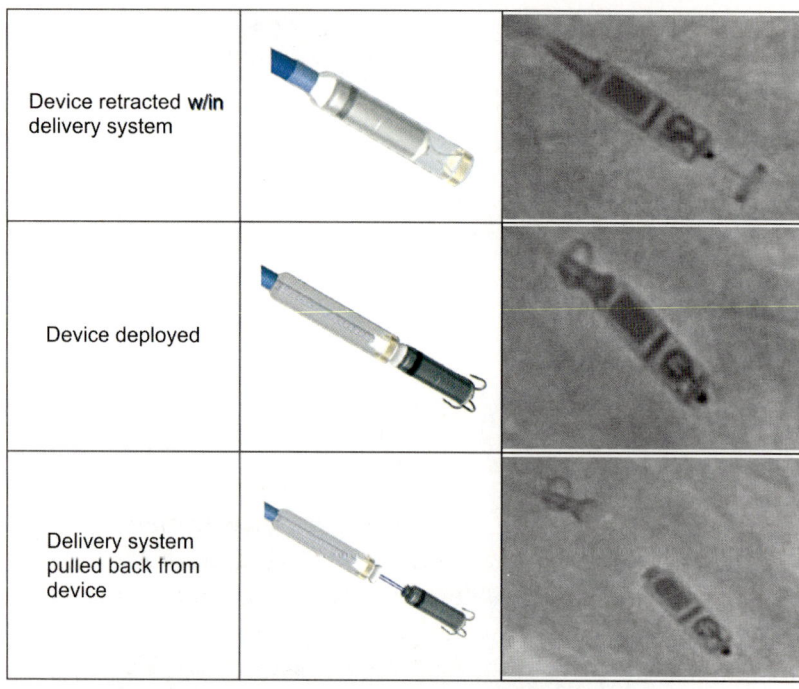

Fig. 5: The implant procedure for the Micra pacemaker.
Courtesy: Medtronic.

2. **Passage of the delivery system into the right ventricle**
   The Delivery system is then flushed continuously and inserted into the introducer. It is then pushed till it reached the right atrium at which stage the introducer is pulled back into the inferior vena cava. The delivery system is the curved using the deflection handle to cross the tricuspid annulus. A counterclockwise rotation might be necessary to aid its passage into the right ventricle. This is done under fluoroscopy guidance and the position confirmed in RAO and LAO projections. Once the device crosses the tricuspid annulus, a clockwise torque is applied to as to direct the device to the right ventricular septum.
3. **Confirming the position in the RV septum**
   Diluted contrast is injected via the delivery system to verify the position of the tip toward the septum. The intention is to avoid the free wall to reduce the risk of free wall perforation.
4. **Deploying the Micra device**
   The first step is to unlock the tether and remove the tether pin once the desired location has been confirmed. The protective sleeve is withdrawn so as to expose the tines. These tines then are released and anchor the device in the trabeculae. Throughout this maneuver, the delivery sheath is kept flexed.

5. **Testing the stability of the device deployment**
   Once the device has been deployed, the pull and hold test is performed by pulling on the tether. Movement of 2 out of the 4 tines ensures that the device is adequately fixed. Subsequently the electrical parameters are tested.
6. **Cutting the tether**
   The tether should then be removed to release the Micra. Once the tether is fully removed, the delivery system is withdrawn from the introducer. The position of the Micra is confirmed in both LAO and RAO views. Subsequently the introducer is removed and hemostasis achieved with application of pressure or a purse string suture.

CURRENT INDICATIONS FOR THE LEADLESS PACEMAKER

The currently available leadless pacemakers are single chamber pacemakers and are so capable of being deployed in single chamber preferably in the right ventricle. Thus they are ideal of patients with atrial fibrillation with complete heart block/slow ventricular rate. Elderly patients with severe morbidity are preferred so as to avoid complications associated with lead implantation.

CLINICAL EXPERIENCE

The Medtronic IDE trial reported around 700 patients who were successfully implanted with Micra transcatheter pacemakers. The success rate was 99.2% with the overall major complication rate being 51% lower that the historical control of leaded systems.[6] Similarly, the Nanostim leadless pacemaker showed promising results with high success rate and low complication rate.[7]

SUMMARY ABOUT LEADLESS PACEMAKER

- The Leadless pacemaker is a capsule shaped device, which houses the lead, battery and the circuitry in a single unit.
- The current devices available for clinical use are Micra from Medtronic and Nanostim from St. Jude Medical.
- Its currently being used for patients with atrial fibrillation as it provides only single chamber pacing.
- It avoids the complications associated with per-venous lead placement.
- It is deployed in the right ventricular septum with the help of a delivery apparatus.
- The clinical data available currently has been promising and may provide dual chamber pacing capabilities in the future.

SUBCUTANEOUS IMPLANTABLE CARDIOVERTER DEFIBRILLATOR (S-ICD)

S-ICDs have been developed with the intention of avoiding complications associated with the ICD leads. Also since the procedure does not need venous access, it does away with the need to do fluoroscopy.

Boston Scientific, Marlborough, MA, develops the current subcutaneous implantable cardioverter defibrillator (S-ICD) used in clinical practice. It uses a pulse generator, which is implanted in the anterior axillary line near the 6th intercostal space. The ICD lead is an 8 cm shocking coil, which is placed parallel and to the left of the sternum. There are 2 sensing electrodes on either side of the coil which as the distal and proximal electrode in relation to the generator. The proximal and distal electrodes and the coil create three different vectors, which allow for sensing and detection of the arrhythmias. The current pulse generator weighs 145 g and has a volume of 69 mL (Fig. 6).

IMPLANT PROCEDURE (FIG. 7)

The greatest clinical experience in around 4000 patients is with a 3-incision technique. The incision for the generator is at the level of the 5th or 6th intercostal space, between the anterior and mid-axillary lines. A 2nd incision (1–1.5 cm) is placed horizontally at the xiphoid directed leftwards. A proprietary tool is used to tunnel the lead from the device pocket to the incision. A similar incision is employed superiorly at the sternomanubrial junction. The lead is then tunneled parallel to the sternum and then anchored at all three incision sites. The whole procedure is based on anatomical landmarks and so does not require fluoroscopy.[8]

Following implantation, defibrillation testing is then performed using 65-J shocks to terminated ventricular fibrillation. The S-ICD delivers nonprogrammable 80-J shocks, so testing at 65 J ensures adequate safety margin.

EFFICACY AND SAFETY OF THE DEVICE

In the largest prospective multicenter evaluation of the safety and efficacy of the device, 304 patients underwent successful implantation and defibrillation testing. There was a 99% complication free rate at the end of 180 days. There were no cases of lead failures, endocarditis, hemopneumothorax. The efficacy of acute conversion of VF with 65J shock was 100%.[9]

The EFFORTLESS S-ICD registry of 472 patients with a mean follow-up of 558 days showed a complication rate of 3% with one hematoma, pneumothorax and one pleural effusion. Eighteen patients (4%) had infection

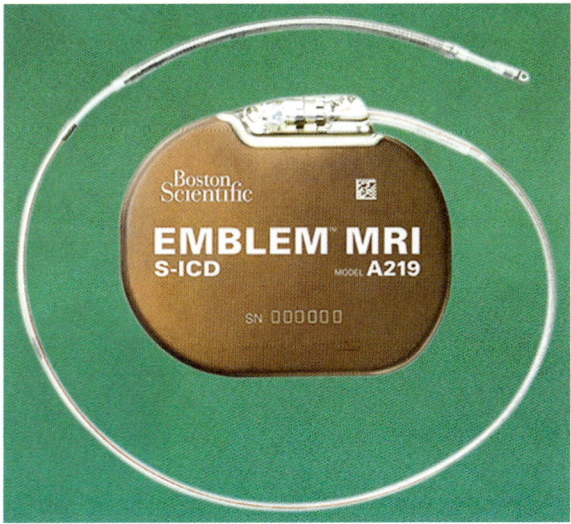

Fig. 6: The subcutaneous implantable cardioverter defibrillator (S-ICD).
Courtesy: Boston Scientific.

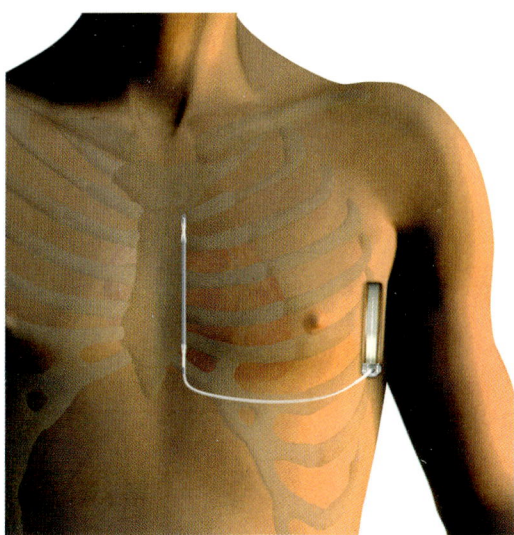

Fig. 7: Placement of the generator in the anterior axillary line and placement of the lead in the left parasternal region.
Courtesy: Boston Scientific.

of which 10 warranted explantation of the device. In this registry the single-shock success rate for VT/VF was 88%.[10]

A 2-year result of a pooled analysis of S-ICD studies and registry confirmed the efficacy of the device in treating VT/VF episodes.[11]

CURRENT INDICATIONS OF THE S-ICD

The device is suitable for patients with poor vascular access or previous infection. Patients who are at infection risk like patients with diabetes, renal failure on dialysis, mechanical valves are more likely to benefit. Patients with genetic channelopathies like long QT syndromes, Brugada syndrome are likely to benefit as there is no need to antitachycardia pacing (ATP) or pacing in these patients.[8,12]

LIMITATIONS OF THE S-ICD

Patients who require chronic pacing due to sinus node and atrioventricular node dysfunction, biventricular pacing for heart failure should not be considered for the S-ICD as the device is not able to support ventricular pacing except for a few seconds following a shock. Similarly, the device is incapable of ATP and so, its role for patients who need ATP to terminate monomorphic VTs will be limited.[8] Most of the trials have reported an infection rate of 5-9%. The other limitations of the device are short (5 years) longevity of the device, lack of remote monitoring capability (which simplifies follow-up).

Over-sensing of T waves and myopotential signals produces most inappropriate S-ICD shocks ranging from 5 to 25%. Pre-implant screening of patients utilizing surface electrodes to avoid T-wave over sensing (in all 3 sensing vectors) prior to device implantation is crucial. The addition of a second tachycardia zone to S-ICD programming may significantly reduce the rate of inappropriate shocks.[8,12]

SUMMARY ABOUT SUBCUTANEOUS ICD

- The subcutaneous ICD were developed in order to overcome problems associated with ICD lead which are seen in as high as 20% of patients on long-term follow-up.
- The S-ICD constitutes a generator, which is implanted in the anterior axillary line in 5-6th intercostal space and the lead, which is placed in the left parasternal region.
- A 3-incision technique is most commonly used to implant the device though a 2-incision technique has also been described.
- The implant procedure does not need fluoroscopy or any venous access to position the leads.
- The current S-ICDs have shown good efficacy and safety in medium term follow-up.
- Though the incidence of inappropriate shocks has ranged from 5 to 20%, its expected that with advances in technology and software, the incidence will decrease in the future.

CONCLUSION

With advances and refinements in technology, the usage of leadless pacemakers and subcutaneous implantable defibrillators will see a rise in the next decade. A proper understanding of its indications, hardware and the implant technique is necessary to provide maximum benefit to the patient. A proper follow-up and optimum programming of each implanted device as per the needs of patient's clinical condition is necessary to derive maximum benefit or the device and optimize its battery life.

REFERENCES

1. Lown B, Kosowsky BD. Artificial cardiac pacemakers. I. N Engl J Med. 1970; 283(17):907-16.
2. Sutton R. The first European journal on cardiac electrophysiology and pacing, the European Journal of Cardiac Pacing and Electrophysiology. Europace. 2011;13(12):1663-4.
3. Ritter P, Duray GZ, Steinwender C, et al. Early performance of a miniaturized leadless cardiac pacemaker: the Micra Transcatheter Pacing Study. Eur Heart J. 2015;36(37):2510-9.
4. El-Chami MF, Roberts PR, Kypta A, et al. How to Implant a Leadless Pacemaker With a Tine-Based Fixation. J Cardiovasc Electrophysiol. 2016;27(12):1495-150.
5. Miller MA, Neuzil P, Dukkipati SR, Reddy VY. Leadless Cardiac Pacemakers: Back to the Future. J Am Coll Cardiol. 2015;66(10):1179-89.
6. Reynolds DW, Ritter P. A Leadless Intracardiac Transcatheter Pacing System. N Engl J Med. 2016;374(26):2604-5.
7. Reddy VY. A Leadless Cardiac Pacemaker. N Engl J Med. 2016;374(6):594.
8. McLeod CJ, Boersma L, Okamura H, Friedman PA. The subcutaneous implantable cardioverter defibrillator: state-of-the-art review. Eur Heart J. 2015. [Epub ahead of print].
9. Weiss R, Knight BP, Gold MR, et al. Safety and efficacy of a totally subcutaneous implantable-cardioverter defibrillator. Circulation. 2013;128(9):944-53.
10. Lambiase PD, Barr C, Theuns DA, et al. Worldwide experience with a totally subcutaneous implantable defibrillator: early results from the EFFORTLESS S-ICD Registry. Eur Heart J. 2014;35(25):1657-65.
11. Burke MC, Gold MR, Knight BP, et al. Safety and Efficacy of the Totally Subcutaneous Implantable Defibrillator: 2-Year Results From a Pooled Analysis of the IDE Study and EFFORTLESS Registry. J Am Coll Cardiol. 2015;65(16):1605-15.
12. Aziz S, Leon AR, El-Chami MF. The subcutaneous defibrillator: a review of the literature. J Am Coll Cardiol. 2014;63(15):1473-9.

Index

A

Absorbable metal stent 17
Absorbable stents 11
Activated clotting time (ACT) 57, 290
Acute coronary syndrome 26, 140
Acute myocardial infarction 11, 118
Acute stent thrombosis 143
Adenosine diphosphate (ADP) antagonists 143
Advanced atherosclerosis 97
Alcohol septal ablation (ASA) 304, 306
American College of Cardiology 141
American Heart Association 141, 305
Amplatzer devices 300
Amplatzer duct 300
Amplatzer septal occluder 289
Amsterdam-Rotterdam (AMRO) trial 111
Anatomy of aortic valve 255
Angiographic binary restenosis 102
Annulus fibrosus 229
Antegrade lumen 56
Antegrade wire dissection and reentry 54
Anterior mitral leaflet (AML) 304
Aortic aneurysm 212
Aortic bifurcation 156
Aortic stenosis 257
Aortitis 60
Aorto-ostial disease 60
Aorto-ostial occlusions 46
Aorto-ostial stent 60
Arterial grafts 116
Asian population criteria 39
Aspiration thrombectomy 142
Atherectomy devices 112
Atherosclerosis 60
Atherosclerotic plaques 122, 181

Atrial fibrillation 328
Autonomic denervation of the donor heart 227

B

β-adrenergic receptor 227
Balloon angioplasty 11
Balloon aortic valvuloplasty 254
    antegrade approach 260
        complications 261
        post-procedure care 260
    consent 256
    indications 254
    pre-catheterization planning 255
    procedure 256
        access 256
        anesthesia 256
        balloon 257
        catheters and wires 257
        steps (retrograde approach) 258
        variations in procedure 259
Balloon diameter 251
Balloon dilatation 100
Balloon mitral valvuloplasty 229
    anatomic considerations 229
    BMV in difficult scenarios 239
        BMV in giant LA/IAS aneurysm 241
        BMV in IVC interruption 241
        BMV in juvenile mitral stenosis 241
        BMV in LA/LAA clot 239
        BMV in pregnancy 242
        BMV in severe subvalvular disease 241
    complications 242
        acute mitral regurgitation 242
        immediate results 244
        long-term results 244

pericardial effusion/tamponade 242
residual atrial septal defect 243
stroke, embolism 243
contraindications 231
historical aspect 229
indications and recommendations 230
patient preparation 232
periprocedural care 231
preprocedural planning 231
role of echocardiography in BMV 231
techniques 233
approach 233
choice of technique 233
crossing the mitral valve 236
dilatation of IAS puncture site 234
inoue balloon technique 233
selection of balloon catheter 234
transseptal puncture 233
vascular access 233
Balloon on antegrade wire 56
Balloon rupture 97
Balloon versus stents 144
Bare metal stents 12
Bifurcation disease 64
Brockenbrough needle 233
Buddy wire 64
Buerger's disease 6

C

Calcified lesions 97
assessment 97
coronary angiography 98
coronary intravascular ultrasound 98
fractional flow reserve 98
lesion preparation 99
optical coherence tomography 98
procedure planning 97
risk assessment 99
treatment 99
Calcified plaque 182
Calcium scoring 216
Cannulation of femoral artery 3
Cardiac CT 211
Cardiac CT angiography 216
Cardiac electrophysiology 328
ablation energy 330
atrial fibrillation ablation 332
catheters 331
mapping techniques 328

CARTO 329
ECVue 330
EnSite velocity 329
focal impulse and rotor
modulation 330
rhythmia system 329
remote navigation systems 334
ventricular tachycardia ablation 333
Cardiac presynaptic sympathetic nerve 227
CA scoring 211
Chordae tendinae 229
Chronic total occlusions 45, 120
access and dual angiography 47
antegrade wire manipulations and
techniques 49
current strategy 50
parallel wire techniques 51
strategy based on wire
advancement 51
wire escalation 49
rationale of the approaches 49
retrograde approach 54
collateral assessment 55
collateral channel navigation 55
crossing the occlusion 55
retrograde wire in the proximal segment and externalization 57
setting up for a CTO case 46
angiographic assessment of CTO
lesion 46
collateral circulation assessment 46
Classic crush technique 84
Closure devices 5
Complications during percutaneous
coronary interventions 162
coronary artery complications 162
arrhythmias 170
coronary and stent thrombosis 165
coronary dissection and abrupt
closure 169
coronary perforation 166
slow/no reflow 162
other complications 174
cerebrovascular events 175
cholesterol crystal embolism
(CCE) 177
contrast-induced nephropathy 174
radiation toxicity 175
retained PCI equipment
components 176

vascular access site related
 complications 170
 access site bleeding and
  hematoma 171
 radial artery access 173
 retroperitoneal bleeding 172
Congenital heart defects (CHDs) 247
Controlled antegrade retrograde
 subintimal tracking (CART) 55
Conventional fluoroscopic methods 60
Coronary angiography 212
 bypass surgery 214
 cardiac MRI 214
 coronary arteries 215
 perfusion 214, 215
 plaque evaluation 213
 stents 212
 viability imaging 215
Coronary artery bypass grafting 11
Coronary artery disease (CAD) 197, 211
Coronary artery dissection 97
Coronary artery fistula 289
Coronary atherectomy 64
Coronary bifurcation lesions 70
 anatomical considerations 71
 classifications 70
 elective double-stent strategy 81
 evidence 75
 indications 81
 provisional side branch stenting
  strategy 75
 stenting strategy 75
 steps 77
  pre-dilatation 77
  SB rewiring or guide wire exchange 78
  stenting the MV across the SB 77
  wiring both the branches 77
 techniques 82
  classical T-stenting 82
  crush technique 82
  nodified T-stenting or minicrush 82
 technique variations 83
  Culotte technique 85
  double kiss step crush technique or
   sleeve technique 83
  internal or reverse crush technique 83
  micro crush technique 84
  simultaneous kissing stents (SKS)
   technique 86
  step crush technique 83
  V-stenting technique 86
Coronary bifurcations 75
Coronary dissections 104
Coronary spasm 104
Coronary stents 11
 first-generation stents 12
 magmaris stent 17
 plain balloon angioplasty 11
 second-generation DES 13
 third-generation stents 14
  bioabsorbable scaffolds 14
  evolution of bioabsorbable stents 15
Coronary wires 206
Crush technique 40
CTO toolbox of guiding wires 52
Culotte technique 86
Cutting balloon angioplasty 100

D

Debulking devices 100
 cutting balloon 100
  clinical evidence 102
  device 100
  mechanism of action 100
 laser atherectomy 110
  clinical evidence 111
  device 110
  mechanism of action 110
 orbital atherectomy 108
  clinical evidence 109
  device 108
  mechanism of action 108
 rotational atherectomy 104
  clinical evidence 106
  complications 106
  device 104
  mechanism of action 105
 scoring balloon 103
  clinical evidence 103
  complications 104
  device 103
  mechanism of action 103
Dedicated bifurcation stent system 90
 advantages 92
 categories 91
 challenges 91
 preliminary clinical results 92

Defibrillation testing 342
Device-assisted dissection and reentry 54
Device entrapment 104
Diabetic autonomic neuropathy 227
Diameter of forearm arteries 27
Diameter of radial arteries 27
Diastolic dysfunction 305
Distal filtration system 125
Donor artery stenosis 208
Donor vessel dissection 57
Donor vessel thrombosis 57
Double balloon technique 230
Double lumen accura balloon catheter 235
Dual antiplatelet therapy (DAPT) 139

E

Elevated pulmonary vascular resistance 229
Embolic protection devices (EPD) 122
Epicardial vessels 305
Ethanol septal ablation (ESA) 305
European Society of Cardiology 41, 197, 315
EuroScore 99
Excel and nobel trials 43
Excisional atherectomy trial 64

F

Femoral access 1
   anatomy of femoral artery 2
   complications 4
      acute arterial thrombosis 4
      arteriovenous fistula 4
      hematoma 4
      pseudoaneurysm 4
      retroperitoneal hematoma 4
   practical landmarks for puncture 2
      bony landmarks 3
      fluoroscopic landmark 3
      maximal pulsation 3
      skin/inguinal crease 2
Fractional flow reserve estimation 197
   FFR in acute coronary syndrome (ACS) 207
   FFR in bifurcation lesions 205
   FFR in graft disease 207
   FFR in intermediate lesion 200
   FFR in left main disease 202
   FFR in multiVessel disease 201
   FFR in serial lesion and diffuse disease 204
   impact of collaterals on the assessment of FFR 208
   pitfalls 199
   technique of FFR estimation 197
Fibrous plaque 182
Fielder family of wires 45
Final kissing balloon inflation (FKI) 80
First septal unit 306
Fractional flow reserve 39
French-guiding catheter 65

G

Gamma cameras 218
Gastroepiploic artery (GEA) 116
Glidesheath slender 30
Glycoprotein 143
Goose-neck snare 293
Graft disease 208

H

High-risk percutaneous coronary interventions 149
   evidence-based observational and registry data 153
   evidence based randomized trial data 154
   evidence of hypotension 150
   extracorporeal membrane oxygenation 156
   fatal ventricular arrhythmias 150
   high-risk PCI criteria 149
   IABP-shock II trial 155
      impella device 155
   intra-aortic balloon counter pulsation 153
   maintenance of end-organ perfusion 152
   mechanical circulatory support (MCS) 150
   optimization of myocardial perfusion 153
   systolic blood pressure 150
   tandem heart 156
Hung's formula 236
Hypertrophic cardiomyopathy 304
   alcohol septal ablation 305
   after the procedure 308

alternative approaches for septal ablation 311
complications 309
criteria for patient selection and anatomical considerations 305
outcome data 309
pathophysiologic mechanism 308
procedure 306
epidemiology 304
pathophysiology 304
Hypoplastic annulus 247

I

Iliac and aortic tortuosity 47
Implantable cardioverter defibrillators 336
Infective endocarditis prophylaxis 253
Inoue balloon catheter 235
Inoue balloon technique 230
Internal crush technique 75
Internal mammary artery (IMA) 116
Internal or reverse crush technique 80
Interventional cardiology 14
Intra-aortic balloon pump 145
intravascular ultrasound (IVUS) 179
   basic interpretation 179
   recent advances in IVUS 187
   recommendations 186
   specific lesion subsets 185
      ACS 186
      bifurcation stenting 185
      identifying vulnerable plaque 186
      left main 185
      ostial lesions 186
   uses 180
      post-PCI assessment 183
      pre-PCI assessment 180
Inverted Cullotte technique 80
Ipsilateral collaterals to the occluded artery 48
Iso-volumetric contraction 153

J

Jugular venous pressure (JVP) 248

K

Kissing balloon inflation 40

L

Late aneurysms 104
Leadless pacemaker 336
   clinical experience 341
   implant procedure 339
      confirming the position in the RV septum 340
      deploying the micra device 340
      passage of the delivery system into the right ventricle 340
      venous access and insertion of the introducer 339
   indications 341
   micra transcatheter pacing system 337
      delivery system 338
      introducer with dilator 338
      leadless pacemaker 337
Leadless system 336
Left circumflex artery 73
Left main coronary intervention 37
   management of LM bifurcation 40
   ostial LM PCI 39
   role of imaging and FFR 39
   trials comparing PCI with CABG 37
Left pulmonary artery (LPA) 247
Left ventricular ejection fraction 37
Left ventricular end-diastolic pressures 305
Limb ischemia 156
Limitations of coronary angiogram 179
Long and tortuous grafts 132
Looped wire in aortic sinus 66
Lumen enlargement 102

M

Major adverse cardiac event 13
MARS pilot registry 32
Medina classification 72
Metallic commissurotomy 230, 233
Miniaturization of hardware 30
Minimum lumen area 39
Mitral leaflets 229
Mitral regurgitation (MR) 305
Mitral stenosis 229
Mitral valve area (MVA) 229
Modified Allen's test 7
Mullins sheath 233
Multitrack technique 233
Multi-vessel coronary artery disease 99

Murray's law 73
Myocardial contrast echocardiography 307
Myocardial ischemia 116
Myocardial territory 75

N

Nanto techniques 51
National cardiovascular registry (NCDR) analysis 116
Native coronary atherosclerosis 122
Native vessel bifurcation stenting 122
Nonadherence to P2Y12 inhibitors 145
Non-Q wave myocardial infarction (MI) 76
Nonsurgical myocardial reduction (NMSR) 305
Non-sustained supraventricular arrhythmias 291
Nordic-Baltic-British left main revascularization study 42
Nordic bifurcation study 76
Nuclear cardiology 218
   myocardial innervation 227
   myocardial ischemia 219, 222
      preparation 221
      principle of MPS 220
      procedure 221
   myocardial viability 225
   scope 218

O

Optical coherence tomography (OCT) 187
   assessment of biovascular scaffolds 193
   basic OCT image interpretation 188
   guidelines 194
   limitations of OCT 193
   rule out geographical miss 191
   uses 188
      post-PCI assessment 191
      pre-PCI assessment 188
Optimal atherectomy trial 64
Ostial lesions 60
   access 61
   classification 60
      aorto-ostial lesions 60
      branch lesions 60
      non aorto-ostial lesions 60
   equipment guiding catheters 62
   fluoroscopic views 61
   lesion preparation 64
   peculiarities and challenges 60
   special situations 65
      coronary spasm 65
      side branch ostial stenosis 67
      technical consideration 66
   stent positioning 64
   wires 63
Ostial stenosis 120

P

Papillary muscles 229
Parkinson's disease 227
Patent ductus arteriosus (PDA) 248
Penetration of the proximal CAP 51
Percutaneous coronary intervention (PCI) 197
Percutaneous transluminal septal myocardial ablation (PTSMA) 305
Percutaneous treatment of mitral valve 311
Periprocedural myocardial infarction 97
Periprocedural thrombotic complications 144
Poly-L-lactic acid (PLLA) 15
Polymer coating 12
Polymeric coated wires 45
Positron emission tomography 218
Post coronary artery bypass grafts 116
   acute myocardial infarction 118
   arterial graft interventions 130
      LIMA graft intervention 130
      LIMA graft restenosis after PTCA 131
      technical aspects of LIMA graft intervention 131
   graft interventions 120
      vein graft interventions 120
   native vessel PCI 120
      aorto-ostial lesions 120
      native vessel CTO 120
   percutaneous coronary interventions 119
   recurrence of ischemia 116
      early 117
      intermediate 117
      late 118
   SVG stenting 123
      adjunctive pharmacotherapy 130
      covered stents 123
      embolic protection devices 123
      intravascular ultrasound 129

selection of EPD 126
SVG CTO 129
technical aspects of SVG PCI 128
treating recurrent ichemia 119
Presynaptic catecholamine 227
Primary angioplasty 136, 138, 145
Proximal optimization technique 78
Proximal subclavian artery stenosis 116
Pulmonary artery (MPA) 247
Pulmonary balloon valvuloplasty 247
  clinical features 248
    cardiac catheterization 249
    echocardiographic findings 249
    electrocardiographic findings 249
    radiological findings 249
    signs 248
    symptoms 248
  differential diagnosis 250
  management 251
    balloon pulmonary valvuloplasty 251
    surgical valvotomy 253
  salient features 253
Pulmonary capillary wedge pressure 156, 229
Pulmonary embolism 315
  classification 315
    high-risk 315
    intermediate 315
    low 315
  management 316
    anticoagulation 316
    indications 318
    oral anticoagulants 317
    parenteral anticoagulation 317
    treatment algorithm 316
    treatment options 316
  percutaneous catheter-directed
      interventions 319
    conventional catheter-directed
        thrombolysis 320
    mechanical thrombus
        fragmentation 321
    pharmacomechanical thrombolysis
        (PMT) 321
    rheolytic thrombectomy 321
    rotational thrombectomy 321
    suction thrombectomy 321
  surgical embolectomy 325
  systemic thrombolysis 318
    contraindications 319

venous filters 322
  indications 322
  procedure 325
  types 322
Pulmonary regurgitation (PR) 251
Pulmonary thromboembolism 212
Pulmonary vascular resistance 289

Q

Quantitative coronary angiography 20

R

Radial access 6
  anatomy of radial artery 6
  complications 9
    bleeding, iatrogenic radial artery
        perforation 9
    forearm hematoma 9
    radial occlusion 9
  modified Allen's test 6
    negative modified Allen's test 6
    positive modified Allen's test 6
  puncture technique 7
    right or left radial approach 8
    ulnar approach 8
Radial artery 116
Radial artery occlusions 34
Radial versus femoral access 141
Ramus intermedius 60
Retrograde wire 56
Rheumatic heart disease 229
Right coronary artery 198
Right internal jugular vein 293
Right ventricular dysfunction 229
Right ventricular (RV) myocardial
    hypertrophy 247
Rotational atherectomy 99
Rubella syndrome 247

S

Saphenous vein 116
Saphenous vein graft (SVG) 116
Scaffold thrombosis 20
Secondary heart field (SHF) 247
Semilunar valve development 247
Septal channel rupture and hematoma 58

Septal puncture 229
Sheath-sizing protocol 28
Sirolimus-eluting stent 38
Slender transradial interventions 30
Small area of myocardium 45
Small radial arteries 27
Stent thrombosis 13
Subcutaneous implantable cardioverter defibrillator 342
    efficacy and safety of the device 342
    implant procedure 342
    indications 344
    limitations 344
Superior pulmonary vein 290
Supraventricular ectopy 291
Surgical myectomy 304
Sympathetic denervation 227
Syntax score 99
Systolic anterior motion (SAM) 304
Szabo technique 66

T

Tandem heart 156
T and protrusion technique 80
T-angulation 73
Target lesion failure 16
Target-lesion revascularization 77
Target vessel 116
Target vessel revascularization 15
Third-generation beta blockers 227
Threatened SB morphologies 74
Transcatheter ablation technology 331
Transcatheter aortic valve implantation 5
Transcatheter aortic valve replacement (TAVR) 263
    balloon-expandable versus self-expanding valves in TAVR 281
    complications 283
        common 283
        infrequent 283
    contraindications 268
        approaches 269
        types of TAVR valves 268
    corevalve pivotal high risk study 278
    current status of evidence 273
    high surgical risk group 274
        partner 1A trial 274
    indication of aortic valve replacement 263
    indications for TAVR 265
        prerequisites 266
    intermediate surgical risk group 279
    low surgical risk group 281
    patient specific selection of TAVR valve 273
        annulus size 273
        risk of annulus rupture 273
        risk of coronary obstruction 273
        valve-in-valve 273
    prohibitive surgical risk (inoperable) group 273
    risk assessment 266
    coreValve pivotal extreme risk ileofemoral study 274
Transcatheter closure of congenital heart defects 289
    atrial septal defect 289
    coronary arterial fistula 299
        complications 301
        procedure 299
    patent ductus arteriosus 295
        contraindications 295
        indications 295
    ruptured sinus of Valsalva aneurysm 297
        complications 299
        procedure 297
    ventricular septal defect 292
        complications 296
        congenital VSDs in adults 292
        post-MI ventricular septal rupture 293
        procedure 293
Transcoronary ablation of septal hypertrophy (TASH) 305
Transesophageal echocardiography 289
Transmitral pressure gradient 236
Transradial access 26
Transradial interventions 27
Transradial (TR) primary angioplasty 26
Transthoracic echocardiogram 307
Transvalvar gradient 257
Traversing the CTO body 51
Tricuspid regurgitation (TR) 249
Tricuspid valve 252
True bifurcation lesion 71

U

Unfractionated heparin 143

V

Valsalva aneurysm 289
Valvuloplasty 229
Vascular complications 31
Vasodilators 130
Venoarterial loop 252
Ventricular septal defect 289
Vessel perforation 97
V-stenting technique 40, 87

W

Wall shear stress 73
Wilkin's score 229
Williams-Beuren syndrome 247

Wizard wire 33
Wood pecking sign 236

X

Xenon chloride 110
Xience arms 16
Xience VR stents 14

Y

Y technique 88

Z

Zotarolimus-eluting stent (ZES) 13